I0131764

Family Stress

Family Stress

Understanding and Helping Families in Diverse Circumstances

Scott S. Hall, Ph.D., CFLE

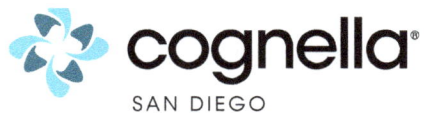

cognella®
SAN DIEGO

Bassim Hamadeh, CEO and Publisher
Amy Smith, Senior Project Editor
Casey Hands, Production Editor
Jess Estrella, Senior Graphic Designer
Kylie Bartolome, Licensing Coordinator
Natalie Piccotti, Director of Marketing
Kassie Graves, Senior Vice President, Editorial
Jamie Giganti, Director of Academic Publishing

Copyright © 2024 by Cognella, Inc. All rights reserved. No part of this publication may be reprinted, repro-
duced, transmitted, or utilized in any form or by any electronic, mechanical, or other means, now known
or hereafter invented, including photocopying, microfilming, and recording, or in any information retrieval
system without the written permission of Cognella, Inc. For inquiries regarding permissions, translations,
foreign rights, audio rights, and any other forms of reproduction, please contact the Cognella Licensing
Department at rights@cognella.com.

Trademark Notice: Product or corporate names may be trademarks or registered trademarks and are used
only for identification and explanation without intent to infringe.

Cover image: Copyright © 2019 iStockphoto LP/Vitalii Bondarenko.
Copyright © 2014 iStockphoto LP/Maxiphoto.
Copyright © 2010 Depositphotos/jordygraph.

Printed in the United States of America.

cognella® | ACADEMIC PUBLISHING
3970 Sorrento Valley Blvd., Ste. 500, San Diego, CA 92121

Brief Contents

Detailed Contents

Preface

What Is This Textbook All About?

This text is designed for undergraduate-level and introductory graduate-level instruction and fits well with courses that focus on various family stressors and challenges. Students preparing to work in helping professions will find the content useful because of its breadth of topics and systematic applications of key theoretical and practical concepts. Many topics are relatable to students' personal and family backgrounds, creating opportunities for reflection and furthering the meaning-making process that cultivates hope and resiliency. While the engaging tone of the chapters is less formal than in some textbooks, the content is explicitly grounded in substantive scholarship.

The main **objectives** of this text are to help students

1. understand a foundation of key concepts of family stress;
2. enhance their abilities to make connections among theory, practice, and diverse family circumstances associated with stress;
3. strengthen resilience regarding their own experiences related to stress and trauma; and
4. sympathize with and empower families from various backgrounds and situations facing stressful circumstances.

The first four chapters introduce theoretical, personal, and professional elements of family stress; they also sensitize students to contextual influences related to gender, ethnicity, sexuality, age, class, religion, and other characteristics that can distinguish the life experiences of diverse families. Subsequent chapters highlight specific topics that illustrate the various foundational and contextual concepts and help prepare students to work with diverse populations in culturally sensitive ways.

Various strategies are included in the text to help students enhance their learning skills and retention:

- The order and pacing of the content and the systematic structure and repetition across chapters help students integrate theory and application.
- Chapter previews highlight the structure and emphases of the chapter, preparing the mind for assimilating the information.

- Questions placed throughout chapters further prime students to associate novel information with what they already know, especially on a personal level.
- Explicit discussion of philosophical assumptions and political ideologies that drive much debate about family topics invites students to analyze the underpinnings of various ideas, identify common ground across viewpoints, and develop an appreciation for competing perspectives.
- **Bolding** is used to highlight key concepts and to anchor readers to summative ideas, making it easier to review a chapter.

Footnotes are used for documenting source materials to enhance the flow of the narrative. For the same reason, sources pertaining to a paragraph or section are often grouped together under a single footnote.

How Can Instructors Use This Textbook in a Course?

Twelve chapters cover a broad array of family stress topics. Chapters are divided into two main parts, each of which could be assigned to a given class period. Instructors could assign a chapter each week and fill in any extra weeks with supplementary readings or experiential learning, or dedicate multiple days to explore certain chapter sections more deeply, especially related to theory, professional issues, or diverse external contexts—although any chapter could be expanded. Chapter content is often dense and includes various interrelated topics, providing ample opportunity to spend more time with and elaborating on a given topic. At the same time, many concepts are touched on only briefly, creating additional opportunities for students or instructors to seek out or provide elaborative content.

Additional resources are included at the end of each chapter, containing various links to videos, websites, and readings that instructors can use to flesh out concepts they wish to highlight and to dictate the pace of the course. Instructional resources include discussion questions and activities that can be used for individual reflection, full-class or small-group interaction, and assignments.

CHAPTER 1

Theoretical Foundations for Understanding Family Stress

About 77% of adults regularly experience physical symptoms caused by stress.[1] Children exposed to traumatic events often develop post-traumatic stress disorder, including 90% of sexually abused children, 77% of children exposed to a school shooting, and 35% of urban youth exposed to community violence.[2]

Chapter Preview

- Stress can make it difficult for families to meet their needs, though it can also promote family flourishing.
- Families are more than just a group of individuals but individuals make up families.
- Family rules, roles, and boundaries are key parts of family patterns that are affected by stressful events or situations and that can also contribute to family stress.
- Central theoretical concepts include elements of resources, perceptions, coping, and environments.
- Daily hassles can have profound effects on family functioning.
- More recent family stress theory includes a focus on families adapting after being in crisis.
- Families can develop resilience to avoid or better cope with crisis.
- A family's internal and external contexts influence stressors and coping.
- Modern perspectives on individual and family functioning emphasize strengths, wellness, and flourishing.
- Childhood trauma can contribute to lifelong patterns of experiencing and coping with stressors.
- An integrated model of family stress will guide the remaining chapters.

What Is This Topic About?

The word "stress" has become a part of our daily vocabulary. We usually use it to describe a negative experience or sensation. It is easy to assume that the term "family stress" means that something is wrong with a family. Is stress really all that bad? Should family stress be avoided? This chapter addresses key terms and concepts related to family stress and includes brief explanations of common family stress theories. Such content helps us realize that understanding and helping families in diverse circumstances is much more intricate and fascinating than some might think.

Part A. Basic Concepts and Theory

What Does It Mean for a Family to Have Stress?

Are you feeling stressed? You are not alone. In our modern era, we better appreciate how **stress** can affect our minds and bodies. Stress can be triggered by a real or perceived threat and activates physiological responses—blood pressure rises, breath accelerates, and hormones get released into the bloodstream. These responses can help us react quickly to a threat, but constant stress wears us out. Medical experts have shown that stress can lead to or worsen a variety of health conditions, including obesity, heart disease, gastrointestinal problems, asthma, Alzheimer's disease, and more. It can consume our thoughts and worries and contribute to mental health problems, such as depression and anxiety. Sorry to start out on such a discouraging note.

But What Is Family *Stress?*
Does family stress simply mean that family members get on our nerves? That could be part of it, but to understand stress on a **family level**, we have to understand what families are all about. You may have already learned that a family can be thought of as a type of system. **Family systems theory** is an important foundation for much of the scholarship on family stress and crisis.[3] We will briefly touch on some key points that you can learn more about or review in another way (e.g., from online sources or an instructor).

Ever watch a group dance routine? One out-of-sync dancer can cause the whole team to lose a competition. Every member plays an important and often unique role in the routine, and one person's mistake can throw everyone else off. Similarly, if a car battery stops working, so will the whole vehicle. There are numerous parts under the hood that can malfunction and affect how well it drives. In some ways, the family system is similar to a team or vehicle. Each family member's attitudes and behaviors affect each of the other members in some way and affect the family as a whole. An angry parent can cause tension in the home, might "forget" to help a child with homework, and avoid communicating directly with a spouse. Each of those reactions can trigger concerns and responses that affect the tone of the family environment, which affects everyone in that environment, including the angry parent. A family is more than just a group of people, it is an entity itself—something unique that is created by the relationships and patterns within the group.

A family unit **functions to meet the needs of each individual**, and each part of the unit contributes to the stability of the family unit. Families benefit by maintaining a sense of **homeostasis**—a balance between the pressure to **resist** change and the pressure to **embrace** change. Change is often resisted for the sake of stability: familiarity is comfortable, routines help address recurring needs, and chaos is problematic. Yet, change must be embraced because life doesn't stand still: children age, the needs of family members alter, and societies shift.

Usually, when we talk about a family system or environment, our focus is on family members who typically live together and have regular if not daily interactions. From a Western perspective especially, that usually means two parents and their children—long referred to as a **nuclear family**—though having only one parent in the home or having children around from other relationships is well within that perspective. Of course, some **extended family** members can live with the nuclear family or otherwise be heavily involved to the point that they regularly influence homeostasis. The family system is often made up of multiple **subsystems**—any pair or combination of certain family members, such as a spousal subsystem, a parent-child subsystem, and a sibling subsystem. Families are also embedded within **larger systems** that influence family patterns and that are likewise influenced by the families within those systems (e.g., neighborhood, community, school district, state, ethnic/cultural group).

Family systems theory highlights **circular** and **reciprocal** processes—instead of one person causing one reaction that leads to one outcome, family members respond back and forth in ways that lack a clear beginning or end. For example, a parent feeling disconnected from a teenage child might impede the child's privacy and pester the child to share more thoughts and feelings. The child feels like the parent is being too nosey and bothersome, so the child becomes even more private and isolated. That pushes the parent to try even harder to get the child to open up, which pushes the child more and more inward (or away from the parent). Each person might blame the other for any tension this causes, but both are actually part of the problem—an example of **circular causality**. When you try to understand what is going on with a family, remember that you are only seeing a portion of a pattern that includes complex causes and influences—the actions of the disconnected parent may not have started this cycle; they are likely part of a pattern that evolved over months or years.

Family patterns related to **rules**, **roles**, and **boundaries** are key to understanding family functioning. The concepts are interconnected and are often made evident in how family members **communicate** with one another and in their daily **routines**.

- What kind of **rules** did you have growing up in a home environment? Were you allowed to use an electronic device during a family meal? Could you stay out as long as you wanted? Were you allowed to raise your voice at a parent? Family systems need rules to **maintain stability and to reach basic goals** such as avoiding starvation, providing a loving environment, and preparing children for independence. Sometimes the rules are clearly spelled out about tasks or appropriate behavior and sometimes they are only hinted at by how others respond to you (e.g., a mother tenses when giving her a hug in public—maybe we aren't supposed to show affection like that). Rules also guide how we verbally communicate and what we are supposed to do to comply with our roles.

- What **roles** did you have growing up in your family environment? Were you the one who took out the garbage, fed the hamster, or cleaned the toilet? Perhaps you were the one who made people laugh, the good listener, or caused all the trouble. The family system needs its members to cover various roles that contribute to **stability and flexibility**— like caregiver, supporter, listener, earner, tension breaker, unifier, and kitchen-floor sweeper. Sometimes roles a subtle. A misbehaving child, for example, can be thought of as playing the role of a **distractor** from parents arguing about their couple relationship problems; the misbehavior triggers the parents to unite and address the misbehavior, which lessens family members' anxiety about the couple not getting along. Sometimes roles that help keep a family stable can ultimately have negative side effects for family members.

- Have you known of a teenager and parent who hung out together as if they were the same age? That might have seemed nice in some ways, but perhaps you had some concerns. Might the parent share information that the child really didn't need to hear (e.g., the parent's sex life or some heavy adult concerns that could stress the child out)? Could the parent have difficulty regaining authority to enforce rules? Family **boundaries** determine who is considered part of the family and how open the family is to letting others freely enter or exit their family context. Some families have complex structures that can lead to **boundary ambiguity** or uncertainty about who is considered family and what can be expected of them—*Is the child from my stepfather's prior relationship really part of my family?* Boundaries also determine the **flow of information** and **levels of emotional interdependence** within the family system and subsystems and between the family and the outside world. Some parents have a very open boundary with their children, giving them an equal vote in family decisions and sharing information that some believe is inappropriate or too stressful for children to hear. Some families share their "business" with anyone outside the home willing to listen, while others are very private. Emotionally, family members can be so close that it is almost as if the boundary between them disappears, and they might struggle with recognizing their individual identities.

What Does This Have to Do With Family Stress?

We tend to understand what it means to say that a person is happy, but what does it mean to say that a *family* is happy? Is there some kind of *group happiness* trait that is different from individual happiness? Do we add up the happiness levels of the individuals to get a total family score? Do we estimate the average happiness across the individuals? Labeling a family with a certain characteristic can be difficult when there are differences among the family members on that characteristic. One way to think about family happiness is whether **all family members** consider themselves to be reasonably happy. If any member is unhappy, can we really say the family itself is happy?

Applying this logic to **general family functioning**, and the idea that a family system functions to meet the needs of all its individuals, we could say that a family is functioning inadequately when the family struggles to meet the needs of every member. Do you see where this is heading regarding family stress?

When addressing topics related to stress, our focus is primarily on the **family as a unit**. We will generally conclude that a family is doing well when all its members are doing well. We assume that how family members interact with one another and with various external systems is highly relevant to the well-being of the family as a whole and to each of its members. But we should remember that individuals are also distinct from their families and make choices that affect individual well-being that arguably have little to do with their current family environment. Family stress theories (and textbook authors) face some tension between the concepts of individuality and the family unit and the extent to which they overlap when explaining family stress. So yes, families can be a source of stress for individuals, but there is so much more going on in a family that gives us fascinating and profound insights into the human condition in the face of life's challenges. Let's get to it!

What Is the Value of Studying Theory?

If you feel intimidated by theory, relax. Theories help us make sense of complexity; they simplify concepts and guide our focus on what arguably matters most for a certain purpose. A theory is more than a guess but less than a complete, fully verifiable, and indisputable answer. Theories are kind of like shortcuts because they abbreviate or symbolize a vast amount of information or processes to help us organize our thoughts and have a common language for discussing a topic. What is great about family stress theory is that it can really help us focus on key ideas that both explain why families struggle and how they can improve their circumstances. We will focus on the more common and practical concepts across a variety of major family stress theories and see how they can be integrated into a single model that will guide us throughout the rest of this book (and maybe even our lives).

Formal theorizing around family stress has tended to increase around major historical events and societal shifts—world wars, major recessions, pandemics, high divorce rates, the rise of the internet and social media, and so on. Several key scholars have come up with theories to guide how we study and help struggling families, one of which was Reuben Hill who is known for his ABCX model of family stress—a foundational model for most family stress theorizing that followed.[4]

What Are the Key Concepts?

Are you hungry? The sensation of feeling hungry is a sign that your body needs nourishment to function well. It pressures you to address that need. If you have food readily available, this sensation is no big deal. You might find some crackers or a cookie to tide you over for a while. If your food is highly nutritious, you might feel better after you eat than you felt before you were hungry. But what happens if you don't have access to any (or enough nutritious) food? Now the feeling of hunger is a big deal, and you are heading toward some serious problems.

Can feeling hungry be a desirable sensation? Have you ever prepared for a feast by eating less ahead of time, knowing that working up an appetite can make the meal more satisfying? Some people purposefully skip meals (fast) for health or religious purposes. The **meaning** of feeling hungry changes when it is something you desire or is linked to some kind of ritual. The meaning of the food we eat to satisfy our hunger can also be important. Think about how terms like "junk food," "organic," and "farm fresh" affect how you think about food and your response to hunger. Advertisements seem to try to convince us that eating a certain brand of food will make us happy or popular.

Some people have insufficient funds for purchasing nutritious food or have difficulty finding food during a natural disaster or food shortage. When one's normal way of obtaining food fails, one may turn to new ways to satisfy that hunger, such as stealing or begging for food. People might find new ways to earn money or tap into government or church resources. While in the process of finding food, one can become overwhelmed by other tasks that pile up (e.g., earning money to pay the rent, attending a mandatory meeting, finding time to sleep). Obviously, if the body goes too long without nourishment, internal organs and muscles deteriorate and long-term health is threatened, making us weaker when facing upcoming challenges. Now consider the case of someone needing to feed a hungry family—this could feel like a burden in the face of difficult circumstances but also as an opportunity to express love and support.

From a family stress conceptual framework, being hungry or having an appetite is analogous to a **stressor**: an **event or situation** that disrupts family patterns and creates pressure on a family system to act or change in some way. Stressors come from within the family itself (e.g., a child gets sick or fails a class) and from outside the family (e.g., problems at work, a major snowstorm, a pandemic). Families ideally respond to stressors in ways that ensure all family members' needs continue to be met.

Can positive events be stressors? Would you consider a wedding a positive event? How about a move to a bigger house in a safer neighborhood? Because these events disrupt normal family patterns and routines, they are indeed stressors. Thus, the term "stressor" is more of a **neutral** concept—it creates pressure to do something, for better or worse. However, stressors differ in their **characteristics**, which can contribute to how they potentially impact a family. A long fast (i.e., missing several meals in a row) is probably more worrisome than a short one. Some key characteristics, inspired by the work of various family stress scholars, are described in Table 1.1.[5]

Similar to the diverse potential connotations and available responses to feeling hungry, whether a stressor is ultimately problematic for families depends largely on several key factors, including the following:

- **Resources:** As food can satisfy the needs signaled by feeling hungry, resources are what a family has available or needs to obtain to address the stressor. These resources can be **tangible** (e.g., money, extended family, tools, community programs) and **intangible** (e.g., knowledge, personality, intelligence, patience, trust in family members). Family resources also include how well the family rules, roles, and boundaries help a family face stressors. Storm damage to a house may not be a big deal to the family of a carpenter, a person with good insurance, or someone who can afford to hire a professional to do repairs. Families lacking such resources could have to tolerate the damage and its consequences for an extended period of time.

- **Perceptions:** As feeling hungry can mean different things depending on motivations and circumstances, the impact of a stressor can also depend on how it is perceived. Do you overreact to little changes? Are you too quick to dismiss the seriousness of someone's concerns? We all construct meaning out of our stressors and that meaning shapes how we respond. For example, you probably react more angrily when someone damages your property on purpose than on accident. You might feel guilty if you lose something of sentimental value, like a gift from a favorite deceased uncle. Reflecting on having successfully dealt with a past stressor can build a family's confidence when facing new stressors.

- **Coping:** As with finding ways to satisfy hunger, coping is a process that involves the use of family resources and the meanings of the stressor. Coping can include **taking direct actions**, like seeking help or learning a new skill; **altering thoughts**, like choosing to view a stressor as a coincidence instead of a punishment for a past misdeed; and **emotional regulation**, like calming one's self to avoid getting overwhelmed with panic. One may need to obtain or develop new resources and different ways of thinking about the situation to better address the stressor. Coping can refer to a minimal adjustment, like grabbing a snack when hungry, or in the case of more disruptive stressors, adapting family behaviors and thoughts to accommodate larger changes, like a parent taking on a second job or coming to terms with having to depend on a public food bank.

Unsuccessful coping, perhaps because of inadequate resources and harmful perceptions, leads to negative outcomes for individuals and families. Sometimes that outcome has interchangeably been referred to as **stress**, **distress**, **strain**, or **crisis** (which can cause confusion when interpreting various theories). Boss suggested that crisis differs from stress; stress is more of a continuous outcome—like a scale from low to high, while crisis is dichotomous—whether or not a family has reached a **state of being** in which the family is unable to meet the needs of its members.[6] The inability to cope with the stressor leads to high levels of stress that push a family into **crisis**. The family might be stuck or blocked from taking healthy actions to reestablish stable functioning (or homeostasis) until they make major changes that require new resources and/or healthier perceptions. The disturbance from a stressor and the experience of being in crisis are considered to have been **managed** when a family is able to successfully cope and minimize stress and avoid or recover from crisis. While a stressor is the event or situation that disrupts normal functioning, stress is the sensation caused by the stressor, depending on the nature of resources, perceptions, and coping. Stressors and crises also have the potential to push a family toward healthier relationships and increased stability if they are well managed.

TABLE 1.1 Characteristics of Stressor (Event or Situation)

Severity	How intense or major is the stressor? Is it more like light rain or like a tornado; more like an argument or like a divorce?
Location of Source	Did the stressor occur within the family or outside the family? Is it more like siblings fighting or like neighbors disturbing your sleep?
Pace of Onset	How gradually or suddenly did the stressor occur? Was it more like a progressive illness or like a broken leg?
Duration	How long did the stressor last? Is it an acute (short-term) stressor or a chronic (long-term) stressor? Is it more like an overdue bill or like being unemployed for a decade?
Predictability	How easy is it to anticipate the stressor? Is it expected or surprising? Is it more like a 16-year-old getting a driver's license or like getting pregnant in one's 40s while using birth control?
Amount of Choice	How much choice did someone have about this stressor occurring? Is it more like leaving a good job for a better job or like being forced to move because the renter decided to sell the apartment?
Cumulation	Is this a single stressor or a pileup of multiple stressors? Is it more like a child gets into one fight at school or like a child gets into one fight at school *and* a big work project is due *and* an ailing parent has a bad fall, all in the same day?
Issues of Quantity	Is the stressor related to having too little or too much of something? Is it more like not having enough water for the family or like having more time than one knows what to do with after retirement?
Clarity	Are the facts surrounding the stressor clear or confusing/ambiguous? Is it more like knowing the expectations for a child's science fair project or like a sick parent deteriorating from an undiagnosed illness?
Potential Trigger	Is the stressor itself the real cause of stress, or does it trigger memories or feelings of the real source of stress? Is it more like the family dog creating a huge mess (and that's all there is to it) or like the death of an old friend that brings back unresolved feelings about a parent's death?

Adapted from: Boss, P. (2002). Family stress management: A contextual approach (2nd ed.). SAGE Publications; Bush, K. R., Price, C. A., Price, S. J., & McKenry, P. C. (2017). Families coping with change: A conceptual overview. In C. A. Price, K. R. Bush, & S. J. Price (Eds.), Families & change: Coping with stressful events and transition (pp. 3–23). SAGE Publications; Hill, R. (1959). Generic features of families under stress. *Social Casework, 39*, 139–150.

Family stress theory that is built upon Hill's classic ABCX framework has organized these concepts with this basic format: "A" is a stressor that pressures families to turn to their "B" resources while being influenced by their "C" perceptions of the stressor, which leads to "X" the level of stress (or crisis) depending on the interaction of "A," "B," and "C." The event or situation is stressful when it creates **hardships**—complications caused by the stressor that puts strain on the family's ability to cope. For example, when a parent is deployed on a military mission away from a family (the stressor), various hardships could arise in the forms of a child acting out because of the parent's absence or the family having to move in with extended family members in tight quarters to help make ends meet. This is perhaps Hill's way of saying that some stressors have more complications than others, depending on the nature of the stressor and the family situation. But remember, sometimes stressors trigger changes that end up benefiting families.

Hill also introduced the **roller-coaster model** that addresses **family adjustment after crisis**. It emphasized that families in crisis can reach a **turning point** that triggers a period of recovery. This recovery can include major reorganizations of family patterns, including roles, rules, and boundaries. Families can recover to **differing levels of functioning**. Some may reach the same level of functioning they had before the event occurred that triggered crisis, some may not quite fully recover to that same level, and some may establish an even better functioning system than before. Experiencing crisis can end up being the best thing that happens to a family in the long run, as painful as the process might be, though families can also become weakened and more vulnerable, just getting by.

What If Each Family Member Has Different Resources and Unique Perceptions?

Remember that when talking about family stress we are focusing on the collective system, but can a *system* really have resources or perceptions? This is a tricky issue that we touched on earlier about individual versus family happiness. In one sense, the system's resources are a collection of what each family member has to offer as a resource. If the family members cooperate and chip in what they can, the system will have greater access to diverse resources. So, does the system itself have any resources outside of that? What do you think? Perhaps when family members are combining their efforts they accomplish more or different types of things than when each member focuses on individual contributions. Perhaps you are familiar with the old *Voltron* cartoon: several people each control robotic creatures that combine to create a giant robot that does things that none of the smaller robotic creatures can do alone.

Something similar can be said about perceptions. To say a family has a certain perception sounds like every member views something the same way. Certainly, that can happen—everyone might be equally annoyed by the neighbor's dog. But what happens when there is disagreement on the perceived causes and meanings of a stressor? Maybe the teenage daughter doesn't mind the barking and thinks the rest of the family is just being snobby. In this case, there are **unshared perceptions**—is that a problem? How might that be a benefit? Either way, it is important to recognize similarities and differences across perceptions when trying to understand processes related to family coping and functioning.

What About the Day-to-Day Things That Get on Our Nerves?

Family stress theory has also incorporated what are sometimes referred to as **daily hassles**— common, regular annoyances.[7] They can be random and unexpected or intentional and anticipated. They can interfere with other activities and plans, as the following examples show:

- Cooking and cleaning can feel burdensome when you would rather visit with a friend.
- Having to respond immediately to a certain text, or hearing a preschooler asking the same question over and over, might get on your nerves.
- A traffic jam can throw off your whole schedule.
- Arguing with others and relationship tension—reportedly two of the most common types of daily hassles—can wear us out.

These relatively minor events add up, sometimes in ways that are even **more difficult** to handle than a larger, single stressor. They can also occur because of major stressors—the death of a spouse could create a need to do more shopping and cleaning that the surviving spouse otherwise wouldn't have had to do alone. Daily hassles can contribute to **vulnerability** to other stressors because one's capacities are already stretched, like physical strength, emotional stability, and the ability to concentrate. Bad weather, a sick child, a late bus, and a misplaced cell phone can add to the complexities and burdens of other daily hassles or stressors.

Many daily hassles are experienced at our places of **employment**: deadlines, chatty coworkers, a grumpy boss, faulty printers, internet outages, employee mistakes—the list is long. However, many common daily hassles occur as part of our **unpaid labor**—tasks associated with maintaining a family and home that are typically unseen by others outside the home. They can be redundant, mundane, and never-really-completed tasks that don't get celebrated. As you might suspect, mothers are prone to report more daily hassles related to the home than fathers, and fathers report more daily hassles related to outside employment than mothers. There are plenty of exceptions and these days the differences aren't as large. Nevertheless, home and workplace are important and common contexts in which daily hassles occur.

But just like with stressors, perceptions and meaning are also integral to the impact of a daily hassle. Some people enjoy cooking a meal for others, viewing it as an act of love. Some people are energized by workplace conflicts, viewing them as interesting opportunities to solve problems or for proving their worth. Daily hassles that end up with a more positive outcome can be referred to as **uplifts**. People tend to feel more uplifted by tasks that are perceived as forms of caring for others. What example first came to mind when you read that about uplifts? What does that tell you about daily hassles?

Improve Your Learning

Without peeking, take a moment to review in your mind (or say out loud) the key concepts from this chapter (this is a proven learning technique). Then review the "Chapter Preview" section at the top and compare. Skim Part A of the chapter with extra attention to the **bolded words**. Skip to the end of the chapter to find more learning resources.

Part B. Theoretical Advancement and Integration

Hill's ABCX model continues to have a major influence in contemporary family stress scholarship. More recent family stress models add a post-crisis and adaptation phase of family stress to explain what happens after a family reaches crisis or bring added attention to influences outside the family that are relevant to family stress. We will briefly explore several examples of theoretical innovation to broaden our understanding of family stress and crisis.

What Has Been Added to the ABCX Concepts of Family Stress Theory?

The **double ABCX** model by Hamilton McCubbin and Joan Patterson incorporates how families cope with crisis by seeking out new resources to add to their earlier resources, are influenced by their perceptions of both the original stressor and now the crisis situation, and have to deal with a **pileup** of new stressors that are created by **unsuccessful coping** attempts and other new stressors that happened to occur with the passage of time.[8] For example, a distressed parent might work late hours to avoid family stress at home, creating new problems of frustration and resentment from family members that linger while in crisis. In the meantime, computers malfunction, grandparents get sick, and the high school has a bomb threat; such pressures pile up while still trying to work through crisis. How well a family **adapts** to this pileup of stressors while in crisis will dictate the overall quality of family functioning along a continuum ranging from **maladaptation** (negative) to **bonadaptation** (positive).

The **family adjustment and adaptation response (FAAR) model** by Joan Patterson similarly has a pre-crisis or adjustment phase and post-crisis or adaptation phase that highlight processes of families trying to balance their demands (stressors) and their capacities (resources).[9] A strong emphasis is placed on the meanings families generate related to their identities and worldviews that influence their demands and capacities. Some other helpful concepts are highlighted in this model:

- **Resilience:** The ability to bounce back from or successfully adapt to difficult circumstances or adversity. A resilient family is less susceptible to reaching a crisis state and is more likely to adapt if it does reach crisis. However, this does not mean a resilient family is free from problems. In fact, some argue that resilience cannot be truly demonstrated until significant challenges occur from which the family actually bounces back.
- **Protective factors:** Mechanisms that help determine whether a family facing risks or stressors will have positive or negative consequences. For example, families who know how to communicate effectively can more easily work together to address a challenge. Families who live in safer neighborhoods can rely more on neighbors for help or are not already drained by living in fear. The more protective factors a family has, the greater the chance of resilience. Protective factors can apply to how well a family normally functions, the suitability of their resources, and the helpfulness of their perceptions.
- **Vulnerability:** A state of family functioning that puts families at higher risks for some stressors and more negative consequences of stressors. A lack of protective factors makes a family more vulnerable and less likely to be resilient.

Pauline Boss's **contextual model of family stress** includes a strong, explicit focus on the contexts inside and outside of the family that influence the ABCX components of family stress.[10] The **internal contexts**, or the ones that families have control over, include the following:

- **Structural context:** Family patterns, such as rules, roles, and boundaries
- **Psychological context:** Family perceptions and definitions related to the stressor

- **Philosophical context:** Family values and belief systems. This might include philosophies about family unity, parental discipline, gender roles, self-sufficiency, fate, and so on.

The contextual model also highlights **external contexts** over which families have no control but that influence the types of stressors families have and how they cope with them:

- **Cultural context:** Social norms and expectations of an ethnic group, region, or mainstream culture, and how one's own subculture is viewed and treated by other groups
- **Historical context:** Time in history when a stressor occurs; how the past has shaped culture and the way families view themselves and others; and major historical events that shape family functioning
- **Economic context:** The overall strength of the economy, unemployment rates and housing prices that contribute to resources and perceptions
- **Developmental context:** Stage of life for each family member and family collectively, needs vary by the age of children and length of a marriage
- **Heredity context:** Inherited traits, abilities, and levels of physical health related to a person's genetic background

Similarly, Jay Mancini and Gary Bowen pointed out that the **community context** in particular, including social networks, has been underappreciated in how it contributes to family functioning.[11] The social and physical infrastructures of communities can influence family and community resiliency. For example, various barriers to building strong connections with fellow community members contribute to feelings of isolation and having fewer resources to turn to. Sometimes communities come together in the face of catastrophe; families that feel a strong sense of community outside themselves can draw from shared meaning with that community to help make sense of stressors. Virtual communities can function similarly.

The **typology model of family adaptation** by Hamilton McCubbin also incorporates the major assumptions of the ABCX model and, like the FAAR model, highlights family protective factors and vulnerability.[12] Families can be classified in a variety of ways based on how they act or organize themselves regarding several key dimensions. The classification—or type—of family is an important factor in how the family copes with stress. Some family types might be more vulnerable to certain problems and are more likely to deal with stressors and crises in certain ways. For example, specific combinations of **family bonding** (closeness, togetherness) and **family flexibility** (compromise, adapting to change) are likely to respond to stressors in distinct ways:

- Low on both bonding and flexibility could mean that family members rely on themselves or others outside the family more than on each other and are unwilling to budge on doing things their own way
- Low on bonding and high on flexibility could mean that members are easygoing about making changes, but their disconnection might mean they get little input from everyone about how to change

- High on bonding and low on flexibility could mean families enjoy being together but have a hard time making group decisions and get stuck doing the same things
- High on both could mean that family members are unified and willing to change and to compromise as needed

While it may seem that high levels of cohesion and flexibility would be ideal, that might not always be the case. For example, because younger children tend to benefit from routines and predictability, being a bit more rigid might serve the needs of the family at that time, whereas a home with adolescents might benefit from high levels of flexibility and giving a bit more space and separation to the adolescents who are working toward independence. Other pairs of dimensions include *coherence* and *hardiness*, *family time* and *routines* and *valuing family time* and *routines*, and *family celebrations* and *family traditions*.

The **family distress model** by Thomas Cornille and Daniel Boroto has a strong focus on the goal-oriented nature of families.[13] The model incorporates therapeutic principles that alter family patterns that contribute to the endurance of illness symptoms. The model is depicted as a flow chart in which the family's stable patterns are disrupted by an event. The key elements include the following:

The family restores stability when it can resolve the disruption by using its normal coping strategies.

Or, the family can seek social support, resolve the disruption in light of their goals, and develop new structures and patterns for family stability.

Otherwise, a family experiences crisis.

Problems are compounded when the family withdraws from social support and becomes completely preoccupied with the stressor, such as dealing with a seriously ill child.

Because of this preoccupation, the family reorganizes around the crisis situation to the point that the crisis situation is helping keep the family together. Rules, roles, and boundaries incorporate the crisis situation to a point that it seems necessary to remain in that situation.

The ways that the family has learned to cope with the crisis situation are difficult to change—even good changes can be scary.

These patterns centered around the crisis situation are now the normal ways of dealing with stressful events, but the family is even more vulnerable when new problems come along.

Reaching outside the family for necessary help is the turning point that can help them function without the crisis situation and establish better family functioning.

How Much Pressure Can a Family Handle?

By now, your initial response to this question should be "it depends." We just focused on a variety of reasons that some families would react differently to, and be differentially affected by, the same stressor. We have also focused on differences in resilience. Some families are particularly strained (overstretched or spread thin) because of insufficient coping capacity, making them even more vulnerable when future stressors arise. You may have noticed that much of this material has skewed toward problems, risks, and negative consequences. In traditional psychology, a person's well-being was generally indicated by an absence of mental, emotional, and, to some degree, physical health problems. Does that mean a fulfilling life is simply about **avoiding or managing challenges** that bring about negative health outcomes?

Scholarship in more recent decades places increasing emphasis on learning from individuals and families who seem to be thriving.

- A **family strengths perspective** presumes that all families have strengths and focuses on what is right with families instead of what is wrong. It also seeks to empower families by emphasizing and honing strengths.
- A **wellness-orientation** focuses on being more than free from health problems but proactively seeking to reach higher goals and fulfillment. Instead of a family just eliminating their internal fighting, the family actively strives toward building strong, intimate relationships that enhance individual and family fulfillment.

Think of the words *survive*, *endure*, and *thrive*—which one sounds most desirable?

Positive psychology has also pushed our thinking toward strengths and wellness. Martin Seligman and others have proposed a concept called **flourishing**.[14] Those who flourish are said to live "**the good life**," which includes experiencing positive emotions, finding great fulfillment in accomplishing meaningful tasks, and connecting deeply with other people. Consequently, people who flourish tend to have fewer problems with health, work, and relationships. Thus, I suggest that **family flourishing** means that the family members are living generally satisfying and fulfilling lives while actively working toward and succeeding in meaningful accomplishments and relationships.

Flourishing families likely handle higher levels of pressure from stressors—that is, are resilient—because they have created or enhanced protective factors and minimized risk factors that affect their vulnerability to stress. While they are not necessarily wealthy, a flourishing family knows how to use its strengths and relationships as resources to successfully cope with challenges and reach its aspirations. Not only that, flourishing families likely **embrace or even introduce certain stressors** into their lives that help them become even stronger and more satisfied—like sacrificing time and goods to serve people in need or going on family outings that push the limits of their skills and trust in one another. Have you witnessed any examples of such families?

What About Families That Create Terrible Environments for Their Members, Especially Children?

Families can be the source of serious **trauma**. Living in fear for one's safety or survival can place a person on constant high alert, which in a sense overloads a person's senses. As will be explored in Chapter 7, child abuse can lead to **child traumatic stress** that lingers in some ways for years and even decades.[15] For example, survivors of child abuse might be extra jumpy with loud noises or sudden movements. They may have difficulty trusting other people because their trust was violated by someone who was supposed to love them. Children can appear distracted (or daydream) at school or act out for attention as ways to cope with their anxiety. Sometimes traumatized children are wrongly assumed to have attention defect hyperactivity disorder or autism because of their learned behavioral tendencies. Some of the ways that children (and adults) **cope with trauma** seem confusing or irrational to observers, but to the victims, their strategies helped them survive or tolerate their erratic circumstances.

Seemingly normal events **trigger fear** because they are reminders of past trauma. A song, a movie, a birthday party, a facial characteristic, a voice—almost anything can be a reminder of anxious times that put the body and mind in a state of high alert. Many survivors of family-related trauma become parents themselves. Try to imagine how many triggers occur while raising children. As has been mentioned repeatedly, some families are more vulnerable than others to various stressors; a history of childhood trauma can contribute to those vulnerabilities. It is also important to remember that many traumatized children show **resilience** and live fulfilling lives, though it might require extra effort to manage anxiety or doubt. Of course, the seriousness and extent of the trauma contribute to the nature of long-term consequences.

How Will These Theories and Concepts Be Used Throughout This Book?

Most of the chapters in this book focus on specific family stressors that can lead to a variety of potential hardships. However, just like with the family system, stressors can be **circular** and **reciprocal**. For example, stressors can lead to an explosive argument, and an explosive argument can be a stressor in itself. Thus, many of our topics are **bidirectional** in nature—they can be thought of as both causes and effects of stressors. The emphasis of this book is on **exploring the stressors** associated with a variety of topics that are typically thought of as challenging and often negative family experiences. However, family stress theory will guide our approach to understanding families' subjective and objective experiences related to stressors and the processes that shape the impact of such experiences, some of which are positive.

Some of the theories and concepts discussed in this chapter probably resonate with you more than others. You have likely also noticed similarities across the theories. Exposure to a variety of theories helps you learn to notice the detail and nuance that appear when different sets of assumptions (or terminology) are used for describing similar ideas. The reality is, no family stress theory can explain or predict everything that families experience because of stressors. But, as discussed, theories can be helpful tools for guiding our attention, communicating about complex things, and determining how to address problems.

For the purposes of this book, however, **I propose a model** that integrates key concepts and ideas from common family stress theories and from contemporary perspectives on family functioning. More than anything, this model visually repackages well-established concepts with some fine-tuning of some definitions. Subsequent book chapters will refer to components of this model to help you master key family stress theory concepts. You will learn to view stressors—including those not explored in this book—in ways that are useful for making sense of their potential impacts on families and for helping families become more resilient.

I call this model the **FSS integrated model (FIM) of family stress and crisis**. The "FSS" refers to different qualities or levels of family functioning, which are key to (1) how vulnerable or strong a family is in the face of stressor events and (2) how families are ultimately affected by the processes of facing and coping with stress and crisis. Graphic depictions of theories help us understand connections across concepts and processes described in a theory, though they inherently oversimplify things. Studying the explanations that accompany the diagram in Figure 1.1 is critical for understanding the theoretical model.

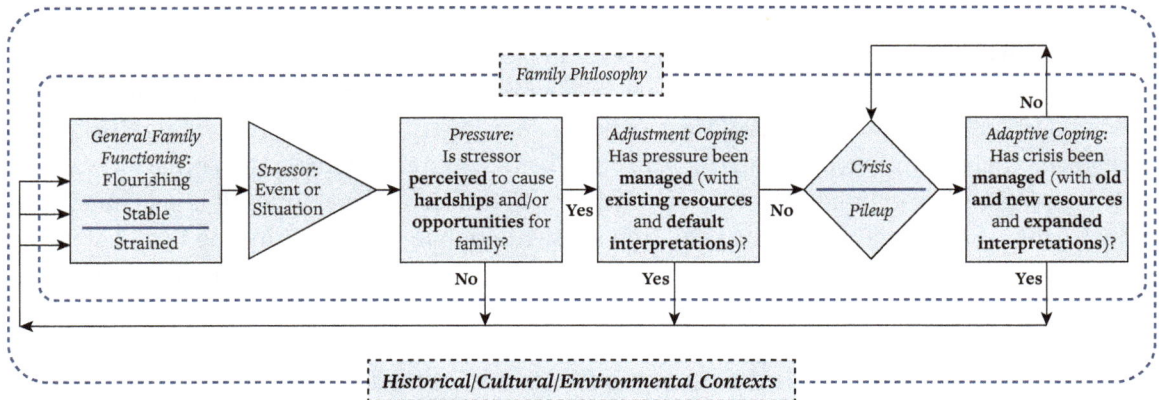

FIGURE 1.1 FIM of Family Stress and Crisis

General family functioning: The overall level of family well-being, including the useful-ness of rules, roles, and boundaries, incorporates vulnerability and protective factors, though no family is immune to struggles. The internal workings of a family set the stage for how a stressor is experienced and interpreted. As the FIM diagram shows, family functioning itself can lead to or cause a stressor and is affected by the other components in the model. Family functioning is embedded within (and influenced by) the internal context of family philos-ophy and external contexts of history, culture, and overall environment—they are depicted with dotted lines (see the following explanations). There are three levels or broad categories of functioning:

- **Strained:** *Overall, family members have their needs met, but just barely.* Family patterns work at a basic level but the family is stretched thin or worn out, so it is more vulnerable to struggling with stressors and reaching crisis, low resilience.
- **Stable:** *Overall, family members have their needs met.* No major issues within the family that threaten well-being, and the family is likely prepared to handle typical stressors pretty well; the family is more reactionary than proactive—like on autopilot until a prob-lem occurs and then reacts to the problem, moderate resilience.
- **Flourishing:** *The family pushes beyond stability to actively strive toward reaching fulfilling goals.* The family is deliberate and intentional in establishing an atmosphere in which all individuals and the collective group thrive (personal fulfillment and deep connections with one another); though still having some level of vulnerability (like every family), it has a high ability to cope with stressor events and may initiate them as ways to help grow and experience "the good life" together, high resilience.

Stressor: *An event or situation that originates from within or from outside the family that disrupts general family functioning.* Stressors can differ in their impacts based on their characteristics, like those described in the table from Part A. **Daily hassles,** as defined earlier, are also types of stressors that apply to this model.

Pressure: *The need to take action or make changes due to disruption caused by a stressor.* Sometimes we use the word "stress" to describe the concept of pressure. Because "stress" is also commonly used to describe a negative psychological or physical outcome of stressors, "pressure" is the preferred term for this part of the model. As shown in the diagram, if the pressure fails to result in any action or changes, the general family functioning should be affected in some way, probably adversely if the disruption is substantial. **Perceptions** of the stressor are important—whether the family considers the stressor noteworthy or problematic helps determine how that pressure is experienced.

- **Hardships:** *The negatively perceived challenges created by the stressor*—which can include the negative consequences of daily hassles.
- **Opportunities:** *The positively perceived challenges created by the stressor* (i.e., opportunities to grow as individuals or strengthen family relationships). In the case of daily hassles, such opportunities could be seen as **uplifts.**

If a stressor is perceived as irrelevant or unthreatening, or is unrecognized as a stressor, the family takes no action and is susceptible to straining their **general family functioning** if indeed the stressor has detrimental impacts on the family. For example, parents might not realize that bullying is contributing to a child developing an eating disorder and dismiss the seriousness of the bullying by just telling the child to toughen up. The eating disorder could eventually lead to child depression and malnutrition, family conflict about eating habits, and parents blaming each other for tension in the home. Families might also fail to recognize stressors that present opportunities for family growth.

Adjustment coping: *The process of using* **existing resources** *in light of the* ***default interpretations*** *the family makes of their stressful circumstances.* Existing resources at the time of the stressor can be tangible and intangible. Default interpretations are the family's typical ways of perceiving things as applied to (1) the perceptions of the stressor (see "pressure"), (2) perceptions of the resources available (e.g., are they recognized as resources? Are they believed to be helpful?), and (3) personal meanings tied to what the family is going through (e.g., how members make sense of the causes and consequences of the stressor). Some families (or family members) who are typically pessimistic or anxious would likely have negative and discouraging default interpretations. As suggested in the diagram, sufficient existing resources and helpful default interpretations would lead to **adjustments** that result in the family having **managed** the pressure in a way that maintains general family functioning at a level that meets family members' needs.

Crisis: A state in which the family is stuck or immobilized, unable to meet the needs of all its members with current resources and default interpretations of the stressful circumstances. The family enters a state of crisis when adjustment coping is insufficient. A family can struggle in a state of crisis for a significant amount of time, creating the opportunity for stressors to pile up and create more vulnerability.

- **Pileup:** *The accumulation of stressors over time, adding to the challenge of coping with any stressor.* Pileup includes (1) the original stressor that eventually led to crisis, (2) new stressors created by unhelpful attempts to cope with the original stressor (e.g., develop a drinking problem), and (3) stressors created by other events that have occurred while trying to cope with the consequences of the original stressor. While stressors can also accumulate prior to or without reaching crisis, the prolonged nature or extra efforts required of dealing with a crisis puts families in a particularly vulnerable state, which the term pileup is used to describe. Simply having multiple, simultaneous stressors can simply be described as such.

Adaptive coping: *The process of using **old and new resources** in light of the family's **expanded interpretations** of their crisis circumstances.* The resources that still exist from when the family experienced the original stressor combine with newly acquired resources that are necessary for the family to **adapt** to crisis and pileup. Expanded interpretations potentially include the combination of (1) lingering default interpretations; (2) initial interpretations of the crisis situation and pileup; (3) new or improved interpretations of the original stressor, the crisis, and pileup; and (4) perceptions of the old and new resources. As suggested in the diagram, sufficient resources and useful interpretations lead to adaptations that result in the family having **managed** crisis in a way that reestablished general family functioning at a level that meets family members' needs. Adaptive coping can require major changes in the organization, patterns, and philosophies of a family, which means there is potential to replace the original family characteristics that contributed to reaching crisis with ones that make the family less vulnerable, more resilient, and more likely to flourish in the future. For example, stressors that trigger **boundary ambiguity** can require adaptation through changing **rules**, **roles**, and **boundaries** (see Chapter 8 for examples).

Family philosophy: *What a family values or believes about families and life in general, what motivates them, what shapes their goals.* Rules, roles, and boundaries reflect the family philosophy—for example, the extent to which roles are gendered, the amounts of disagreement or individuality that are tolerated or encouraged, and ways that children should honor parental authority. This **internal family context** influences all the components mentioned earlier, especially when subjective meaning is relevant. Thus, the family philosophy can be thought of as the foundational belief system that influences how families perceive and interpret stressors, resources, their ability to cope with pressure or crisis, and the characteristics of their general family functioning. Sometimes adaptive coping requires that the family philosophy be revised to make it compatible with new rules, roles, and boundaries.

Historical/cultural/environmental contexts: *The larger-scale influences from outside the family that potentially impact all other components of the model.* **External contexts** can impact the types of stressors families face (e.g., discrimination), the resources they are likely to have at their disposal (e.g., earning opportunities, extended family involvement), and interpretations of the stressor and its consequences (e.g., feeling victimized and taking it personally). External contexts influence perceptions and interpretations through their influence on shaping the family philosophy. For example, families with members from a historically marginalized cultural heritage, who are guided by isolating cultural beliefs about self-sufficiency, or who live in an unsafe neighborhood could be more vulnerable to negative impacts of stressors. In short, this part of the model is a reminder that families function within larger contexts that can make major differences related to facing and dealing with daily and major stressful events.

Do You Want to Learn More?

Without peeking, take a moment to review in your mind (or say out loud) the key concepts from this chapter (this is a proven learning technique). Then review the "Chapter Preview" section at the top and compare. Skim Part B of the chapter with extra attention to the **bolded words**.

We have only touched on a portion of information related to some elements of this topic. **What really sparked your interest? What do you wish was covered more thoroughly?** Consider taking some time to further deepen your understanding of family stress concepts and processes. The following are a variety of resources that you might find helpful and some references directly or indirectly referred to in this chapter. In theory, you will have a great time.

Videos

(Use links or do searches with the key words provided.)

- *Mind Matters: Family Systems* (2.5 mins). Sober College. https://www.youtube.com/watch?v=yBjOpDKHWOM
- *Family Reaction to Stressful Events* (27 mins). Douglas Murphy, The Bowen Center, https://www.youtube.com/watch?v=KGDPjWRvSss
- *Raising Resilient Teens: The ABCX Model* (4 mins). Professor Jarom Petersen. https://www.youtube.com/watch?v=-VeexQUhU7I
- *Voltron: Master of the Universe* (1.5 mins). IMDB. https://www.imdb.com/video/vi1585823001/?ref_=tt_vi_i_2
- *How Childhood Trauma Affects Health Across a Lifetime* (16 mins). Pediatrician Nadine Burke Harris, TED Talk. https://www.ted.com/talks/nadine_burke_harris_how_childhood_trauma_affects_health_across_a_lifetime?language=en
- *Through Our Eyes: Children, Violence, and Trauma—Introduction* (8 mins). Office of Victims of Crime. https://www.youtube.com/watch?app=desktop&v=z8vZxDa2KPM

Websites

- National Child Traumatic Stress Network. https://www.nctsn.org
- PositivePsychology.com. https://positivepsychology.com
- The American Institute of Stress. https://www.stress.org/

Readings (Articles, Books, Book Chapters)

- Boss, P. (2002). *Family stress management: A contextual approach* (2nd ed.). SAGE Publications.
- Cornillo, T. A., & Boroto, D., R. (1992). The family distress model: A conceptual and clinical application of Reiss' strong bonds finding. *Contemporary Family Therapy*, 14, 181–198. https://doi.org/10.1007/BF00901503

- McCubbin, H. (1988). *Family types and family strengths: A life-span and ecological perspective.* Burgess Publishing.
- McCubbin, H., & Patterson, J. (1983). The family stress process: The double ABCX model of adjustment and adaptation. *Marriage & Family Review, 6,* 7–37. https://doi.org/10.1300/J002v06n01_02
- Patterson, J. (2002). Integrating family resilience and family stress theory. *Journal of Marriage and the Family, 64,* 349–360. https://doi.org/10.1111/j.1741-3737.2002.00349.x
- Whitchurch, G. G., & Constantine, L. L. (2009). Systems theory. In P. Boss, W. J. Doherty, R. LaRossa, W. R. Schumm, & S. K. Steinmetz (Eds), *Sourcebook of family theories and methods* (pp. 325–355). Springer. https://doi.org/10.1007/978-0-387-85764-0_14

Notes

1   The American Institute of Stress. (n.d.). *What is stress?* https://www.stress.org/daily-life

2   National Council for Mental Wellbeing. (2022, February 4). *How to manage trauma infographic.* (https://www.thenationalcouncil.org/topics/trauma-informed-care/trauma-infographic/

3   The Bowen Center for the Study of Families (n.d.). *Introduction to the eight concepts.* https://www.thebowencenter.org/introduction-eight-concepts; Whitchurch, G. G., & Constantine, L. L. (2009). Systems theory. In P. Boss, W. J. Doherty, R. LaRossa, W. R. Schumm, & S. K. Steinmetz (Eds), *Sourcebook of family theories and methods* (pp. 325–355). Springer. https://doi.org/10.1007/978-0-387-85764-0_14

4   Hill, R. (1949). *Families under stress.* Greenwood.

5   Boss, P. (2002). *Family stress management: A contextual approach* (2nd ed.). SAGE Publications; Bush, K. R., Price, C. A., Price, S. J., & McKenry, P. C., (2017). Families coping with change: A conceptual overview. In C. A. Price, K. R. Bush, & S. J. Price (Eds.), *Families & change: Coping with stressful events and transition* (pp. 3–23). SAGE Publications; Hill, R. (1959). Generic features of families under stress. *Social Casework, 39,* 139–150.

6   Boss, P. (2002). *Family stress management: A contextual approach* (2nd ed.). SAGE Publications.

7   Repetti, R. L., & Wood., J. (1997). Families accommodating to chronic stress. In B. H. Gottlieb (Ed.), *Coping with chronic stress* (pp. 191–220). Plenum Press; Wheaton, B. (1996). The domains and boundaries of stress concepts. In H. B. Kaplan (Ed.), *Psychosocial stress: Perspectives on structure, theory, life-course and methods* (pp. 29–70). Academic Press.

8   McCubbin, H., & Patterson, J. (1983). The family stress process: The double ABCX model of adjustment and adaptation. *Marriage & Family Review, 6,* 7–37. https://doi.org/10.1300/J002v06n01_02

9   Patterson, J. (2002). Integrating family resilience and family stress theory. *Journal of Marriage and the Family, 64,* 349–360. https://doi.org/10.1111/j.1741-3737.2002.00349.x

10 Boss, P. (2002). *Family stress management: A contextual approach* (2nd ed.). SAGE Publications.

11 Mancini, J. A., & Bowen, G. (2009). Community resilience: A social organization theory of action and change. In J. A. Mancini & K. A. Roberto (Eds.), *Pathways of human development: Explorations of change* (pp. 245–265). Lexington Books.

12 McCubbin, H. (1988). *Family types and family strengths: A life-span and ecological perspective.* Burgess Publishing.

13 Cornillo, T. A., & Boroto, D., R. (1992). The family distress model: A conceptual and clinical application of Reiss' strong bonds finding. *Contemporary Family Therapy, 14,* 181–198. https://doi.org/10.1007/BF00901503

14 Courtney E., & Ackerman, C. E. (n.d.). *Flourishing in positive psychology: Definition + 8 practical tips.* PositivePsychology.com. https://positivepsychology.com/flourishing

15 The American Institute of Stress. (n.d.). *What is child trauma?* https://www.nctsn.org/what-is-child-trauma

CHAPTER 2

Theoretical Elaboration of Personal and Professional Contexts of Family Stress

Research has shown that individuals over the age of 50 who report high levels of stress and negative beliefs about aging experienced about three times more physical symptoms than similar individuals with high stress levels but who report more positive beliefs about aging.[1]

Chapter Preview

- Subjective meaning plays a profound role in how we address family stressors.
- Family philosophy and cultural forces contribute to how we interpret our circumstances.
- Common cognitive biases can skew our perceptions in unhelpful ways.
- Conservative and liberal ideologies are based on similar and different foundations of morality.
- Political ideologies have fundamentally different views regarding changing family norms; these views can shape perceptions related to family stress.
- Professionals can encourage families to consider certain cognitive and behavioral coping strategies.
- Motivational interviewing is an approach that can help professionals understand families and cultivate families' motivation to make changes.
- Self-care is an important element of avoiding job burnout and personal stress when working with families in crisis.

What Is This Topic About?

Our minds are extremely powerful when it comes to how we experience—or construct—our reality. Whether in our personal or professional life, paying attention to how our minds guide **our interpretations of our circumstances** helps us understand ourselves, our family members, and those we help. We can learn to be open to others' perspectives and experiences. We can also learn to use our minds to think about stressful situations in diverse ways. Most of the chapters ahead of us highlight specific stressors and the various ways they affect families. The importance of resources and perceptions reoccur throughout the chapters in the context of helping families as a professional. This chapter lays the groundwork for contemplating those reoccurring segments. First, let us revisit the importance of the personal meanings we assign to our stressful circumstances and to family life in general.

Part A. Personal Context and Considerations

Even though a family as a unit can have shared perceptions among its members of a stressor, families are made up of individuals who each form personal meanings about family experiences—that includes you. We all have our own feelings, beliefs, and opinions about families and what it means to experience family stress. You are also part of the human race that has all sorts of interesting and curious ways of interpreting the world. The concepts that follow further highlight the important functions of perceptions throughout the coping process and clarify why you are likely to have differing opinions with someone down the street—or with someone in your own family. Family units are likely to differ from one another in their philosophies for similar reasons.

How Is Personal Meaning Related to Family Stress?

What does earning a college degree mean to you? Would you be the first to do so in your family? Do you already have a job lined up once you verify your diploma? Have you defied major odds throughout your degree? Will anyone you care about treat you differently with a degree? Do you feel like you finally jumped through enough hoops to satisfy a pointless expectation? Are you continuing on to an advanced degree? These questions highlight some factors that can shape the meanings of this specific event, sometimes subtly and sometimes dramatically. Why is **meaning** so flexible?

Similarly, a parent's reaction to a child's messiness can depend on the meaning of the mess and the circumstances surrounding it. Does the parent believe the child did it on purpose? Does that parent believe that such behavior is expected of a child of that age? Did the child make a mess of something the parent highly values? Is the parent embarrassed by the mess? Is the child perceived to have some kind of developmental delay or abnormality? Is the parent perceived by others as being competent? So many possibilities.

Isn't it fascinating that people can have such different perceptions and interpretations of the *same* incident? Perhaps you find it frustrating at times. But is it only **circumstances** that matter for meaning? It has been said that "perception is reality." Consider: in an analysis of over 28,000 U.S. adults over a 9-year period, people who reported high levels of stress were no more likely to have died than those who reported low or no stress.[2] Similarly, those who believed that stress had hurt their health were no more likely to have died than those who didn't believe stress hurt their health. However, people who reported the combination of high levels of stress *and* the belief that the stress hurt their health were more likely than everyone else to have died (while accounting for all sorts of other health behaviors and circumstances). It was projected that 20,000 extra deaths potentially occurred each year of the study because people believed their stress affected them negatively. Did that get your attention?

Philosophies abound about what is real. Our amazing minds seem to have the capacity to help us make **order out of complexity**. The mind edits what we observe into something we can label, categorize, and judge in ways that facilitate easier decision-making. Subjective understanding of reality contributes profoundly to how

- **families** make sense of stressors, assess their resources, and cope with stressors and crisis;
- **you** make sense of **your** family stressors, assess your resources, and cope with stressors and crisis;
- **you** make sense of a family you intend to help as a **professional** (or out of the goodness of your heart);
- **you** decide how to best **help** a given family; and
- **all of us** interact with others who view things differently.

Let's explore why meaning can be so personal and have profound implications for family stressors.

When Is a Problem a Problem?

Remember that the **pressure** caused by a stressor can be perceived as a **hardship** or **opportunity** (or **hassle** or **uplift**), or both at the same time. People who underestimate the family disruption caused by a stressor could respond too passively and increase the risk of family strain. Overestimating the disruption can lead to unnecessary anxiety and hastily altering patterns that actually work well for the family. Striving for realistic **appraisals** of a stressful situation can help us avoid feeling overconfident or overwhelmed. Our situational interpretations affect our emotions and our will to endure. Though some situations are indeed dire and require major responses regardless of what we think about them, our thoughts nevertheless impact how we experience stressors. For example, here are some stressors with different ways of thinking about them:

- **You just hurt your back:** "Of course this happened to me; now I'm going to be slowed up at work!" "Looks like I need to strengthen my core muscles." "I have been looking forward to getting a massage anyway!"

- **He forgot his wife's birthday; she is upset:** "She is way too sensitive about these things." "I have such a horrible memory; I will never get this right." "I need to do something special to make it up to her and it could end up bringing us closer."
- **Her daughter just said she wants to drop out of high school:** "People will think I'm a failure as a parent." "This is probably just a phase she is going through." "Maybe I can help her brainstorm ideas to support her in becoming who she wants to be someday."
- **Your parent is experiencing hearing loss:** (now you come up with some different ways of thinking about it).

We often embrace assumptions and interpretations that make us feel better about ourselves—though some of us have learned to think very negatively about ourselves. But was it the truth? We arguably **construct narratives** or stories about ourselves and our families that include overgeneralizations and exaggerations (e.g., I have always had bad luck; my family rules the neighborhood; he is the jealous type). Much of this construction process might happen without our direct awareness. Our personal narratives can be reflected in how we dress, the media we consume, and the overall identity we portray. A history of **trauma** can also contribute to skewed beliefs about our value and abilities. Unfortunately, these narratives can trap us into seeing just a narrow version of ourselves and our capacities—like developing a reputation that is difficult to change.

For example, you might think of yourself as having always been the quiet kid in school—sitting on the sidelines watching others live more interesting lives and that is how you describe yourself to others. But when you really think about it, you can remember times and places in which you were more of the center of attention or had people admire you—almost as if you had a different personality. The "quiet kid" narrative is incomplete and misleading, but for whatever reason, it became the version you hold onto, and it could dampen your confidence in social situations. Conversely, a narrative about being a family that knows how to work together through adversity could also be an oversimplification but can fuel confidence and trust when a family needs extra cooperation. In other words, we as individuals and families play a large role in constructing our past and current realities. Yes, there is an objective reality—the family dog was actually hit by a car and died—but a multitude of assumptions, reconstructed memories, current attitudes, and philosophies impact our perceived realities in ways that help us make sense of our circumstances. We and our families can choose to view things in certain ways and alter our narratives to expand our interpretations of our circumstances and generate new ways of coping.

What Shapes Our Narratives and Other Perceptions?

A **family philosophy** (see Chapter 1) is a key source of how we learn to view things and to construct our **narratives**. You might have heard statements that reveal family ideals or beliefs, like, "Our family doesn't quit!," or "We need to be good examples of our religious faith," or "In this life, you have to fight for everything you get." What other examples come to mind? Some families clearly prioritize what they value most in life: peace, togetherness, unity, money, comfort, freedom, excitement, and so on. Some clearly articulate their assumptions that shape how they interpret their experiences: "Nothing ever goes right for us," "We are very blessed," "People are just jealous of us," "Everyone thinks they are better than us," and so forth. Whether or not they are made obvious to others or themselves, families have philosophies about human nature, families, society, and culture that guide their interpretations of experiences. And, of course, as individual family members, we might adjust our philosophies based on other experiences and social influences.

Our **cultural heritage** can also shape how we view things through both its influence on shaping family philosophy and its direct influence on individuals. Cultural and other external contexts potentially benefit or hamper our perceptions, depending on the situation. For example, cultures vary in their beliefs about **mastery**—how much of life we can control.[3] Western cultures tend to lean toward a high mastery belief system:

- Good decisions and actions are rewarded, and bad ones get what they deserve.
- Following procedures lead to predictable outcomes.
- The physical environment is something that can be manipulated to serve human purposes.

Such an orientation can bring confidence and comfort to those required to follow orders or who undergo a medical procedure. Some other, particularly Eastern cultures, lean more toward fate and passivity than mastery:

- Natural disasters happen when they happen, and we are at their mercy.
- There is little point in resisting when you have no power to change a situation.
- Fate has determined our circumstances.

Such an orientation can bring peace when people truly are helpless and out of control—such as Jewish victims held in Nazi concentration camps. We will focus more on culture in Chapter 3.

What Else Shapes Our Thinking?

Evolutionary psychology has long proposed that we naturally have biases that have aided with survival and adaptation but can also contribute to unhelpful interpretations of our situations and of other peoples' perspectives. An online search will lead you to lists of the top 5, 10, 12, 20, and even 50 **cognitive biases**.[4] They all may be worth investigating regardless of how many there really are; you will find some additional resources at the end of this chapter for that purpose. Table 2.1 includes just a few to illustrate the commonality and power of biases and their potential relevance for interpreting stressors or understanding people we try to help.

TABLE 2.1 Select Cognitive Biases

Name	Description	Relevance to Stressor?
Blind Spot Bias	We see biased perceptions in others better than we see them in ourselves.	Think about what this means for how we judge others' perceptions and regarding the rest of the biases in this table.
Confirmation Bias	We recognize and remember things that confirm what we already believe or feel strongly about and dismiss things that don't.	Think about which types of stressors we might perceive as a big deal or who we think caused them.
Self-Serving Bias	When we fail, it is because of the situation or someone else, but we should get credit for when we succeed.	Think about what we might overlook about ourselves when viewing a stressor.
False Consensus	We assume that more people agree with us than actually do.	Think about how this fits with the idea that family members can have differing perceptions of the same stressor.
Anchoring	When making decisions we tend to rely on the first information we received.	Think about how first impressions of a stressor—or of someone facing a stressor—might steer us away from a deeper understanding of the situation.
Reactance	We tend to resist or do the opposite of what someone tells us to do, especially when we see it as a threat to our freedom.	Think about how this applies to family coping and to trying to help a family cope.
Sunk Cost Fallacy	We struggle to give up on something in which we have already invested, even when it is better for us to do so.	Think about how some families might struggle with giving up certain rules or ways of doing things that are holding them back.
In-Group Favoritism	We have more favorable perceptions of people who belong to the same group (race, religion, fans of a sports team, political party) than of those outside the group.	Think about how this push us to view certain people as hostile or enemies.

Adapted from: Dwyer, C., (2018, September 7). 12 common bases that affect how we make everyday decisions: Make sure that the decisions that matter are not made based on bias. *Psychology Today.* https://www.psychologytoday.com/us/blog/thoughts-thinking/201809/12-common-biases-affect-how-we-make-everyday-decisions; Hallman, C. (n.d.). 50 cognitive biases to be aware of so you can be the very best version of you. *Titlemax.* https://www.titlemax.com/discovery-center/lifestyle/50-cognitive-biases-to-be-aware-of-so-you-can-be-the-very-best-version-of-you.

As we become aware of such biases, it is probably easier to see them in others than in ourselves (see "blind spot bias"). That's a start. While our biases won't always lead us in the wrong direction, making the effort to evaluate our biases could help us avoid misunderstandings as we cope with family stressors or simply interact with fellow beings. Some suggestions for **evaluating our biases** include the following:

- Be humble enough to realize you have biases.
- Recognize that nobody has a perfect memory and that biases shape our memories without us realizing it.

- Look for evidence that supports an assumption and evidence that refutes an assumption with equal sincerity and rigor.
- Seek influence from others who have different opinions than you.
- Ask genuine questions about things you think you already know the answers to.

When we work to manage our biases, we become less prone to skipping important steps of discovery. We are more open to diverse perspectives. In short, we are better able to more fully assess our own stressors and resources, understand how family members assess them, and help family members and clients evaluate their perceptions in ways that bring further insight into coping with stressors.

What About Political Bias?

That's an intriguing question. Political bias can also influence what we perceive to be problems, why such problems exist, and how to solve them. This kind of bias seems most relevant to the topic of family stress when our focus is on the **larger external contexts** in which families function—especially when evaluating whether particular social trends are conducive to either family vulnerability or resiliency. Political bias can also help shape the **family philosophy**, be a source of conflicting perceptions within a family (see examples in Chapter 6), and influence the types of solutions that families and their professional helpers are open to.

It seems evident that in the United States (though not exclusively), political tensions are high and **polarizing**—people taking sides in more extreme ways against one another. Writing about politics is challenging because complex ideas and institutions are easily oversimplified and mischaracterized. The biases mentioned earlier also promote misunderstandings and hostility around political topics and public figures. An all too common technique used in presenting political arguments is the **straw man fallacy**: to present an opponent's argument in an exaggerated and misleading way that is much easier to argue against than the real argument. Sometimes this is unintentional because we parrot back what we have heard from some sources without taking the time to really investigate the original argument. Other times, people know exactly what they are doing. The descriptions that follow are genuine attempts to avoid any sense of a straw man fallacy—they are intended to describe perspectives from the viewpoint of people who hold the perspectives. They are also generalities—some subtleties and variations can be difficult to articulate briefly and lack relevance to our purpose, which is to have a basic understanding of how major political ideologies shape our perceptions related to family stress. Such perceptions shape our interpretations of stressors, including their causes, consequences, and solutions, especially when we consider the roles of the broader society.

Our attention is on **political ideology**, which is not the same thing as a **political party**, though there is considerable overlap. Political ideology is a foundational **worldview** that influences our interpretations of reality, our opinions on social and economic matters, and our voting patterns. As we focus on ideology, think more about a **continuum of conservative to liberal perspectives** in a broad sense more than on Republicans and Democrats or any particular politician. What do you believe your ideological perspective is?

The prominent moral psychologist and cofounder of the Heterodox Academy for viewpoint diversity, Jonathan Haidt, argues that morality **"binds and blinds."**[5] Research consistently shows that humans have strong tendencies toward grouping themselves and defending their groups. We easily form an *us versus them* mentality and judge people outside our groups more harshly (despite polls that say both conservatives and liberals equally claim to judge people across all ideologies fairly). Some even think of others with different views as enemies or evil and treat them as such.[6] A polarizing approach to viewpoints can become a barrier toward mutual trust among struggling families, neighbors, and professionals.

Our focus is primarily on social conservatism and liberalism and not the complete details of any political platform. We emphasize how political ideologies align with or inform perspectives and values related to family issues.[7] Being able to objectively evaluate political ideologies might require us to **guard against** our binding and blinding tendencies.

First, imagine you observe the following exchange on an elementary school playground:

> A group of children is playing dodgeball (two teams of 10 players each trying to hit opponents with a bouncy ball to get the other team members "out"). Three other children are sitting and just watching the game. One is in a wheelchair, one is much smaller than all the other children, and one has significant mental delays. An approaching teacher tells the children to stop playing for a moment. "Hey, everybody, how about letting these other children play?" says the teacher, pointing to the three children watching. Some of the other children protest, saying that those other three would mess up the game because they aren't able to play the right way. The teacher says they should change the rules of the game to be more accommodating. Maybe everyone should throw underhand, and everyone should be a certain distance away from each other before throwing the ball. Maybe use a lighter ball that glides slower.
>
> A second teacher who had overheard part of the conversation approaches the group and asks the first teacher, "Hey, um, why are you trying to get the children to change the rules?" The first teacher argues that it is unfair for these three children to be left out; it isn't their fault that they are a little different. It is important for everyone to feel included. The second teacher agrees that it is nice for everyone to feel included, but it is also important to honor the rules of the game because they are there for specific purposes that make the game what it is. The game teaches the children important life lessons about teamwork, winning and losing with dignity, and how to play by and enforce rules. The vast majority of the children are getting needed exercise and enhancing skills of strategy and hand-eye coordination. In real life, things aren't always fair, and that's an important lesson too.
>
> The first teacher counters, saying, "That's true, but by changing the game, you are also teaching compassion, which is even more important. Creativity and personal expression also increase because they are not bound by one set of rules. The game is not more important than individual children—nobody should be left out."

"I see your point, but by changing the game that much, it isn't dodgeball any-more, and then nobody has the opportunity to actually play dodgeball and get all the benefits that come with it," argues the second teacher. "The children are free to invent or play a different game, but it would be better to leave dodgeball the way it is and let each child choose what to play." The first teacher continues to disagree, arguing that getting rid of dodgeball would be better than leaving any children out, while the second argues that dodgeball has important benefits for the children overall.

Which teacher do you find yourself siding with based on the arguments? Does each teacher's argument have some logic to it? Can each argument be motivated by genuine and positive desires for the children? Do your feelings about dodgeball affect your opinion (you can choose another example for the analogy—dodgeball isn't the point)? What values or principles would you say the first teacher prioritizes? How about the second teacher? Like any analogy, this has its flaws, but it introduces some key differences in ideological perspectives.

What Assumptions About People Relate to Our Political Biases?

The economist and social theorist Thomas Sowell argued that for centuries philosophers have debated over two visions of human nature and society along a spectrum of **social constraint**.[8] In brief, the more conservative, **constrained vision** highlights the limits and pitfalls of human nature: we have (1) underlying selfish motives that help us survive and preserve our own well-being, (2) a hunger for power and esteem from others, and (3) strong tendencies toward self-deception (e.g., rationalizing, biases, lying to ourselves). Long-standing religious and social customs, sexual mores, respect for the rule of law, and the family unit (especially marriage) are assumed to be time-tested and systematically created means to counter those elements of our nature and promote positive behavior and societal order. We should be concerned when the few in power push to redesign society, especially in ways that are incompatible with human nature; the inherently flawed human reasoning and utopian aspirations of such leaders could damage important societal traditions and institutions and introduce unforeseen societal consequences (or repeat problems from that past that were due to such changes). If change is needed, it best occurs incrementally while adjusting to feedback from societal trends and the evaluation of their broad consequences.

The more liberal, **unconstrained vision** highlights the potential for human nature to be flexible or to change: social circumstances shape human nature so traditions and institutions become irrelevant as the world changes and they stifle progress. Hence, past oppressive regimes and practices that were once thought to be influenced by human nature have lessened over time in some places (e.g., slavery). Current traditions and institutions must be proven to show their value to society. Constantly striving toward a world that is free of suffering and injustices requires big changes that are driven by social policies. Conservatives are less optimistic about dramatic changes to human nature, and they value safeguards (**constraints**) to maintain social stability; liberals are less convinced that human nature is as set or rigid, and they value **less constraint** or social safeguards and are prone to see them as unnecessary or unfair. Such assumptions about human nature seem to be evident in ideological disagreements related to issues of sex, gender, and family. Can you think of any?

How Do Perspectives on Morality Relate to Political Bias?

Jonathan Haidt and colleagues similarly proposed key spectrums or dimensions along which ideological perspectives vary.[9] They also generally integrate the issue of social constraint but with added nuance. Their **moral foundations theory** is based on years of cross-cultural and historical study and data analysis. Throughout history, various types of moralities have tended to facilitate cooperative living in societies. They identified six foundations of morality (what we view to be good, especially for a society):

- **Care (vs. harm):** kindness, gentleness, and nurturing, concern about suffering and harm
- **Liberty (vs. oppression):** resentment toward domination, bullies, and restricting of liberties
- **Fairness (vs. cheating):** a sense of proportionality—you should get what you deserve or earn, no freeloading or cheating; do your part
- **Loyalty (vs. betrayal):** loyalty to a group, self-sacrifice, and duty for the sake of the group—patriotism
- **Authority (vs. subversion):** order, hierarchy, leadership, and followership, respect for traditions and institutions that enforce order and stability
- **Sanctity (vs. degradation):** caution around sources of disgust (a natural reaction to signs of contamination), purity and sacredness of body or what is put into the body, controlling our natural, carnal urges

Extensive research shows that people with a more **liberal** ideology tend to value the **care** foundation the most, followed closely by **liberty** and then **fairness.** The other three tend to be valued much less as forms of morality. People with a more **conservative** ideology highly value **all six** of the foundations about the same (so it will require a bit more space to describe them here). Though generally high on the care foundation, they appear more willing than liberals to compromise a bit on care for the sake of supporting other foundations if they believe it results in the greater good. They also tend to rate the **fairness** foundation a bit higher than liberals.

Overall, the most sacred social value from a liberal perspective is **to care for victims of oppression.** This can represent a mentality of supporting the underdog and a focus on those on the fringes of a society. It may require changing social systems and institutions to make things more **equal.** This perspective is clearly evident in liberal politics that focus on **underrepresented** or **marginalized groups** of people (and families), often associated with gender, race, class, and sexual identity issues. An ideal society is one in which everyone has equal rights to express themselves as they want (but without harming others), that fosters **creativity** and **diversity**, and in which people voluntarily band together to **change things for the better.** For highly progressive liberals especially, a key indicator of such a society would be **minimal if any differences** among demographic groups of people—be it across gender, race, sexual identities, immigration status, and so forth. Liberals are prone to interpret problems related to the family as largely **stemming**

from economic factors beyond the family's control. Thus, liberals are generally open to greater governmental control of the economy.

Overall, the most sacred social value from a conservative perspective is to **preserve traditions and institutions that sustain a moral community**. This can represent resistance to quick societal changes that threaten how social **stability** is maintained. Humans need social structure to help them **overcome** some harmful, natural tendencies and to live in more **dignified** ways (control over carnal urges). Many **traditions** and **institutions** exist to help promote and enforce cooperation and good behavior for the sake of the community. **Loyalty** and **sacrifice** are necessary and helpful for people to build meaningful social connections and preserve order; this helps counter risks of isolation and depression. **Social change should be gradual at best** and guard against unintended consequences for society and families. For highly **traditional** conservatives especially, an ideal society would support and promote a strong marriage and family ethic that includes some gendered family roles, parents instilled with **authority** who **sacrifice** for their children, and (for more religious conservatives) that yields to **God's ways** rather than to our limited human understandings. Conservatives are prone to interpret problems related to the family as largely **stemming from changing cultural norms, values, and policies** that enable if not celebrate less stable family forms (e.g., single parent) and a lack of personal discipline and effort.

For those whose conservatism is largely shaped by **religion**, their arguments for what is best for families and societies can be rooted in beliefs about what a higher power has dictated to be righteous living. Those whose conservatism is more rooted in a philosophy or their interpretation of scientific findings tend to reach similar conclusions but may justify them differently. Those who are conservative based primarily on **economic issues** tend to be less passionate about social issues that are seemingly inconsequential to the economy, and the way they live their lives may not apply the same way to the moral foundations. While many liberals are religious (though a disproportionally smaller group than among conservatives), liberals as a whole view religious traditions and institutions as being too rigid to accommodate social change. **Culture** can also play a role in diverse perspectives within a political group: whereas 89% of Democrats in recent years agreed that it is unnecessary to believe in God to be a moral person, only 44% of Black Democrats agreed with that statement.[10] As opposed to aligning predominantly with a conservative or liberal ideology, many people consider themselves ideological **centrists** who align more on some issues with conservatives and more on others with liberals, and who might take a more middle-ground approach to disagreements.

Did you find yourself thinking or muttering "yeah, but …" at any point while reading about these ideologies? Maybe you thought something like, "I'm liberal and I don't believe that," or "I'm conservative and think that too." Here are some things to keep in mind:

- These are generalities and based on average differences or tendencies; you may not be average, so to speak.
- Like so many of us, the political label you apply to yourself may have much to do with the people you get along with or the political party that shares your viewpoint on a very specific issue you care deeply about.
- Political party platforms and strategies change, and some politicians espouse positions that have little to do with the foundations of liberal and conservative ideologies.

- Media portrayals of political or ideological positions arguably focus more on public figures with more extreme positions, which can skew our perceptions of people who vote for the same candidates.

People with differing ideologies can share some of the same ideas about families but have different perspectives on **causes, consequences, and solutions** related to family stressors. Regardless of disagreements, people can **minimize polarization** within and between families and among service providers by seeking to understand where each other is coming from and respecting the foundations for their arguments. Seeing others as erring on the side of the moral foundations that they believe bring about the greater good is a gracious attitude that de-escalates unwarranted conflict. People can work together to find common ground and to broaden each other's perspectives in ways that lead to useful interventions and policies (or to fewer interventions and policies that cause more harm than good). Despite their differences, conservative and liberal families actually report similar lifestyles. Though conservatives are a bit more likely to be married, both groups tend to do several things at least weekly together: eat dinner, do chores, attend family members' activities or events, do family activities (like a movie), and have arguments.[11] Much more could be said about ideologies, politics, and family issues—feel free to do some additional exploration on your own. Just look out for straw man fallacies and all sorts of biases that create distortions.

Improve Your Learning

Without peeking, take a moment to review in your mind (or say out loud) the key concepts from this chapter (this is a proven learning technique). Then review the "Chapter Preview" section at the top and compare. Skim Part A of the chapter with extra attention to the **bolded words.** Skip to the end of the chapter to find more learning resources.

Part B. Professional Context and Considerations

The lines between personal and professional identities and roles are not always firm. Professionals are also people who construct their narratives and are subject to cognitive biases and political ideologies. Furthermore, the coping strategies that follow apply to professionals dealing with their own professional (or personal) stressors and to the families they assist. Here we continue to establish a basic foundation for applying theoretical concepts to helping families cope with stressors. Later chapters will reference this foundation and add some topic-specific suggestions for working with families.

How Can Meaning Contribute to Coping?

Theory helps us make sense of what we observe about families. The theoretical foundations from Chapter 1 can guide you in your quest to make a difference in people's lives—including your own. You may have opportunities to help families build **resiliency** and to cultivate **flourishing**.

The **FSS integrated model (FIM) of family stress and crisis** helps explain why certain family characteristics and processes could contribute to positive and negative outcomes of stressors.

As a reminder, the **stressor** (event or situation) triggers a sense of **pressure** that requires **coping** activities to ensure that the pressure is **managed** before the family becomes overwhelmed and reaches **crisis**. **Resources** and **perceptions** (or **interpretations**) are primary influences on how the family copes with a stressor and the ultimate impact of that stressor on family functioning. As indicated in the **FIM diagram** in the previous chapter, perceptions of whether or not the stressor causes pressure on the family can lead to inaction that potentially strains the family. Perceptions also differ as to whether that pressure to change is viewed negatively (as a **hardship** or **hassle**) or positively (as an **opportunity** or **uplift**). Such perceptions interact with other interpretations of the stressor-induced circumstances and of family resources, leading to coping that helps the family **adjust** to the stressor or eventually **adapt** to crisis; both of these stages of coping impact general family functioning, possibly for the better. Perceptions are influenced at least in part by **family philosophy** and **historical/cultural/environmental contexts**.

Coping can also include forming or changing our thoughts. Making **meanings** out of our circumstances is an active process, though we may not always be aware of it. Can you think of a time in which you talked yourself into doing something? In some way, you helped yourself think differently about someone or a situation—perhaps as being less intimidating than at first glance. Paying attention to how we and family members think about a stressor—and helping others do the same—can foster successful family coping.

What Are Some Helpful Thinking Strategies?

Psychological research has identified at least nine common **cognitive reactions** we can have when we encounter stressful circumstances.[12] While they might be natural inclinations for many of us, they can also be learned responses based on our past experiences or future intentions. They can also be unlearned when needed.

- **Rumination:** persistent focus on one's feelings and thoughts about the event, not getting a mental break from it
- **Catastrophizing:** focusing on the exaggerated disastrous effects of the event
- **Self-blame:** placing the blame for the event or situation on one's self
- **Other-blame:** placing the blame for the event or situation on someone else or on one's environment
- **Putting into perspective:** brushing off the seriousness of the event, including thinking about worse events as a way to not overreact to the current event
- **Positive refocusing:** distracting one's self from concerns about the current event by thinking of things that bring positivity and joy
- **Positive reappraisal:** choosing to view the event in a more positive way—it creates opportunity instead of just hardship
- **Acceptance:** coming to terms with the reality of the situation and accepting that the event has happened
- **Refocus on planning:** focusing on the steps required to manage the event or situation

These reactions can be thought of as **cognitive coping strategies.** Generally speaking, **rumination** and **catastrophizing** seem to put us at greater risk for negative outcomes, such as depression or anxiety. **Blaming one's self or someone else** could have mixed effects—self-blame can fuel or confirm self-doubt and discouragement, though some people may feel empowered with a sense of control over their circumstances by taking the blame. Similarly, blaming others can be a way to lessen our own sense of shame or insecurity, though it might also foster negative feelings toward someone else and distract from more positive strategies. Blame is a risky and controversial concept—it might help people make sense of their situations, but it connotes a presence of resentment that could embitter and weigh someone down (though some people seem energized by their anger). **Putting into perspective** can help a problem feel manageable, though it might be risky to overly **minimize** the seriousness of the situation or of one's role in it—like being in **denial**. Denial has been shown to perhaps help people in the short term create more time for themselves to accept a harsh reality, but long-term denial can be a major barrier to making needed changes.

Positive refocusing helps us manage our emotions and avoid getting overwhelmed with negativity. **Positive reappraisals** have the potential to increase our hope and energy toward addressing a challenge, though the reappraisals need to be seen as at least plausible if not convincing. Also referred to as **reframing**, we can choose to reappraise a situation in a more positive manner—such as by

- looking at the bright side (e.g., "at least I will get to spend more time at home with this cutback of work hours"),
- making the situation seem more normal (e.g., "it's normal for employers to have to make cuts; it's nothing personal"),
- giving someone the benefit of the doubt (e.g., "Dave was under a lot of pressure when he told me about the cuts, he didn't mean to sound impatient with me"), and
- seeing new opportunities (e.g., "I think I will finally get that degree I always wanted so I can get long-term, stable employment").

Acceptance and **refocusing on planning** are similar approaches toward getting beyond ruminating or catastrophizing. They help us establish a foundation of reality that becomes a basis for moving forward.

Can We _Really_ Change Our Long-Established Thinking Patterns?

What do you think? Do you have an example one way or another? There is good reason to believe the answer is yes. A key part of **cognitive behavior therapy** (**CBT**)—which has an impressive success rate for treating anxiety, depression, and anger control issues—is **cognitive restructuring**.[13] This involves a process of learning to identify negative thinking that dampens our moods and to challenge those thoughts by gathering and evaluating legitimate evidence that contradicts the thoughts. We can learn to see the inaccuracy of catastrophizing a minor incident, to avoid needlessly taking personal offense, to cease expecting near perfection from ourselves or others, or to define ourselves by more than just a single incident. In short, we can

- catch ourselves thinking in ways that make us feel discouraged or immobilized to act,
- question the validity of the thoughts by thinking of or looking for exceptions, and
- replace the thoughts with something that is more accurate and encouraging.

Finding real evidence is important; we need to be convincing to ourselves. There are many CBT-based self-help books out there and good CBT therapists. You might consider looking into it (see resources at end of chapter).

Practicing **mindfulness** also involves our thoughts and has become increasingly popular as a stress-coping strategy.[14] In brief, being mindful means focusing on the here and now—it is a way to stop ruminating about things that bring us stress. It can be a slow, deliberate process that helps us appreciate something we enjoy and give us a break from other concerns. A mindful hike would include paying close attention to your surroundings, looking for all the details you can take in while feeling lost in the moment. **Mindful breathing** is a form of meditation that helps us become more aware of our thoughts from an objective standpoint—letting our thoughts come as they do without judging them or reacting to them but also not lingering on them but returning to an intentional focus on our breathing. This process can ease our minds, relieve our bodies from tension related to our worries, and ultimately energize us toward facing our stressors. Look into it if you haven't already.

How Can We Help Others Put These Things Into Practice?

As a professional (or a friend/family member), focusing on the words people use to describe themselves, families, and situations can tip you off about their potentially skewed interpretations and negative cognitive coping strategies. Are they catastrophizing or self-blaming? Avoid assuming that the way you understand the situation is the way anyone else understands it. Seek to understand how family members make sense of their perceived realities by asking **thoughtful questions** and **listening attentively** (see the following discussion on **motivational interviewing**). Once someone feels understood, you might help them do some cognitive restructuring. Help them recall and look for evidence that challenges their negative thinking. Help them evaluate their resources in ways they might have overlooked—some people don't realize all the resources they have available to them (including their strengths) or how best to use them.

What Is Motivational Interviewing?

Based largely on work by William Miller, motivational interviewing is an approach toward helping people make changes, especially when people lack the motivation to do so on their own.[15] This collaborative, nonthreatening approach values client autonomy and perspectives. Encouraging clients to talk about change is a key step toward motivating change. Good listening skills can help draw out the client's goals and realization about the changes needed to accomplish those goals. The **OARS** interviewing framework can help guide your efforts to understand the perceptions of people you assist. Table 2.2 includes information about the four parts of this framework.

TABLE 2.2 Components and an Application of Motivational Interviewing

OARS Components	Description/Example	Purpose
Open-ended questions	Questions that invite longer, more detailed responses ("What did it mean to you to watch your child suffer like that?")	Gets at information that can build momentum toward wanting to make changes. Gives clients autonomy to explain things in their own words.
Affirmations	Genuine statements that highlight the client's strengths ("I can see that you keeping calm really helped give your family hope.")	Build confidence in clients' own abilities, reframe an issue in a more positive light, and help build positive connections between the interviewer and client.
Reflections	Statements that indicate that the interviewer has been listening carefully, has empathy for the client, and brings attention to the benefits of change ("It sounds like that was very painful. I can see why your family wasn't happy about that.")	Strengthen trust and connection with interviewer and highlight client's underlying desires for things to be different.
Summaries	Statements that summarize large portions of the discussion, or the full discussion ("What I'm understanding is that you feel … because … but are concerned about … though you ultimately want to. … Did I miss anything?")	Demonstrates understanding of the client's situation; brings attention to certain information that the interviewer can highlight to help empower and encourage change.

Adapted from: Motivational Interviewing Network of Trainers (n.d.). Home page. https://motivationalinterviewing.org/

What About Behavior Change as a Form of Coping?

Indeed, changing our thinking alone might be insufficient for coping successfully with stressors, though it's importance can easily be overlooked in our desire to "do something about" a situation. A key form of **behavioral coping** involves seeking formal and informal support from others. **Formal support networks**—including human services agencies, health providers, educators, school systems, and afterschool programs—are specifically created to provide professional services.[16] Such forms of support address a family's lack of resources needed to cope with stressors and have the ultimate goal of **empowering families** to become more self-reliant. However, we often turn first to our **informal support** networks, those who are chosen or emerge more naturally such as friends, extended family, coworkers, neighbors, and church communities. These groups can assist with doing physical tasks, gathering or sharing information, providing emotional support, and fostering needed companionship. Ideally, formal support networks help families form, strengthen, and transition to their informal networks that can offer more personal, affordable, long-term support. Building trusting, reciprocating informal networks can help buffer families from the effects of future stressors and foster resiliency.

Within the home, fortifying strong family bonds and a spirit of mutual support can facilitate effective coping behaviors that occur as a family unit or any given subsystem (e.g., siblings, parent-child). McCubbin and Patterson from Chapter 1 suggested that families dealing with crisis need to **consolidate** as a durable unit by doing the following:[17]

- **Synergizing:** Coordinating the awareness of each individual's needs, perceptions, and resources and pulling together as a unit to work through crisis and attending to each other's perspectives while "getting on the same page."
- **Interfacing:** Improving the fit between the family's restructuring and the community norms and resources; this could mean moving to a different community that is more compatible with the family's rules and philosophy (e.g., leaving a neighborhood with a heavy gang presence for one that supports parental authority and cooperation).
- **Compromising:** Be willing to accept less-than-perfect solutions to consolidating around family needs and community fit; having everyone be equally satisfied with the results of synergizing and interfacing is not always possible, but needed improvement can still occur.
- **System maintenance:** Continue to attend to everyday needs and build morale in the home while in the process of making adaptations because of a crisis; avoid extra strain caused by neglecting the "little things" while focusing on the major stressors.

Other common behavioral coping strategies focus on enhancing overall emotional and physical health to help prevent becoming overwhelmed. This can include meditation, deep breathing, journaling, talking with a friend or professional, taking a break (removing self from the situation for a while), practicing forgiveness, regular exercise or sports participation, healthy eating, sufficient sleep, and avoiding unnecessary substances that create chemical dependency. You know, the things we are supposed to be doing anyway.

Though the synergizing process involves unifying perceptions and resources, that does not mean that forcing all family members to cope the same way with a situation is a good idea. Everyone choosing to have the exact same cognitions or behavioral responses is probably not necessary, even though having different perspectives could lead to arguments and misunderstandings. Nevertheless, family members benefit when they work to **appreciate** where each other is coming from and realize that having different ways of coping is **normal**. The constant tug between individuals and the family unit can be a tricky balance and involves **compromise**. Ideally, personal coping preferences don't undermine family coping overall. Yet, having different types of cognitive and behavioral responses to the same situation could be an **asset** for families, giving the family more options for expanding their interpretations and having a broader array of behavioral techniques to choose from (this last sentence is an example of **reframing** by me, the author).

How Should Professionals Care for Themselves While Assisting Others With Coping?

You might be wondering how professionals (or others) are affected by assisting families in crisis. Indeed, there is some cause for concern. Like with any work, professionals feel **pressure** to complete their tasks on time and with quality results, and some tasks are especially challenging. While working with people as individuals or as families can feel very rewarding, it is often difficult; humans and human relationships are complex. When people look to you as their problem solver—even when your goal is to empower them to solve their own problems—it is easy to become burdened with worry and obligation. That is good—at least to the extent that it shows you are a caring individual. It is bad when it wears you down and you can no longer meet your own personal and family needs, let alone help someone else do the same.

Self-care is an important practice for preventing and countering professional stressors. What you learned about risk and protective factors, vulnerability and resiliency, and adjustment and adaptive coping also applies to you in your professional (or voluntary) efforts to help families. As with any profession, taking on too much work mixed with insufficient resources can lead to **burnout**—*I can't do this anymore.* When the work involves families that have experienced trauma, we are at risk of experiencing **compassion fatigue**, which comes from psychologically taking upon ourselves the suffering of distressed or traumatized families we help.[18] We might extend so much empathy that we seemingly run out of empathy to give and become a bit jaded. We might consequently feel excessively tired, on edge, and depressed, and lose the satisfaction of helping others.

We also need to be aware of our potential for **secondary** or **vicarious trauma**.[19] Specifically, listening to others' trauma can be traumatizing in itself. Our vivid imaginations can make us feel as if we are in danger, especially when we replay traumatic images over and over in our heads (even if they aren't of our own experiences). Our senses get put on high alert, and if they stay there too long we can become **anxious and worn down**. If what we hear reminds us of our **own past trauma**, we could experience strong feelings and even flashbacks that induce a crisis-like state—immobilized to help others meet their needs and possibly meet our own needs. People who have experienced family trauma sometimes go into helping professions because they have great empathy and understanding to share with others. That can be a good thing, but they need to be sure they have made substantial strides in confronting their trauma and in coping with its aftereffects.

Being resilient when our own trauma is triggered helps us meet our obligations to ourselves and to others. Psychotherapists commonly also receive therapy for this very reason; there is nothing wrong with seeking extra help to be empowered as a competent professional or well-functioning individual. If you find yourself consumed with strong emotions, feeling burned out or powerless, being highly irritable, being full of cynicism, having the urge to avoid others, and even experiencing physical symptoms that seem to lack an obvious cause (e.g., fatigue, stomachaches, headaches), you might be taking too much of your work home with you. Caring individuals must learn the delicate **balance** between genuinely investing themselves in helping others and being able to set those investments aside and focus on other important things in their lives. Have you seen anyone do that successfully?

What Can We Do to Avoid Negative Outcomes Like Burning Out?

The cognitive and behavioral coping strategies already mentioned certainly apply to professionals. Additionally, working in an **agency** can provide important sources of formal and informal social support. Supervisors should be looking out for your welfare and will need to receive honest self-assessments from you. Coworkers can empathize with your circumstances and help you feel understood and confident. Some companies provide other self-care resources that help employees relax, clear their heads, and strengthen connections with colleagues such as recreation or exercise equipment, retreats, and parties. Take advantage of those when you can. Keep in mind that it is **not selfish** to make sure you are healthy and happy, especially when your goal is to be an effective helper to others.

The National Center on Safe Supportive Learning Environments created a "Secondary Traumatic Stress and Self-Care Packet" that includes a thorough assessment tool that could also be used as helpful lists of recommendations for how to prevent or minimize problems like burnout, secondary trauma, and compassion fatigue.[20] What do you think would be most helpful for you?

Physical Self-Care

- Eat regularly (e.g., breakfast and lunch)
- Eat healthfully
- Exercise or go to the gym
- Lift weights
- Practice martial arts
- Get regular medical care for prevention
- Get medical care when needed
- Take time off when you are sick
- Get massages or other bodywork
- Do physical activity that is fun for you
- Take time to be sexual
- Get enough sleep
- Wear clothes you like
- Take vacations
- Take day trips or mini-vacations
- Get away from stressful technology, such as pagers, faxes, telephones, and email

Psychological Self-Care

- Make time for self-reflection
- Go to see a psychotherapist or counselor for yourself
- Write in a journal
- Read literature unrelated to work
- Do something at which you are a beginner
- Take a step to decrease stress in your life
- Notice your inner experience—your dreams, thoughts, imagery, and feelings

- Let others know different aspects of you
- Engage your intelligence in a new area—go to an art museum, performance, sports event, exhibit, or other cultural event
- Practice receiving from others
- Be curious
- Say no sometimes to extra responsibilities
- Spend time outdoors

Emotional Self-Care

- Spend time with others whose company you enjoy
- Stay in contact with important people in your life
- Treat yourself kindly (supportive inner dialogue or self-talk)
- Feel proud of yourself
- Reread favorite books, review favorite movies
- Identify and seek out comforting activities, objects, people, relationships, places
- Allow yourself to cry
- Find things that make you laugh
- Express your outrage in a constructive way
- Play with children

Spiritual Self-Care

- Make time for prayer, meditation, and reflection
- Spend time in nature
- Participate in a spiritual gathering, community, or group
- Be open to inspiration
- Cherish your optimism and hope
- Be aware of nontangible (nonmaterial) aspects of life
- Be open to mystery, to not knowing
- Identify what is meaningful to you and notice its place in your life
- Sing
- Express gratitude
- Celebrate milestones with rituals that are meaningful to you
- Remember and memorialize loved ones who have died
- Nurture others
- Have awe-filled experiences
- Contribute to or participate in causes you believe in
- Read inspirational literature
- Listen to inspiring music

Workplace or Professional Self-Care

- Take time to eat lunch
- Take time to chat with coworkers

- Make time to complete tasks
- Identify projects or tasks that are exciting, growth promoting, and rewarding for you
- Pursue regular learning and professional development
- Get support from colleagues

I suspect you can find something in these lists to try out when you need a little self-care. Some of these may require specific planning to ensure they happen on a regular basis. As we invest in ourselves across these different realms, we also model to the individuals and families we help ways to live that foster resilience and increase chances for flourishing.

Do You Want to Learn More?

Without peeking, take a moment to review in your mind (or say out loud) the key concepts from this chapter (this is a proven learning technique). Then review the "Chapter Preview" section at the top and compare. Skim Part B of the chapter with extra attention to the **bolded words**.

We have only touched on a portion of information related to some elements of this topic. What really sparked your interest? What do you wish was covered more thoroughly? Consider taking some time to further deepen your understanding of personal and professional issues related to helping families cope with stressors. The following are a variety of resources that you might find helpful, and some references directly or indirectly referred to in this chapter. Don't interpret my invitation as a guilt trip (unless it works).

Videos

(Use links or do searches with the key words provided)
- *How to Make Better Decisions: 10 Cognitive Biases and How to Outsmart Them* (8 mins). The Art of Improvement. https://www.youtube.com/watch?v=ZhYO68O2jWU
- *The Moral Roots of Liberals and Conservatives, Jonathan Haidt* (19 mins). TED-Ed Talk. https://www.youtube.com/watch?v=8SOQduoLgRw&t=981s
- *What Is Mindfulness?* (5 mins). Psych Hub. https://www.youtube.com/watch?v=7-1Y6IbAxdM
- *Lifting the Burden in Motivational Interviewing, William Miller* (2 mins). Psychwire. https://www.youtube.com/watch?v=SsNgZ47o2I4

Websites

- Hallman, C. (n.d.). 50 cognitive biases to be aware of so you can be the very best version of you. Titlemax. https://www.titlemax.com/discovery-center/lifestyle/50-cognitive-biases-to-be-aware-of-so-you-can-be-the-very-best-version-of-you/
- Moral Foundations.org. https://moralfoundations.org/
- Motivational Interviewing Network of Trainers. https://motivationalinterviewing.org/

- *Psychology Today.* (n.d.). *Cognitive behavioral therapy.* https://www.psychologytoday.com/us/basics/cognitive-behavioral-therapy
- The Heterodox Academy (Mission: To improve the quality of research and education in universities by increasing open inquiry, viewpoint diversity, and constructive disagreement.) https://heterodoxacademy.org/

Readings (Articles, Books, Book Chapters)

- Gillihan, S. (2018). *Cognitive behavioral therapy made simple: 10 strategies for managing anxiety, depression, anger, panic, and worry.* Althea Press.
- Haidt, J., (2012). *The righteous mind: Why good people are divided by politics and religion.* Vintage Books.
- National Center on Safe Supportive Learning Environments. (n.d.). *Secondary traumatic stress and self-care package.* https://safesupportivelearning.ed.gov/sites/default/files/TSS_Building_Handout_2secondary_trauma.pdf
- Sowell, T. (2007). *A conflict of visions: Ideological origins of political struggles.* Basic Books.

Notes

1   Witzel, D. D., Turner, S. G., & Hooker, K. (2022). Self-perceptions of aging moderate associations of within- and between-persons perceived stress and physical health symptoms. *The Journals of Gerontology. Series B, Psychological Sciences and Social Sciences, 77*(4), 641–651. https://doi.org/10.1093/geronb/gbab228

2   Keller, A., Litzelman, K., Wisk, L. E., Maddox, T., Cheng, E. R., Creswell, P. D., & Witt, W. P. (2012). Does the perception that stress affects health matter? The association with health and mortality. *Health Psychology, 31*(5), 677–684. https://doi.org/10.1037/a0026743

3   Boss, P. (2002). *Family stress management: A contextual approach* (2nd ed.). SAGE Publishing.

4   Dwyer, C., (2018, September 7). 12 common bases that affect how we make everyday decisions: Make sure that the decisions that matter are not made based on bias. *Psychology Today.* https://www.psychologytoday.com/us/blog/thoughts-thinking/201809/12-common-biases-affect-how-we-make-everyday-decisions; Hallman, C. (n.d.). 50 cognitive biases to be aware of so you can be the very best version of you. Titlemax. https://www.titlemax.com/discovery-center/lifestyle/50-cognitive-biases-to-be-aware-of-so-you-can-be-the-very-best-version-of-you

5   Haidt, J., (2012). *The righteous mind: Why good people are divided by politics and religion.* Vintage Books.

6   Edsal, T. B. (2019, March 13). No hate left behind: Lethal partisanship is taking us into dangerous territory. *New York Times.* https://www.nytimes.com/2019/03/13/opinion/hate-politics.html

7   Brueck, H., & Lopez, C. (2020, October 27). These key psychological differences can determine whether you're liberal or conservative. *Business Insider.* https://www.businessinsider.com/psychological-differences-between-conservatives-and-liberals-2018-2; Glenn, N. (2000). Who's who in the family wars: A characterization of the major ideological factions. In N. Benokraits (Ed.), *Feuds about families: Conservative, centrist, liberal, and feminist perspectives* (pp. 2–13). Pearson Publishing.

8   Sowell, T. (2007). *A conflict of visions: Ideological origins of political struggles.* Basic Books.

9   Haidt, J., (2012). *The righteous mind: Why good people are divided by politics and religion.* Vintage Books.; Moral Foundations.org. https://moralfoundations.org

10 Pew Research Center. (2019, December 17). In a politically polarized era, sharp divides in both partisan coalitions. https://www.pewresearch.org/politics/2019/12/17/in-a-politically-polarized-era-sharp-divides-in-both-partisan-coalitions

11 Collins, L. M. (2015, November 17). Liberals and conservatives disagree about marriage, but have similar family lives, survey finds. *Deseret News* (*Salt Lake City, Utah: 1964*). https://www.deseret.com/2015/11/17/20598348/liberals-and-conservatives-disagree-about-marriage-but-have-similar-family-lives-survey-finds

12 Hall, S. S., & Adams, R. A. (2011). Cognitive coping strategies of newlyweds adjusting to marriage. *Marriage & Family Review, 47,* 311–325. https://doi.org/10.1080/01494929.2011.594217; Garnefski, N. (2006). Relationships between cognitive emotion regulation strategies and depressive symptoms: A comparative study of five specific samples. *Personality and Individual Differences, 40,* 1659–1669. https://doi.org/10.1016/j.paid.2005.12.009

13 Gillihan, S. (2018). *Cognitive behavioral therapy made simple: 10 strategies for managing anxiety, depression, anger, panic, and worry.* Althea Press.; *Psychology Today.* (n.d.). Cognitive behavioral therapy. https://www.psychology-today.com/us/basics/cognitive-behavioral-therapy

14 Mindful.org. (2020, July 8). What is mindfulness? https://www.mindful.org/what-is-mindfulness

15 Motivational Interviewing Network of Trainers (n.d.). Home page. https://motivationalinterviewing.org/

16 Bowen, G. L., Martin, J. A., Mancini, J. A, & Nelson, J. P. (2000). Community capacity: Antecedents and consequences. *Journal of Community Practice, 8,* 1–21. https://doi.org/10.1300/J125v08n02_01

17 McCubbin, H., & Patterson, J. (1983). The family stress process: The double ABCX model of adjustment and adaptation. *Marriage & Family Review, 6,* 7–37. https://doi.org/10.1300/J002v06n01_02

18 Clay, R. A. (2022, July 11). Are you experiencing compassion fatigue? APA. https://www.apa.org/topics/covid-19/compassion-fatigue

19 Office of Victims of Crime. (n/d). What is vicarious trauma? https://ovc.ojp.gov/program/vtt/what-is-vicarious-trauma

20 National Center on Safe Supportive Learning Environments. (n.d.). Secondary traumatic stress and self-care package. https://safesupportivelearning.ed.gov/sites/default/files/TSS_Building_Handout_2secondary_trauma.pdf

CHAPTER 3

Theoretical Elaboration of Diverse External Contexts of Family Stress

Characteristics of children who have ever been threatened or injured with a weapon at school: 29% of transgender youth, 16% of gay and lesbian youth, and 7% of straight youth.[1]

Chapter Preview

- Cultural contexts that influence family functioning reflect how groups of people adapt to their environment.
- Ecological theory illustrates how families interact with other layers of the environment to produce unique family experiences and social norms.
- Community types—urban, suburban, rural—have some unique cultural elements that contribute to family stressors.
- Establishing a sense of community within neighborhoods can foster family resilience.
- Immigrant families face unique circumstances that shape family stressors.
- Gender differences and gendered experiences can contribute to how family members experience and cope with stressors.
- Minority stress refers to stressors associated with having a specific minority status within a broader society.
- Minority stressors commonly focus on issues related to belonging, stereotypes, and opportunity.
- Families of diverse genders, ethnicities, sexual orientations, and religious groups are prone to experiencing some similar and some unique stressors.
- Cultural competence is important for professionals who work with families.

What Is This Topic About?

Most of us don't live in a literal bubble—we navigate through layers of influence that shape us on a daily basis. As shown in the **FSS integrated model (FIM) of family stress and crisis diagram**, larger **external contexts** impact family philosophy and all other parts of the model (e.g., the nature of the stressors we encounter, the resources we have available to us, the meanings we construct regarding the stressor, and overall family functioning). This chapter highlights external contexts and further lays a foundation for a more nuanced understanding of topics appearing in subsequent chapters. You will become more attuned to the complexities of diverse family circumstances that are shaped at least in part by external contexts. We also explore unique elements of family stress due to minority status within larger social contexts.

This chapter alludes to numerous hotly debated ideas that deserve more attention than can be provided here. If any of them pique your interest, I encourage you to seek out multiple, diverse sources of information and use your best judgment about their validity, looking for how ideology informs what you find and how you interpret it. Certain terminology and ways of framing issues can be controversial and evoke strong feelings. My approach is to address concepts at a basic though meaningfully nuanced level, trying to present them from a neutral and not overly political perspective. That is a difficult task and is only one way of approaching these subjects. The main goal is to emphasize **likely stressors** for families that share certain characteristics or circumstances, not necessarily whether such stress is rational or justifiable. Because meaning is so important in family stress theory, I try to **honor diverse perceptions** of families rather than critique the accuracy of such perceptions.

Part A: Diverse External Contexts of Stressors

How Do External Contexts Influence Family Stress?

In Chapters 1 and 2, we highlighted the internal family context of **family philosophy** as a key element of perceptions, interpretations, and meaning making, all of which are important elements of the **FIM framework**. Our subjective realities influence how we interpret our stressors, the relevance of our resources, and how we cope with stressors. We discussed how our perceptions are influenced by psychological and political biases and by our families' values. However, the meanings and influences of our individual traits and immediate circumstances, and the nature of the stressors we encounter, also depend somewhat on **external contexts**—things over which we have little control, including our genetics, inherited traits and disabilities, and circumstances outside the home, often related to culture.

What External Contexts Are Relevant to Family Stress?
Urie Bronfenbrenner's **ecological theory** helps sensitize us to various external contexts that can influence daily life and thus pertain to family stressors.[2] In short, families interact within

multiple levels of environmental systems such as neighborhoods, school districts, communities, religious and political institutions, and social and cultural norms (including customs and traditions). Each of these levels continually interacts with one another to create unique sets of circumstances that influence our **individual development** and **social change**. Family stressors can have different implications based on unique combinations of environmental influence. For example, imagine:

> A child with a cognitive disability is born in the United States in the early 21st century. The child lives in a state that prioritizes funding for disabilities and in a community that welcomes diverse children. The child has a mother who is a special ed teacher, and the family has a clean, spacious home. The child later attends a specialized school with numerous resources for children with disabilities. How differently would this child's family experience disability-related stressors if one or two of the environmental circumstances were different (e.g., born 200 years ago, a school system incapable of making accommodations for the child, disadvantaged neighborhood)?

The ecological theory also asserts that we do more than simply respond to external contexts—we also shape them. Parents can influence school and workplace policies and neighborhoods contribute to a city's reputation and attractiveness to various visitors or investors. Families and professionals can be important advocates for larger systemic changes that benefit families. Appreciating **connections between larger, often cultural contexts and family experiences** helps us better understand why certain families are more vulnerable to specific stressors, why they might cope with them differently, and what to consider when helping diverse families. Let's proceed with some examples.

How Does Culture Influence Family Stressors?

Culture is a broad, external context with various facets and meanings.[3] Specifically, culture forms when a group of people accumulate and share their knowledge and discoveries about their surroundings. Distinct cultures evolve when groups lack access to one another due to distance and geographical barriers. **Conventions and social innovations** that help groups adapt to their physical surrounding, coordinate the group's efforts to maximize efficiency, and address social conflict become part of that culture. Culture can spread quickly across a group due to a seemingly natural propensity for humans to imitate one another. (Next time you go somewhere and see multiple lines of people, notice how many wait in a longer line for no apparent reason other than because it is the first thing they see other people do.) Groups likewise borrow ideas from each other when they do come in contact.

Some elements of culture are more arbitrary (or random) but require social agreement and institutional structure to create social harmony and conformity. For example, it is interesting to me that in only some languages the same word is used to describe a type of fruit and a color (orange). Such a pattern may not be particularly important for survival but having a shared language within a group promotes unity.

The direct impact of culture on families can be difficult to observe. Cultural influences can be like **background** noise that we grow accustomed to—it affects how we hear things, but we don't always notice it. We tend to notice it more when the noise dramatically changes—or in other words, when we are surrounded by a different cultural context. The United States brings together many cultural groups (e.g., ethnicities, religions) with various histories of in-group and between-group interactions that contribute to what it means to be part of a given culture and to be an American. Families often draw strength from their cultural identities and through bonding within a cultural group, but **groupishness** can also create bias and favoritism that foster stressors associated with cultural clashes among groups of families.

How Do Societal Norms Affect Family Stressors?

The direct impact of societal norms on families can be subtle. However, mass media and the virtual world make social norms easier to identify and to spread. Norms are interconnected with various social institutions like government, economic systems (e.g., capitalism, socialism), law enforcement, educational systems, health care, mass media, ethnic culture, religion (or religious groups), workplace culture, and the family as an organizational structure.

Societal and institutional norms impact the meanings that individuals and families construct out of their experiences—they are **benchmarks** against which they compare themselves. *Are we an unusual family? Are we being treated fairly? Do we have the comforts we need to be happy? Is this a normal thing to be going through?* Subjectively, interpretations of family stressors depend somewhat on how families view themselves and their circumstances relative to what seems normal or typical in their environments. Objectively, families that have values and customs that **clash** with surrounding social norms can experience stressors of social isolation and less access to preferred goods and services less commonly found in mainstream society. As we seek to understand and help families cope with stressors, and if we advocate for the welfare of families in general, we need to analyze how social norms contribute to family vulnerability/resiliency and coping.

How Does Life in Big Cities and Small Towns Differ Regarding Family Stressors?

Cultural and social norms and institutions vary within the same country, state, or region. **Community type** is a common distinguisher of such variation. Specifically, urban (higher **population density**), suburban (moderate density), and rural (lower density) communities tend to differ in ways that could contribute to experiencing family stressors. The importance of the community context was introduced in Chapter 1. We focused on communities contributing to feelings of isolation or as a resource when facing a challenge.

Around half of the U.S. population lives in urban (big city) locations, about 30% live in suburban areas, and 20% in rural areas. **Rural** communities are often spread out, sometimes with small-town hubs. Rural families are more at risk of feeling isolated and having less access to health-care and other service providers. Travel to obtain services can be more difficult for poorer families or families with fewer childcare options. The following are some common differences across these community types that could apply to a given family within such contexts.[4] Think about how each one might be relevant to family stressors:

- **Demographics:** Rural areas have the lowest proportions of racial minorities (21% compared to 56% in urban and 32% suburban). However, Black and Hispanic populations seem to be increasing in rural areas as some families migrate away from the fast-paced life of bigger cities. Overall, however, population growth has been slower in rural areas, and people tend to remain there longer. Tribes of Indigenous peoples often also live in more rural areas. Children in rural areas are somewhat more likely to live with cohabiting parents and less likely to live in single-parent households than urban children (though living with married parents is most common in all areas). Lesbian, gay, bisexual, and transgender (LGBT) family members in rural areas might be at greater risk of a lack of family and social support.
- **Attitudes toward the area:** When asked if people would move away from their community if they could, urban adults are the most interested (37%), followed by suburban (34%), and rural (25%) adults; having family in the area is the top reason for not moving. The pace of lifestyle in each area likely attracts different types of families. Some rural communities pride themselves on being close-knit and supportive.
- **Values:** About 62% of urban residents lean Democrat, while about 54% of rural residents lean Republican (suburban residents are split fairly equally). However, rural Republicans are more likely than urban Republicans to oppose same-sex marriage, while rural Democrats are less likely than urban Democrats to favor high immigration numbers. Most residents think that others don't understand the unique problems faced in their community type (65% of urban, 79% of rural, 52% of suburban adults believe this). Over half of rural and urban residents believe that the two community types differ in what people value.
- **Problems:** About half of rural and urban residents say drug problems are a major issue in their community; problems with affordable housing, crime, poverty, and quality of education are more commonly mentioned by urban residents; problems with public transportation, availability of jobs, and higher speed internet are more commonly mentioned by rural residents. Rural areas often lack access to social services and center-based childcare.
- **Health risks:** Rural areas have fewer physicians, medical specialists, and dentists. Overall, rural residents tend to report having poorer overall health, are more likely to have physical limitations that impede employment and housework, and have a higher death rate due to substance use. Rural residents are slightly more likely to smoke or binge drink, to have chronic health conditions, and to be uninsured.

How Are Neighborhoods Important Types of External Contexts?

Neighborhoods can also have their own culture of sorts. What was your neighborhood like growing up? Did you know your neighbors? Were you welcome in their homes? Would you trust them in your home? Could you have turned to them for help? Were any of them hostile or dangerous? Did you feel safe in your neighborhood after dark? Did you feel good about yourself being there? Did it bring you hope? What was stressful about it?

Neighborhood communities can contribute to the **vulnerability** and **resilience** of families. On the positive side, a **sense of community** is characterized by personally identifying with the community in a way that fosters pride, fellowship, loyalty, and a shared responsibility to look out for one another.[5] This sense of community is cultivated when

- neighbors remain for long periods of time (not many move-ins and move-outs);
- crime rates and other dangers are low;
- neighbors perceive each other as being friendly, which can bolster participation at community events;
- the physical built environment is conducive to walking and encountering others (sidewalks or paths, low-traffic areas, conveniently placed parks); and
- formal and informal networks are abundant (see Chapter 2).

Being surrounded by trusted and supportive people can be a major **protective factor** for families. Conversely, unfriendly and dangerous neighborhoods have been shown to contribute to family stressors connected to higher depression rates, family conflict, and harsher parenting styles. Parents also face pressure in deciding just how closely to monitor their children. Families are important **mediators** of the impact of neighborhoods on children, meaning that they can use their resources and perceptions to lessen or worsen the effects of neighborhood influences on children. Can you think of examples of that happening?

How Does Immigrant Status Affect Family Stressors?

Much of what contributes to unique stressors for immigrants relates to other topics in this chapter—ethnicity, culture, and minority status. Disentangling these elements from one another is difficult. However, the **act of immigrating** to another country can create stressors from adjusting to cultural and language differences, perceptions and treatment from natives, and economic demands. Aside from debates about documentation (legal) status and ideological views about how undocumented should be socially and legally regarded, families facing legal consequences of their immigration status clearly have additional stressors related to **secrecy and fear of deportation**. How might those stressors affect daily life?

Scholars have pointed out important considerations when trying to understand and address family stress from an immigration standpoint.[6] On the positive side, children with at least one immigrant parent (compared to having no immigrant parents) are more likely to go to college regardless of parental resources. Motives for immigration could be a factor in the emphasis on education. Some immigrants have escaped high-risk circumstances in countries with civil wars, unstable democracies, and high poverty rates. The **resilience** they established from earlier stressors might help them confront new immigration-type stressors. Hispanic immigrants are especially known for having a strong emphasis on family, education, and religion as coping resources.

Immigrant families can face some unique challenges based on certain circumstances. For example, those who have **family members "back home"** face separation anxieties and worry. Immigrant parents face decisions about how much to **acculturate** into their new country, sometimes feeling torn about their children seemingly abandoning their cultural heritage. A family's cultural norms could conflict with mainstream norms (e.g., gender roles in marriage, parental discipline techniques) adding stressors related to fitting in.

Some particular **vulnerabilities** are more common among immigrant families. For example, they may face challenges due to their **minority status**, including discrimination and stigma (see Part B). Attitudes and stereotyping aimed at immigrant families tend to worsen during negative economic shifts and higher unemployment rates—particularly toward Hispanic immigrants in the United States with ambiguous documentation status. Employers can also exploit undocumented immigrant laborers with low wages and dangerous or unhealthy work conditions since such employees won't risk publicly complaining and drawing attention to their own legal status. When **language barriers** exist, immigrants may struggle to get access to social and health services; they might also heavily rely on their children (who more easily pick up the language) to translate for them, which empowers children in ways that could potentially impede healthy development and disrupt more normative rules, roles, and boundaries in the home.

How Do Our Genes and Inherited Traits Function as External Contexts?

Though **nature-nurture** continues to be somewhat unclear, we know that our personalities, intelligence, talents, and identities are shaped by genes passed down through the generations. As of now, we have little control over our genetic makeup or the traits we inherit, or the broad cultural norms and societal conventions that influence how such traits shape our lives. Thus, our genetic inheritance is part of our external context. In light of family stress theory, genetic traits can function as important resources and inform our perceptions; they can also be thought of as vulnerabilities or protective factors for our individual and family functioning. Differing perceptions of how and why gender, sexuality, and race influence a person's behavior, attitudes, and perspectives can contribute to friction inside and outside the home. Individuals and families can be viewed and treated differently (including by professional helpers) based on beliefs about biological traits, which can be a source of external pressure.

How Relevant Is Our Gender?

Why might boys and girls, men and women, or fathers and mothers experience stressors differently? What it means to be male or female, especially regarding masculinity and femininity, is more than just a biological issue. Nevertheless, to the extent that most people fit broad categories of boy/girl (or man/women) based on biological traits and long-standing social understandings of maleness and femaleness, we would suspect some commonality in how gender contributes to ways in which families experience stressors. For our purposes, "gender differences" is defined as **average differences between males and females as groups** based on the conventional categorization of male and female. Issues related to nonbinary conceptualizations of gender and to sexual orientation appear in Part B.

Our focus is on understanding **why and how gender might contribute to family stressors**, not to provide comprehensively nuanced ideas about the causes of gender differences. Highlighting gender differences is fraught with metaphorical landmines. Gender differences are easily over- and understated. **Ideological biases** can inform our perspectives on gender—conservatives seem to err more on the side of nature and liberals seem to err more on the side of nurture (though it is possible that most people regardless of ideology don't lean either way). Nevertheless, gendered social norms and personal tendencies can contribute to a family's vulnerabilities and protective factors, interpretations of stressors, and the use of coping resources. Gender differences within families can contribute to diverse perspectives that create friction—*Why doesn't that stress you out? You think WHAT will help!?* However, gender differences are sometimes minor or nonexistent. While understanding gender tendencies can help us make sense of a family's perceptions and stressful circumstances, being **cautious** with our assumptions about gender for a given family is also prudent.

Researchers have provided useful summaries of the more consistent differences, when there are any, between men and women in psychological research across cultures.[7] Table 3.1 highlights average differences that could be relevant to perceiving and experiencing family stressors in diverse ways. Think about how gender differences could contribute to (1) how men and women interpret stressors differently, (2) some different psychological and social resources that men and women might prefer to turn to when coping with stress, and (3) distinct solutions men and women might come up with to maintain or improve family functioning. The comparisons in the table highlight which group is more likely to have higher levels of a characteristic, which is not the same thing as saying that a majority of either group has a given characteristic (e.g., women as a group may be more extroverted than men, but that doesn't necessarily mean that most women are extroverts).

TABLE 3.1 Summary of Average Differences Between Women and Men

Category	Women (Higher/More)	Men (Higher/More)
Personality	Agreeableness, empathy/compassion, extraversion, conscientiousness (self-discipline, planner)	Sensation seeking, decisiveness, physical aggression, competitiveness (with a strong win-lose mentality), risk-taking
Emotions/ Emotional Expression	Intensity of emotions (except perhaps anger), depression and intense positive emotions, shame and guilt, openly express emotions, cry	Emotional regulation, intense anger, openly express anger
Attitudes	Acceptance of diverse perspectives, more sensitive to shame and thus attuned to doing the "right thing"	Openness to casual sex and pornography, accepting of aggression to solve problems
Social	Extroverted, sensitive to social rejection (could play into prioritizing others above themselves, which can lead to stress and resentment), intimate friendships, providing care for family	Introverted, isolated, narcissistic, domineering
Interests/Values	Working with people more than things, family and community involvement, wide set of interests, religious, liking school	Working with things more than people, preference for full-time work so as to make an impact and have a higher income

(Continued)

Category	Women (Higher/More)	Men (Higher/More)
Risk/Protective Factors	Depression, perceive an environment as hazardous and risky for injury, deep social connections with others	Learning disabilities, attention deficit hyperactivity disorder, problems with alcoholism/binge drinking and death by suicide, constructive thinking and cognitive flexibility that helps with problem-solving and mood regulation, self-esteem
Coping	Seek out help, ruminate, self-reflection	Fix things on their own, substance usage, emotional regulation

Adapted from: Ellis, L. (2011). Identifying and explaining apparent universal sex differences in cognition and behavior. *Personality and Individual Differences, 51*, 552–561. https://doi.org/10.1016/j.paid.2011.04.004; Hyde, J. S. (2014). Gender similarities and differences. *Annual Review of Psychology, 65*, 373–398. https://doi.org/10.1146/annurev-psych-010213-115057; Pinker, S. (2017, October 10). His standards or hers? How men and women define success. Institute for Family Studies. https://ifstudies.org/blog/his-standards-or-hers-how-men-and-women-define-success; Schmitt, D. P. (2014). The evolution of culturally-variable sex differences: Men and women are not always different, but when they are … it appears not to result from patriarchy or sex role socialization. In V. A. Weekes-Shackelford & T. K. Shackelford (Eds.), *The evolution of sexuality* (pp. 221–256). New York: Springer.

Of course, individual tendencies would only be part of what distinguishes how gender shapes families. As noted with the **ecological theory**, the external gender context should **interact** with other contexts to influence a given situation. For example:

- The scent of a newborn has been found to stimulate more aggression in women but block aggression in men, suggesting that some biological-based triggers could mix with larger gender norms to promote certain behavior.
- Psychological gender differences are largest in societies in the most gender-equal countries (e.g., Netherlands, Sweden), suggesting interconnections among personal characteristics, the presence of gendered norms, and broader cultural influences.
- Being religious tends to lessen personality-based gender differences by promoting agree-ableness and countering narcissism and social dominance in men, though it also tends to promote a more gendered division of work and family roles.

How Relevant Is Our Ethnicity?

Race and ethnicity are related concepts over which there is much technical nuance and philosophical debate. As we continue to focus on contexts external to families, the emphasis here is on groups of families based on (typically) having certain physical characteristics (e.g., skin color) and shared cultural and historical identities—or **ethnic groups**. The contexts of culture, social norms, community type, neighborhood, and immigration status often have different connotations for distinct ethnic groups, especially regarding minority status. Our ethnicity, as influenced by our physical characteristics interacting with historical and social norms regarding racial groups, inform the meanings families make about their stressful circumstances, the resources they have available to them, and ultimately the level of family functioning. For example, Native American families have a long legacy of trauma that contributes to highly valuing their unique cultural heritage as a source of resilience.[8] They tend to emphasize values of community and cooperation and have strong deference toward older family members and tribal leaders. When navigating mainstream school systems, Native American families can struggle with teachers interpreting their children's soft-spoken (out of respect), noncompetitive demeanors as disinterest. Children can feel caught between different sets of values at home and school, potentially creating friction in the family

Just as our multiple external contexts interact to create various combinations of influence, so do our own personal characteristics. Our gender, ethnicity, sexual orientation, and social class can **intersect** to produce distinct social implications for families. For example, a Black lesbian could be subject to unique challenges for her gender, ethnicity, and sexual orientation—and the intersection of the three can create unique circumstances. She may face racism differently as a lesbian and face discrimination based on her sexual orientation differently as a Black woman. Disentangling the exact reasons why certain people face unique challenges can be complicated, more so when economic circumstances and community types are also thrown into the mix. Some of the differences for ethnic groups could arguably be a function of poverty when those groups have disproportionately high poverty rates (often for complex reasons having to do with minority status, which will be discussed in Part B and in the next chapter).

Improve Your Learning

Without peeking, take a moment to review in your mind (or say out loud) the key concepts from this chapter (this is a proven learning technique). Then review the "Chapter Preview" section at the top and compare. Skim Part A of the chapter with extra attention to the **bolded words**. Skip to the end of the chapter to find more learning resources.

Part B. External Context and Minority Stress

What Is Unique About Family Stressors Based on Minority Status?

Were you ever made fun of for being different? Maybe you were even persecuted for it. Many of us have characteristics or perspectives that put us in a minority position at times. A helpful definition of **minority** appears in the *Encyclopedia of Critical Psychology* as follows:[9]

> A minority or minority group is a subgroup of the population with unique social, religious, ethnic, racial, and/or other characteristics that differ from those of a majority group. The term usually refers to any group that is subjected to oppression and discrimination by those in more powerful social positions, whether or not the group is a numerical minority. Examples of groups that have been labeled minorities include African Americans, women, and immigrants, among others.

The **minority stress model** can help us understand why being part of a minority group based on race/ethnicity, gender, social class, sexual orientation, and religion is conducive to some unique types of family stressors and distinct elements of coping with those stressors.[10] On average, members of ethnic and sexual minority groups are at higher risk for **health problems**. This has caused scholars to study the potential disadvantages of minority groups that can account for extra or unique sources of stress and strain. Some have focused on processes related to **identity development**, which is largely based on how we compare ourselves to others and how we believe others perceive us. Seeing negative portrayals of people like us in popular media, or having other reasons to believe some facet of our identities is looked down upon, can hinder developing positive perceptions of the self. The more **salient** (prominent or important) a particular facet of our identity is to us (e.g., one's Polynesian ancestry, one's blindness, one's Buddhist worldview), the more stress we feel when that facet is the target of ridicule or exclusion. Common hardships associated with minority stress consist of the following:

- **Internalizing negative social attitudes:** Observing and then internalizing negative perceptions to the point of feeling insecure and even preferring a different identity.
- **Stigma or the expectation of being rejected**: This can include fears of having job applications rejected because of one's race or gender, worries about being bullied because of one's sexual or gender identity, and concerns over losing friend or family support because of one's religious membership.
- **Discrimination**: Mistreatment from others, including being passed over for a promotion because of one's sexual orientation, being rejected for housing because of one's race, and being relegated to a remedial math class because one looks poor.
- **Concealment**: When possible, trying to hide one's minority status to avoid stigma and discrimination, such as pretending not to be gay, avoiding talking about one's religious affiliation, and hiding learning disabilities.

Think about the extra amount of emotional and physical energy and focus it would require to worry about yourself or a family member being rejected and mistreated, facing obstacles you know others don't have to, trying to build confidence in light of negative social perceptions, or maintaining hidden elements of who you are. Minority families can also feel pressure to **represent their identity group positively** to help counter misconceptions and negative stereotypes—some of which popular media portrays. Though some families embrace such pressure, they might refrain from admitting personal struggles and feel drained from always being on "their best behavior." Even seemingly trivial things like difficulty in finding appetizing food, effective hair products, or religious materials require extra effort and are reminders of being **outside the mainstream**. Discrimination can lead to feelings of **powerlessness** over one's future. Feeling compelled to conceal one's identity can create anxiety over being **discovered**. What would it be like if you believed that the discovery of your identity (or the identity of a family member) could lead to harassment, injury, or even death? Concealment also limits the amount of support people can openly access to cope with minority stress. Chronic minority stress can leave families with less "fuel left in the tank" (coping capacity) for daily hassles and more typical family stressors, increasing their **vulnerability**.

How Is Coping Affected by Minority Status?

Sources of minority stress can lead to having fewer **resources** to help cope with stressors. For example, discrimination can limit access to **economic security** (e.g., education, employment, stable housing, savings). Sexual and gender minorities in particular might lack **family support**. Thus, **solidarity** from a minority community can be an important protective factor for minority families. People within a cohesive group are also more likely to compare themselves with each other and **rely less on the attitudes and perceptions of mainstream society** to define them. Being surrounded by others who are similar can provide an escape from stigma and create opportunities to create alternative values and structures that solidify the group's culture. However, by virtue of being small in number (in some cases), **finding others** in a given setting who truly relate and empathize can require extra effort.

Perceptions and interpretations also have some unique elements when focusing on minority stress.[11] Regardless of the actual motivation, simply perceiving that an action is motivated by discrimination (e.g., job loss, violence, vandalism) brings additional stress in that it fuels or **validates concerns** about threats based on their minority status. While experiencing or perceiving prejudice from a majority group can feel distressing and disempowering, it can also **galvanize** or solidify the unity within a minority group. Some families take pride in and draw strength from feeling distinct or "special." A possible side effect of bolstering a group's solidarity is elevated **resentment** toward the majority or other minority groups. Perceptions of hostility from members of different ethnic, sexual orientation, and religious groups, regardless of intention, intensify the effects of stressors created through social interaction.

On the more hopeful side, identifying with a minority group can cultivate **greater purpose** when families feel attached to meaningful cultural legacies. Strength gained through coping with minority stress and a stronger need to form an identity rooted in meaningful connections with others can facilitate protective factors that members of majority groups feel less pressure to develop. Some scholars are concerned that pointing out any positive results of discrimination or other victimization places a **double burden on victims** to make the most of their situation—that it signals a reluctance to condemn or stop discrimination.[12] Others argue that downplaying how victims draw strength from adversity would be less empowering and could discourage important coping mechanisms. What do you think?

What Are Some Unique Minority Stress Issues for Diverse Types of Minority Groups?

While groups of people or families share certain characteristics that tend to be used to define them, one should be cautious about overgeneralizing or assuming that every family with such characteristics is similar. Nevertheless, understanding how experiences and perceptions can differ across diverse populations and family types can sensitize us to our own assumptions about families and stressors that might not apply to particular situations.

How Does Minority Stress Relate to Gender?

Gender minorities are typically thought to include women and people who do not conform to socially expected gender norms, often called gender-nonconforming individuals (some of whom might be transgender). From a mainstream **feminist perspective**, women can be thought of as a disadvantaged group because of cultural and legal norms that limit **equal access** to societal services and benefits and that stigmatize some lifestyle options (e.g., employment of choice, sexual behaviors). The extent to which women in the United States are currently disadvantaged is more debatable than it used to be and is far less the case than in some other places in the world.

When it comes to stress, research tends to suggest that stress differences for men and women have more to do with the **types of stressors and coping strategies** rather than the absolute amounts of stress experienced. For example, the American Psychological Association conducts an annual national survey and found that on average, men and women report similar amounts of overall stress (4.6 vs. 5.0, respectively, on a scale from 1–10).[13] Common, average gender differences they have found include the following:

- Women feel more stress when they think about terrorism, international conflicts, the economy, and family relationships than men.
- Men feel more stress when they think about work responsibilities than women.
- Women are more likely than men to say a lack of willpower contributes to taking better care of themselves and that the biggest sources for increasing willpower would be having more energy, confidence, encouragement from friends, time, and help with chores.
- Men are slightly more likely than women to say that having more money would increase their willpower to care for themselves.
- Women and men differ in many of the ways they report trying to manage their stress as seen in Figure 3.1 (which includes only the largest differences as reported in the 2010 report).

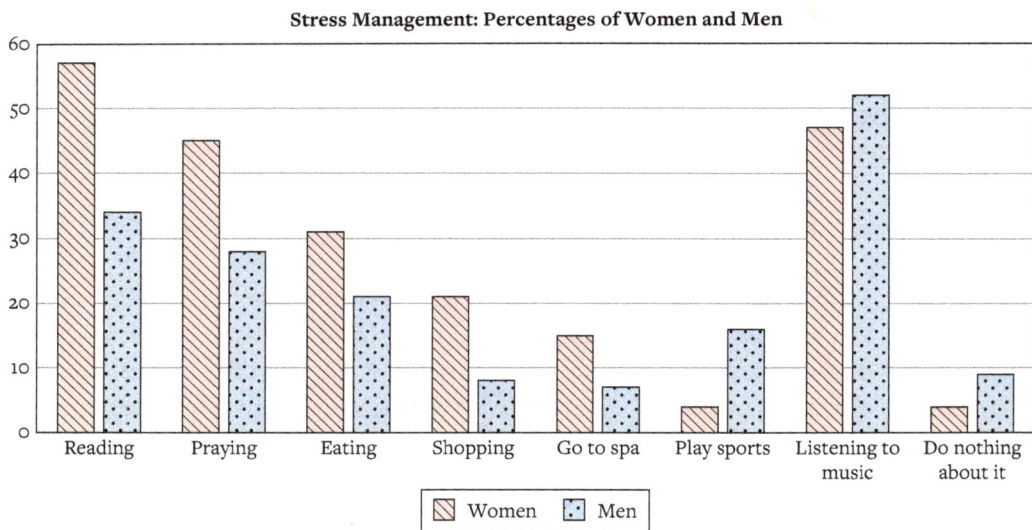

FIGURE 3.1 Stress Management: Percentages of Women and Men

Intense interviews with diverse samples of men and women in New York City produced a similar finding.[14] Specifically, women overall reported more stress related to caring for others, managing social networks, and receiving inferior services (e.g., from a mechanic). Men reported more stress due to having been denied bank loans, being hassled by police, receiving stronger legal penalties because of their gender, and having had a teacher discourage them from seeking higher education. Women tended to feel a lower sense of control over their circumstances but received more social support than men. When thinking about all the factors in the **FIM framework** (e.g., resources, perception, risk/protective factors, internal and external contexts), why might it be difficult to conclude that males or females experience worse outcomes from experiencing stressors?

Western cultures appear increasingly open to gender nonconformity. Today's adolescents and young adults as a whole are freer to explore their gender identities to the point of avoiding strict categorizations of masculinity and femininity, or male and female. Terms like **nonbinary**, **gender fluid**, and **genderqueer** have entered into mainstream vocabulary, though significant ideological pushback still exists. The social environment in which people feel that their gender identity is different from conventional norms would contribute to the types of stressors one might have. What concerns might a parent have whose child wants to go to school dressed in a gender-non-conforming way? Why might it be difficult for a parent to decide whether to allow or encourage such behavior? These are extra pressures that such families face.

What About Transgender as a Type of Gender Nonconformity?

Transgender issues have become highly visual. In some ways, they represent gender nonconformity in that transgender is typically defined as one's gender identity differing from one's assigned sex based on reproductive organs at birth. At the same time, someone who is transgender can express very conventional (conforming) masculine or feminine characteristics that correspond with their gender identity. Aside from some of the nuances of transgender issues and controversies, our focus is primarily on how families that include at least one transgender person—or who confront the possibility of a family member identifying as transgender—create unique family stressors.

From a parent's perspective, having a trans child can create stress associated with fears about how the child will be treated by others. According to the Centers for Disease Control and Prevention, trans youth are much more likely than other students to be bullied at schools (43% vs. 18%), be threatened or hurt with a weapon while at school (29% vs. 7%), and to attempt suicide (29% vs. 7%).[15] **Bullying** is a stressor that can lead to health problems and alcohol use during adolescence. Even when peers are supportive, their parents may not be, leading to the trans child being **excluded** from spending time in classmates' homes or attending parties. Extended family members, and even others in the home, may not support the child or efforts by the parents that affirm the child's trans identity.

Andrew Solomon's in-depth interviews of families facing transgender issues and of specialized medical professionals provide much insight on this topic.[16] Common parental pressures include (many of these can apply to **siblings'** stressors also):

- Having to confront their own worldviews and beliefs about gender, which can require much mental and emotional exertion

- Deciding whether to accept the child's claims about having a trans identity given the age and creativity of the child (e.g., referring to the child by the child's preferred gender identity, using the child's preferred pronouns or desired name, allowing the child to wear gender-nonconforming attire)
- Feeling the loss of the child they had envisioned with a specific future, and, in more extreme cases, actually rejecting and disowning the child
- Their own parents and other relatives or a church community encouraging them to disrupt any of the child's attempts to adopt a trans identity
- Dealing with potential disagreement between parents and other family members on any of these issues, and being negatively judged by other parents and associates
- Feeling some personal rejection (parents of the sex that their child transitions away from have felt some personal rejection and even a loss of bond they might have felt because of being the same sex)
- Adjusting to referring to a child as a daughter or son when used to the opposite title (which could be a constant reminder of uneasy feelings)
- Potentially finding the money for expensive treatments and surgeries not necessarily covered by insurance

Solomon also noted that parents who seek out information and advice about transgender children will likely feel frustrated at what they find. They might hear that most children grow out of a desire to change their gender, that fads in high school and college create temporary pressure or incentive to have unconventional identities, and that some people regret having transitioned and feel even worse. They might also find that such claims are not universally accepted and that debates on such issues can be influenced by **ideological differences**. Getting clarity from doctors may not help much either; knowledge about the causes of trans identity is limited and politically charged. From his observations, Solomon concluded that accomplished academics with personal integrity, and the activists who attack them, "seem to imply that universals exist in a field of highly varied stories" (p. 632). In other words, individual cases vary enough that assuming there are universal causes and consequences of transgender identity and associated outcomes is unproductive.

Perhaps the biggest challenge for parents and transgender youth, however, is dealing with decisions about the **timing** of a physical transition. Generally speaking, beginning hormone treatments prior to puberty is more likely to achieve the desired physical results. Yet, the child is young and still establishing an identity. Acting "too soon" on largely irreversible changes risks children having regrets about transitioning later on. Can you imagine how stressful such a decision could be for a parent and child?

What About an Adult Family Member Who Is Trans?

The minority stressors mentioned earlier, and some of the stressors faced by children exploring a trans identity, also apply to adults who make transitions. Additionally, people who are deeply unsatisfied with their bodies may not take good care of them and suffer the consequences, and pressure to conceal one's desired (or sensed) identity can be draining. Such negative outcomes **become potential hardships** for their families who are concerned about the adult, though some family members also feel shame and embarrassment and ultimately distance themselves. Some adults who physically transition feel a loss of not being able to be **reproductive** within their gender identities (e.g., a trans woman who would like to birth a child).

Trans parents might also worry about being **rejected** by their children. Even if the children appear accepting, parents might fret over whether their children will be bullied or wish they had their "mother (or father) back." Having a spouse transition can also be a significant stressor. *Is this the same person I committed to in the marriage ceremony? Am I physically attracted to my spouse?* Some couples seem to make it work but there isn't much data from which to draw conclusions about the success rates of such relationships.

How Does Minority Stress Relate to Ethnicity?

Being a member of an ethnic minority group is typically difficult to hide. Thus, when people are treated poorly, wondering whether the treatment was **ethnically motivated** is itself a stressor. Pew Research Center data from the United States indicate that about 65% of Black adults report incidents of people having suspicion about them because of their race.[17] Sizable proportions of Asian (34%) and Hispanic (37%) adults report the same. While only 25% of White adults report being victims of suspicion due to their race, 45% of White adults report feeling that others assumed they were racist or prejudiced because of their race (compared to 21%–25% of racial minority groups). As family stress theory reminds us, **perceptions and interpretations** are key factors in how families experience and cope with stress, so actual or perceived negative attitudes or behaviors create or **reinforce concerns** about raising a family in a socially or physically hostile environment.

Poverty is one of the biggest stressors for some ethnic minority groups, and minority stress is typically thought to be a significant factor in creating and maintaining income disparities across some ethnic groups. According to the U.S. Census Bureau, Hispanic, Black, and Native American families have higher average poverty rates than White and Asian families, though the higher rates have been lowering and converging in the last decade.[18] Median household income (combined income of the earners in a household) also differs by ethnicity (2019 numbers): Asian being the highest ($98,000), followed by White ($76,000), Hispanic ($56,000), and Black ($45,000). We will focus more on poverty stressors and income disparities in Chapter 4, but a key takeaway here is that some stressors that are more common among ethnic minority families are also more common among **impoverished families** of any ethnic background. Determining whether ethnicity (e.g., cultural values, minority stress) or poverty/social class—or a particular combination of both—is the driving factor of some family stressors is tricky.

Below are some other examples of stressors that tend to be **disproportionately associated** with ethnic minority group families in the United States.[19] They should not be thought of as stereotypes but tendencies to be aware of that could apply to a given family with such a heritage. Only some ethnic groups are included for illustrative purposes. Experiences can depend on the **recency of immigration** (when applicable) and the **social class** to which a family belongs (see Chapter 4).

- Black (or African American) families are disproportionally likely to experience stressors of teenage mothers and single-mother-headed households. Besides the economic pressures, raising children alone (or with inconsistent contributions from a partner) has its own challenges (see Chapter 8). While attitudes toward single parenthood tend to be more affirming across Black families, Black single mothers can feel pressure to live up to cultural expectations of being a "strong woman," which can contribute to hiding vulnerability and the need for help. With a long history of racial segregation and discrimination, some Black families struggle to trust mainstream institutions and professionals. For example, teenage girls and women may avoid seeking sufficient sexual, prenatal, and postnatal health care, putting themselves and their children at higher health risks. Black men in particular might distrust White police officers, especially when high profile cases of White officers using excessive force toward—including shooting—Black men. Some Black parents feel ignored by their children's teachers or school administrators or overly blamed for their children's struggles. Despite some of these extra challenges, Black youth are known for their relatively high self-esteem, perhaps as a result of intentional parenting and community socialization to promote a resilient ethnic identity to help cope with minority stress. Support from **fictive kin**—people who take on family roles but who are not technically related—are a common protective factor.

- Hispanic/Latino (or Hispanic-American) families share some similarities with Black families. They disproportionately have a high rate of single-mother households and live in higher crime neighborhoods with more exposure to hostile police encounters. Some issues mentioned earlier regarding **immigration** can apply to Hispanic families in general. They tend to be education-oriented but language barriers (when applicable) can make it more difficult for parents to advocate for their children; sometimes teachers view their bilingual children as less competent than native English speakers and expect less of them. A strong sense of family unity can compel children to put family needs ahead of schoolwork, which can create stress. They can also feel torn about their children speaking English—it is a useful resource but can also symbolize a barrier toward valuing their ethnic heritage. Living in communities with other Hispanic families is a way such families might choose to develop resilience through the familiarity of customs, food, and cooperation with one another, particularly for immigrants.

- Asian (or Asian American) families are less likely than other ethnic minority groups to struggle with poverty, but some subgroups are at greater risk than others. **Immigration** status can also differentiate the kinds of stressors Asian families encounter. Sources of minority stress often involve perceptions from other people. Asian adults have especially felt like they have been subject to slurs and jokes. During the early stages of the COVID-19 pandemic particularly, some Asian families were harassed as if they shared responsibility for the spreading of the novel coronavirus. Because Asian families are perceived to be well educated, hardworking, and prosperous—a "model minority" some say—those who struggle might feel extra pressure to hide their so-called weaknesses and are easily overlooked by government and social services that focus on helping disadvantaged families. Overall, Asian families indeed highly value and invest in their children's education, which can foster resiliency in the face of economic challenges. This can also place high pressure on children to succeed educationally and participate less in leisure and sports than many of their peers.

How Does Minority Stress Relate to Sexual Orientation?

Sexual minority groups based on sexual orientation are prone to experience discrimination and stigma, though lesbian, gay, and bisexual (LGB) individuals are perceived much more favorably in the United States than in the past. Minority stress varies based on the social norms and attitudes of where (and when) sexual minorities live. Nevertheless, **identity concealment** can be a key issue for families with LGB individuals that contributes to stressors in the workplace, neighborhood, and educational and other social environments. What comes to mind?

Like with any general group, subgroups of sexual minorities have some distinct circumstances. For example, about one third of sexual minorities are also ethnic minorities, who are also more likely to have children than White sexual minorities. Furthermore, the "lesbian, gay, bisexual, transgender, and queer or questioning (LGBTQ) community" is a **group of diverse people** with some distinct challenges.[20] For instance, some bisexual and transsexual individuals feel stigmatized by gay and lesbian individuals. Some LGB advocates express concern about a movement to separate gender completely from one's biology, which others interpret as being anti-trans.

Scholars have identified that families that include LGB members face minority stress related to parenting and couple relationships.[21] Common pressures for parents of LGB children include the following:

- Heterosexual parents can struggle with relating to their children's feelings and concerns, even to the point of ignoring the concerns or rejecting the children. Some parents feel guilty about the perceived possibility that they did "something wrong" to cause the sexual orientation.
- Learning about the unique needs of LGB youth can take added time and effort regardless of a parent's comfort level.
- Parents who feel the need to mourn over their child's orientation (i.e., mourn over the perceived loss of certain hopes and expectations they've long had for a child) might feel unable to express themselves without hurting a child's feelings. Children might feel upset or rejected by a parent's initial negative emotional response when the child "comes out" to them, which could lead to feelings of guilt on both sides.
- Parents might feel embarrassed or judged in public when their children nonconform to heterosexual norms.
- Parents likely worry about their children being excluded from peers' social events or facing bullying and threats to their safety. Children who suffer from rejection and discrimination have more mental health problems (including suicidal ideation and substance issues). Exposure to negative public comments and to news about policies perceived as anti-LGB(T) fuels thoughts of rejection.
- Children sometimes try to spare their parents' stress by not notifying them about bullying, which adds feelings of isolation for the children and confusion for the parents.

Same-sex couples and LGB parents also face some fairly unique pressures, including the following:

- Stigma and discrimination could threaten the couple's relationship stability by prompting couples to question their relationship legitimacy and commitment (though sometimes couples respond to stigma by reinforcing their commitment).
- The typical processes of LGB couples becoming parents include the use of assisted reproductive technology, adoption, and one or more partners having already had a child (usually from a former heterosexual relationship). Such processes typically include their own sets of financial and relationship stressors (see also Chapter 5). Any thoughts as to what they might be?
- When becoming parents, some same-sex couples lose support and affirmation from family members (though the opposite also happens).
- Same-sex couples who conceal their relationship can experience various pressures. Fears of family rejection are stressful. When only one partner conceals the relationship, the other partner would have to assist with the secrecy against one's own desires; the couple's relationship could suffer from the partners' conflicting perspectives. Having to keep track of the circumstances in which one should pretend and deny is stressful. A partner's internalization of negativity toward LGB people can interfere with identity security, which is important for relationship intimacy.

Families with LGB members tend to rely heavily upon **family and other social support** to help cope with minority stress. Some also find strength in **religion**.[22] While religion is often thought of as adversarial toward LGB people, and the most outspoken opponents of same-sex marriage have been religiously motivated, it also appears to be a **potential protective factor**. Data from over 73,000 middle and high school students in Utah showed that while LGBT youth were more likely to be bullied, depressed, and suicidal than other youth, LGBT youth who were members of the largest local religion (the Church of Jesus Christ of Latter-Day Saints, or "Mormons") were less depressed and suicidal than the other LGBT youth (and nonreligious LGBT youth were more depressed than religious LGBT youth). LGBT youth in general were more likely to be nonreligious, report higher family conflict, not live with both a mother and father, and have drug use in the family home. These factors generally corresponded to higher rates of depression and suicidality and were also less present in homes of members of the Church of Jesus Christ of Latter-Day Saints, suggesting some noteworthy connections between family and religious factors in risk and resiliency.

How Does Minority Stress Relate to Religious Groups?
Families who are members of minority religious groups (relative to the mainstream culture) can experience minority stress related to **ignorance and misunderstandings** and to **hostility and discrimination** like other types of minorities. For example, Equal Employment Opportunity Commission data indicates that thousands of workplace religious discrimination claims are filed every year (which have increased by 25% over the past 20 years).[23] **Concealing** one's religion is

more difficult for some groups based on religious clothing, uniqueness of customs, and desire to demonstrate one's religious affiliation. Scholars have highlighted some other potential stressors for religious minority families.[24]

- Like with some other minority groups, parents are often concerned about how their children will be treated at school. Children can be made to feel like outsiders when they dress differently, avoid participating in holiday or patriotic celebrations or rituals, and when people verbalize hurtful misconceptions about them. Extracurricular and community events tend to be scheduled on Saturdays and Sundays, days that are considered holy enough by some groups to avoid such activities, adding to more isolation and feeling like outsiders. Parents might have to work harder to console their children and prepare them for being different from others.
- Family rules, roles, and boundaries that are shaped by religion might clash with other families in the neighborhood, school district, or larger region. For example, Orthodox Jewish families who seek to assimilate into a Christian or secular culture may find themselves acting contrary to Jewish conventions, creating potential guilt and distress. Amish families have lifestyles that fit poorly with mainstream cultures, and even though they might benefit from living in tight-knit communities, some families feel disconnected from the world in ways that contribute to a sense of being outcasts.
- Families who are more open about their religion feel greater stress when they experience religious discrimination. Families might feel the need to refute negative mainstream assumptions and portrayals of their religion by outwardly showcasing its positive effects on their lives, which can be tiring. People associating one's religion with negative events can also be painful, such as for Muslim families when their religion was linked with violence and anti-Americanism after 9/11.

Religion for many families is a central part of how they make meaning from their experiences—including stressors—and can inspire attitudes, beliefs, and behaviors that act as **protective factors**. Like with any kind of identity, the contexts surrounding the religious (or nonreligious) nature of a family affect how religion shapes experiences inside and outside of the family.

What Does All This Mean for You?

Take a few moments to ponder the following:

- How have you been feeling while engaging with this information? Why?
- Which topics can you personally relate to?
- Did you grow up in a neighborhood or community that heavily influenced family stressors?
- What other examples have come to mind that illustrate similar or diverse ways that families experience minority stress?
- How can being part of a minority group contribute to promoting family flourishing?

Your insights can be valuable to your personal life, your family relationships, and your professional roles. Consider the elements of the **FIM framework** and other family stress concepts. As a person of influence, you can help guide people through the coping processes and ideally help foster a **flourishing** life. However, take care to avoid letting your personal interpretations push you toward **assuming** too much about somebody else's circumstances, perceptions, and motivations. Always be ready to address issues that might be hard for you to face because of your own history and be sure to **practice good self-care** (Chapter 2).

Effectively working with a variety of families requires **cultural competence**. The National Association of Social Workers code of ethics highlights elements of cultural competence that you might find useful. Specifically (emphasis added):[25]

1. Demonstrate understanding of culture and its function in human behavior and society, recognizing the strengths that exist in all cultures.
2. Demonstrate knowledge that guides practice with clients of various cultures and be able to demonstrate skills in the provision of culturally informed services that empower marginalized individuals and groups ... take[ing] action against oppression, racism, discrimination, and inequities, and acknowledge personal privilege.
3. Demonstrate awareness and cultural humility by engaging in critical self-reflection (understanding their own bias and engaging in self-correction), recognizing clients as experts of their own culture, committing to lifelong learning, and holding institutions accountable for advancing cultural humility.
4. Obtain education about and demonstrate understanding of the nature of social diversity and oppression with respect to race, ethnicity, national origin, color, sex, sexual orientation, gender identity or expression, age, marital status, political belief, religion, immigration status, and mental or physical ability.
5. [When providing electronic-based services] be aware of cultural and socioeconomic differences among clients' use of and access to electronic technology and seek to prevent such potential barriers ... [assessing] cultural, environmental, economic, mental or physical ability, linguistic, and other issues that may affect the delivery or use of these services.

In short, understand the **relevance** of culture and membership in a disadvantaged group to how families experience stress. Learn through your own study of scholarly literature and from communicating with diverse kinds of families about the best ways to accommodate their unique perspectives, values, and family processes. Implement what you learn.

Improve Your Learning

Without peeking, take a moment to review in your mind (or say out loud) the key concepts from this chapter (this is a proven learning technique). Then review the "Chapter Preview" section at the top and compare. Skim Part B of the chapter with extra attention to the **bolded words**.

Do You Want to Learn More?

We have only touched on a portion of information related to some elements of this topic. **What really sparked your interest? What do you wish was covered more thoroughly?** Consider taking some time to further deepen your understanding of personal and professional issues related to helping families cope with stressors. The following are a variety of resources that you might find helpful, and some references directly or indirectly referred to in this chapter. Assimilate with the rest of the students by investigating some of them—don't be left out.

Videos

(Use links or do searches with the key words provided)
- Why Millennials Are Moving Away From Large Urban Centers (7 mins). *PBS NewsHour.* https://www.youtube.com/watch?v=mjZu5AU3NYI
- Hiding in Plain Sight—My Life as an Undocumented American (10 mins). Leezia Dhalla TEDxSanAntonio. https://www.youtube.com/watch?v=tBoBC3nBoFs
- I'm the Daughter of Immigrants. I Never Felt Like I Could Be a Kid: Throwback Thursday (4 mins). *Washington Post.* https://www.youtube.com/watch?v=LdzpR-sQn0w
- *Place Matters, Joint Center for Political and Economic Studies. Social Determinants of Health* (11 mins). Intercultural Productions. https://www.youtube.com/watch?v=y1SeLM2crUs
- Sex Differences, Human Nature, & Identity Politics (Pt. 1), Stephen Pinker (35 mins). The Rubin Report. https://www.youtube.com/watch?v=sYf6dD4N86E
- *Minority Stress* (2 mins). ACON Health. https://www.youtube.com/watch?v=PI1eNnV9_po
- *Racism and Mental Health* (4 mins). Psych Hub. https://www.youtube.com/watch?v=aV4Hk4PQ4Tc

Websites

- Parker, K., Horowitz, J. M., Brown, A., Fry, R., Cohn, D., & Igielnik, R. (2018, May 22). What unites and divides urban, suburban and rural communities. Pew Research Center. https://www.pewresearch.org/social-trends/2018/05/22/what-unites-and-divides-urban-suburban-and-rural-communities/
- Pinker, S. (2017, October 10). His standards or hers? How men and women define success. Institute for Family Studies. https://ifstudies.org/blog/his-standards-or-hers-how-men-and-women-define-success
- United States Census Bureau. (2022). Race and poverty: US Census Bureau, current population survey. https://www.census.gov/programs-surveys/cps.html

Readings (Articles, Books, Book Chapters)

- Bronfenbrenner, U. (1986). Ecology of the family as a context for human development: Research perspectives. *Developmental Psychology, 22*, 723–742. https://doi.org/10.1037/0012-1649.22.6.723
- Lefevor, G. T., Davis, E. B., Paiz, J. Y., & Smack, A. C. P. (2021). The relationship between religiousness and health among sexual minorities: A meta-analysis. *Psychological Bulletin, 147*(7), 647–666. https://doi.org/10.1037/bul0000321
- Marks, L. D., Dollahite, D. C., & Young, K. P. (2019). Struggles experienced by religious minority families in the United States. *Psychology of Religion and Spirituality, 11*(3), 247–256. https://doi.org/10.1037/rel0000214
- Meyer, I. H. (2003). Prejudice, social stress, and mental health in lesbian, gay and bisexual populations: Conceptual issues and research evidence. *Psychological Bulletin, 129*, 674–697. https://doi.org/10.1037/0033-2909.129.5.674
- Schmitt, D. P. (2014). The evolution of culturally-variable sex differences: Men and women are not always different, but when they are … it appears not to result from patriarchy or sex role socialization. In V. A. Weekes-Shackelford & T. K. Shackelford (Eds.), *The evolution of sexuality* (pp. 221–256). Springer.
- Solomon, A. (2012). *Far from the tree: Parents, children, and the search for identity.* Scribner.

Notes

1   Centers for Disease Control and Prevention. (n.d.). Adolescent and school health. https://www.cdc.gov/healthyyouth/data/yrbs/reports_factsheet_publications.htm

2   Bronfenbrenner, U. (1979). *The ecology of human development: Experiments by nature and design.* Cambridge University Press.; Bronfenbrenner, U. (1986). Ecology of the family as a context for human development: Research perspectives. *Developmental Psychology, 22*, 723–742. https://doi.org/10.1037/0012-1649.22.6.723

3   Pinker, S. (2016). *The blank slate: The modern denial of human nature.* Viking.

4   National Council on Family Relations. (n.d.). Family focus. https://www.ncfr.org/ncfr-report/focus; Parker, K., Horowitz, J. M., Brown, A., Fry, R., Cohn, D., & Igielnik, R. (2018, May 22). What unites and divides urban, suburban and rural communities. Pew Research Center. https://www.pewresearch.org/social-trends/2018/05/22/what-unites-and-divides-urban-suburban-and-rural-communities

5   Mancini, J. A., & Bowen, G. (2009). Community resilience: A social organization theory of action and change. In J. A. Mancini & K. A. Roberto (Eds.), *Pathways of human development: Explorations of change* (pp. 245–265). Lexington Books.

6   Lauderdale, M. K., & Heckman, S. J. (2017). Family background and higher education attainment among children of immigrants. *Journal of Family and Economic Issues, 38*(3), 327–337. https://doi.org/10.1007/s10834-017-9537-4; National Council on Family Relations (n.d.). Family focus. https://www.ncfr.org/ncfr-report/focus; Parra-Cardona, J. R., Cordova, D., Holtrop, K., Villarruel, F., & Wieling, E., (2008). Shared ancestry, evolving stories: Similar and contrasting life experiences described by foreign born and U.S. born Latino parents. *Family Process, 47*, 157–172. https://doi.org/10.1111/j.1545-5300.2008.00244.x

7   Ellis, L. (2011). Identifying and explaining apparent universal sex differences in cognition and behavior. *Personality and Individual Differences, 51*, 552–561. https://doi.org/10.1016/j.paid.2011.04.004; Hyde, J. S. (2014).

Gender similarities and differences. *Annual Review of Psychology, 65,* 373–398. https://doi.org/10.1146/annurev-psych-010213-115057; Pinker, S. (2017, October 10). His standards or hers? How men and women define success. Institute for Family Studies. https://ifstudies.org/blog/his-standards-or-hers-how-men-and-women-define-success; Schmitt, D.P. (2014). The evolution of culturally-variable sex differences: Men and women are not always different, but when they are ... it appears not to result from patriarchy or sex role socialization. In V. A. Weekes-Shackelford & T. K. Shackelford (Eds.), *The evolution of sexuality* (pp. 221–256). Springer.

8 Vang, C. T. (2010). *An educational psychology of methods in Multicultural education.* Peter Lang.

9 Perkins, K., & Wiley, S. (2014). Minorities. In *Encyclopedia of critical psychology* (pp. 1192–1195). Springer. https://doi.org/10.1007/978-1-4614-5583-7_188

10 Meyer, I. H. (2003). Prejudice, social stress, and mental health in lesbian, gay and bisexual populations: Conceptual issues and research evidence. *Psychological Bulletin, 129,* 674–697. https://doi.org/10.1037/0033-2909.129.5.674

11 Chan, N. K. M., & Jasso, F. (2021). From inter-racial solidarity to action: Minority linked fate and African American, Latina/o, and Asian American political participation. *Political Behavior,* 1–23. https://doi.org/10.1007/s11109-021-09750-6; Gaskin, A. (2015, August). Racial socialization: Ways parents can teach their children about race. APA. https://www.apa.org/pi/families/resources/newsletter/2015/08/racial-socialization; Sawyer, P. J., Major, B., Casad, B. J., Townsend, S. S. M., & Mendes, W. B. (2012). Discrimination and the stress response: Psychological and physiological consequences of anticipating prejudice in interethnic interactions. *American Journal of Public Health, 102*(5), 1020–1026. https://doi.org/10.2105/AJPH.2011.300620

12 Frost, D. M. (2014). Redemptive framings of minority stress and their association with closeness in same-sex relationships. *Journal of Couple & Relationship Therapy, 13*(3), 219–239. https://doi.org/10.1080/15332691.2013.871616

13 American Psychological Association. (n.d.). *Stress in America.* https://www.apa.org/news/press/releases/stress

14 Meyer, I. H., Schwartz, S., & Frost, D. M. (2008). Social patterning of stress and coping: Does disadvantaged social status confer more stress and fewer coping resources? *Social Science Medicine, 67*(3), 368–379. https://doi.org/10.1016/j.socscimed.2008.03.012

15 Centers for Disease Control and Prevention (n.d.). *Adolescent and school health.* https://www.cdc.gov/healthyyouth/data/yrbs/reports_factsheet_publications.htm

16 Solomon, A. (2012). *Far from the tree: Parents, children, and the search for identity.* Scribner.

17 Pew Research Center. (2019, April 9). Race in America 2019. https://www.pewresearch.org/social-trends/2019/04/09/race-in-america-2019

18 United States Census Bureau. (2022). Race and poverty: US Census Bureau, current population survey. https://www.census.gov/programs-surveys/cps.html

19 Roy, R. N., James, A. G., & Brown, T. L. (2021). Racial/ethnic minority families. *Journal of Family and Economic Issues, 42,* 84–100 (2021). https://doi-org.proxy.bsu.edu/10.1007/s10834-020-09712-w; National Council on Family Relations (n.d.). Family focus. https://www.ncfr.org/ncfr-report/focus

20 Formby, E. (2017). *Exploring LGBT spaces and communities: Contrasting identities, belongings and wellbeing.* Routledge.

21 Mereish, E. H., Miranda, R., Jr., Liu, Y., & Hawthorne, D. J. (2021). A daily diary study of minority stress and negative and positive affect among racially diverse sexual minority adolescents. *Journal of Counseling Psychology, 68*(6), 670–681. https://doi.org/10.1037/cou0000556; National Council on Family Relations. (n.d.). Family focus. https://www.ncfr.org/ncfr-report/focus; Prendergast, S., & MacPhee, D. (2018). Family resilience amid stigma and discrimination: A conceptual model for families headed by same-sex parents. *Family Relations, 67*(1), 26–40. https://doi.org/10.1111/fare.12296; Solomon, A. (2012). *Far from the tree: Parents, children, and the search for identity.* Scribner.

22 Dyer, J. Goodman, M., & Wood, D. S. (2021). Religion and sexual orientation as predictors of Utah youth suicidality. *BYU Studies.* https://foundations.prod.brigham-young.psdops.com/0000017b-88a0-dafa-adff-eaeb8cd40001/religion-and-sexual-orientation-as-predictors-of-utah-youth-suicidality; Lefevor, G. T., Davis, E. B., Paiz, J. Y., & Smack, A. C. P. (2021). The relationship between religiousness and health among sexual minorities: A meta-analysis. *Psychological Bulletin, 147*(7), 647–666. https://doi.org/10.1037/bul0000321; McGraw, J. S., Docherty, M., Chinn, J. R., & Mahoney, A. (2021). Family, faith, and suicidal thoughts and behaviors (STBs) among LGBTQ youth in Utah. *Psychology of Sexual Orientation and Gender Diversity.* Advance online publication. https://doi.org/10.1037/sgd0000517

23 Equal Employment Opportunity Commission. (2020). Charge statistics FY 1997 through FY 2016. https://www.eeoc.gov/eeoc/statistics/enforcement/charges.cfm

24 Haque, A., Tubbs, C. Y., Kahumoku-Fessler, E. P., & Brown, M. D. (2019). Microaggressions and Islamophobia: Experiences of Muslims across the United States and clinical implications. *Journal of Marital and Family Therapy, 45*(1), 76–91. https://doi.org/10.1111/jmft.12339; Marks, L. D., Dollahite, D. C., & Young, K. P. (2019). Struggles experienced by religious minority families in the United States. *Psychology of Religion and Spirituality, 11*(3), 247–256. https://doi.org/10.1037/rel0000214; Parent, M. C., Brewster, M. E., Cook, S. W., & Harmon, K. A. (2018). Is minority stress in the eye of the beholder? A test of minority stress theory with Christians. *Journal of Religion and Health, 57*(5), 1690–1701. https://doi.org/10.1007/s10943-017-0550-6; Štekovič, M. (2012). Crossing cultural frontiers: Representations of the Amish in American culture. *Acta Neophilologica, 45*(1–2). https://doi.org/10.4312/an.45.1-2.19-31

25 National Association of Social Workers. (n.d.). Read the code of ethics. https://www.socialworkers.org/About/Ethics/Code-of-Ethics/Code-of-Ethics-English

Image Credits

Fig. 3.1: Source: Adapted from https://www.apa.org/news/press/releases/stress/2010/national-report.pdf.

CHAPTER 4

Economic and Financial Contexts of Family Stress

In 2020, the median income of households headed by married couples between the ages of 35 and 44 was $115,000; the median income of households led by single mothers of the same age was $46,500.[1]

Chapter Preview

- The extent to which families have responsibility for and control over their financial situations is a fundamental debate along some ideological lines.
- The family context, including family philosophy, shapes family members' financial literacy and behavior.
- The economy is an important context for influencing financial family stressors.
- Issues related to inflation and debt affect most families but in diverse ways.
- Work-family conflict, family caregiving, and retirement occur within a larger economic context in which families find different ways to meet their needs.
- Real income gaps and perceptions of economic inequality create family stress.
- Poverty places stress on parents, which then impacts children because of family conflicts and less investment in children.
- Stressors associated with poverty include disadvantaged living environments, food instability, homelessness, and class discrimination.
- Differences in age, gender, ethnicity, education levels, and marital status are interrelated factors in experiencing financial anxiety and stress.
- A master table is presented that summarizes key concepts in previous chapters related to helping families with stressors.

What Is This Topic About?

Prior chapters have explained the importance of external contexts on family stressors and coping. The economy is a central element of such contexts and influences all elements of the **FSS integrated model (FIM) of family stress and crisis framework**. Regardless of their level of wealth or poverty, all families have stressors related to accessing and managing economic resources to meet certain goals. Some families face chronic financial stressors that contribute to their overall vulnerability to other stressors. Subjective perceptions of fairness also impact how we experience economic stressors.

What Are the Assumptions?

Until we reach a point at which food, clothing, and shelter are no longer necessary for our survival, we have to find ways to meet our **basic needs**. Consider the following:

- Who is **responsible** for meeting a person's needs? Who is responsible for meeting a family's needs?
- How much **control** do we have over our individual and our family's economic circumstances? Who or what else might limit some of that control?

Such questions can foster intense debate about personal accountability, government involvement, inequality of opportunity and ability, and basic human rights. Our assumptions about responsibility and control over our economic circumstances contribute to how families experience and respond to economic stressors, and how helpers—perhaps you—perceive such families.

In Chapter 2, you encountered the moral foundations of political ideologies. You may recall that the foundation of **fairness** tends to be somewhat more highly valued by conservatives than liberals, particularly the element of proportionality—people should get what they earn: no freeloaders. Conversely, the **care** foundation is what tends to be valued above all by liberals—harm should be alleviated as much as possible. While both these foundations are highly valued by both conservative and liberal ideologies, conservatives seem to err more on the fairness side and liberals on the care side when the foundations are at seeming odds with one another.

When it comes to issues of family financial hardship, conservatives may focus more on **the decisions family members make** that contribute to their problems and that could lead to them changing their circumstances; liberals may focus more on how to **provide the resources families need** to compensate for their circumstances, particularly through **government programs and policies**. Conservatives tend to express concern about any programs and policies that could discourage heads of households from earning a living through their own efforts, which would undermine people's sense of worth, punish those who work hard, and ultimately destabilize a healthy economy for all. Liberals tend to express concern that without such intervention innocent children are punished and kept in a cycle of poverty that should not exist in a wealthy society, which hurts the economy overall. What is each perspective right about? What are they wrong about? What are the consequences of erring too far on one side or the other?

As you engage with the rest of the chapter, remember the key elements of family stress theories (e.g., stressors, resources, perceptions, coping, and crisis) and consider the following:

- What economic stressors do families have besides simply not having enough money?
- Why might some families in similar economic circumstances flourish while others are strained?
- How do the various pieces of information throughout the chapter fit together to help explain why each family might be affected differently by economic stressors?
- What experiences have you had or observed that help you relate to specific concepts?
- How might the ideological perspectives influence how people (including you) think about potential causes of and solutions to families' economic struggles?

Part A. Normative Economic Family Stressors

We all have "normal" family stressors related to our economic circumstances. In this section, we focus on several common family stressors that most families face, while keeping in mind that some families are highly vulnerable to experiencing crisis as a result of such stressors. Fortunately, some families are highly resilient and able to cope with stressors in ways that promote family flourishing.

Why Do Families Experience Economic Stressors?

I know what you are thinking—families have economic stress because they don't have enough money. True enough. But is that all there is to it? Certainly, families face daily decisions about their budget and spending habits that have real consequences for their financial future. Some dread the topic of money and avoid mentioning it at all costs; some see money as simply a means to enable activities that lead to a satisfying life, and some see it as validating one's importance or power. The value of a dollar is more than its objective worth as currency; its subjective value depends on the different meanings we as individuals, families, and cultures assign to having it. Such meanings can contribute to our earning, saving, and spending habits, each of which contributes to family stress.

How Does the Family Context Affect Economic Stressors?

Part of the **family philosophy** context includes attitudes and values related to money. You might hear phrases like, "it's only money," "money doesn't grow on trees," "mo money, mo problems," or "the best things in life are free." Family philosophy about money and the "stuff" money can buy shapes family rules, roles, and boundaries related to finances. Did you have any rules growing up about how to use money?

Within the family context, seemingly smaller but common money-related challenges at home can be impactful. Family philosophy can contribute to how family members respond to them. Consider how each of the following scenarios can put pressure on family members:

- Siblings believe that a parent spends more money on one child's birthday presents than another's.
- Two parents disagree on whether to pay children for doing chores.
- Spouses or romantic partners have vastly different saving and spending styles.
- One set of grandparents takes the children on expensive vacations while the other(s) can't afford to do so.
- An uncle comes to visit and asks to borrow money to help him make an investment on a "can't miss" business deal.
- (Come up with a scenario on your own).

Family philosophy and other socialization processes within the family also contribute to what is often referred to as **financial literacy**—our understanding of finances and skills related to personal money management, budgeting, and investing. The family context has been shown to influence its members' financial attitudes and activities—sometimes unintentionally. Key forms of **socialization** appear to be:[2]

- **Parental modeling**: Children observe parents' day-to-day financial behaviors such as paying bills and buying groceries. Young adults commonly report that they imitate what they saw from their parents from years past. Even though some financial socialization happens through peers, work experience, school programs, and the media, young adults report that they learned the most about finances from their parents (though some wished their parents had taught them more about money).
- **Discussions/communication**: Generally speaking, having parent-child financial discussions has been linked to more positive and healthy attitudes, knowledge, and behavior when children reach young adulthood. For some families, money is a taboo topic, which could end up impairing their children.
- **Experiential learning**: Parents who provide and monitor children's hands-on experiences with money tend to produce good results. Adolescents had more positive perceptions and knowledge of banks when a parent had previously taken them to a bank. Adolescents with a savings account were more financially independent as young adults, regardless of family wealth, personal employment, and education level. Young adults who had had a childhood allowance reported less financial worry, and adolescents with a history of earning money tended to demonstrate healthier financial behavior. It is important to note that not all families have the same opportunities to provide such experiential learning; parents with a higher socioeconomic background especially have been shown to demonstrate modeling, communication, and experiential learning.
- **Parenting quality**: Perhaps more indirectly, the quality of parent-child interaction is an important part of financial socialization. A high level of parenting caring was linked to less adolescent materialism (the importance of having material things). Authoritative parenting (supportive, warm, high expectations) was linked to adolescent and adult money saving. Monitoring childhood spending behavior was linked to feeling confident about money management and less financial worry during young adulthood. Overall, as

with any socialization efforts, a positive parent-child relationship contributes to more successful financial socialization.

Poor financial literacy, problematic spending habits, an uninspiring work ethic, and a lack of opportunity to gain early financial experience (because of poverty or other barriers) can create family economic stressors. They also hamper a family's ability to cope with financial stressors, especially when they foster passivity, contention, and shame. However, families are also embedded within **larger systems** that influence their circumstances and behaviors related to economic stressors.

How Does the Economy Influence Family Stress?

The nature and condition of the local and broader economies have profound effects on families. An **economy** is essentially a region's cumulative wealth and resources. Major economic recessions threaten the earning and spending power of families by no fault of their own. The Great Recession around 2009 in the United States and the challenges for the global economy from the COVID-19 pandemic are recent examples of such. Even more typical shifts in an economy can put significant pressure on families. For example, insurance companies make changes in what they cover and the share they require consumers to pay; property taxes can increase based on nearby developments or local policy changes. What is it about the economy that can lead to feelings of powerlessness? Why would those feelings matter?

How Does Inflation Influence Family Stress?

What happens when things get more expensive but your earnings stay the same? Oftentimes, wages increase to match the rising costs of goods and services so inflation itself may not be a hardship. Otherwise, not being able to keep up with rising costs can cause anxiety and worry about the future.

When a family lives from paycheck to paycheck, rising costs can be a huge source of insecurity and stress.[3] Purchasing the **necessities** may feel insurmountable, and families may **cut back on other expenses** they are accustomed to or had been looking forward to (e.g., vacationing, upgrading a vehicle, home improvement, a new outfit). Higher costs can magnify existing anger and resentment employed parents have about their salaries, possibly creating negative feelings about their place of employment and devaluing the positive aspects of a job. With inflation comes greater **uncertainty** about the future and a sense of having diminished control over financial circumstances. Such concerns take their toll on mental health.

Sometimes the rise in the costs of certain goods and services is more relevant to certain families. The surges in gas prices in 2008, 2012, and 2022 in the United States would seemingly hit families harder who rely on longer commutes. Gas price increases also contributed to rising costs in transporting goods, in flights, and some services (e.g., trash removal), making things harder on low-income families especially. Similar rises and consequences have occurred with housing prices. Price increases produce pressure not only by **diminishing buying power** but also through the psychological strain of **feeling helpless** about changing the situation. Even for those who feel less discouraged and more prone to act, change may require much time and other resources (e.g., getting a degree, job training, applying for public assistance) that stretch the family's capacities and create new pressures, though ideally fostering greater resilience and family flourishing.

How Does Debt Influence Family Stress?

Debt itself is a good example of a stressor—something that disrupts the system and thus pressures the family to respond. In this case, having to pay back the debt is the pressure. On the positive side, debt enables families to purchase large items too expensive to pay for all at once, such as a car or house. It also enables many to go to college and increase their earning potential. As with any stressor, having the resources and perceptions to adequality cope with debt (i.e., make the monthly payment while being able to afford to meet other needs) means that debt could end up being **a helpful stressor**. Are you eager to go out and get a loan now?

Difficulty in paying off debts likely induces family hardships.[4] What's the first example that comes to mind? The accumulation of student loans, a 30-year mortgage, an upside-down car loan (you owe more than the car is worth), and maxed-out credit cards can feel threatening. Debt can seem like a never-ending burden that restricts freedom and the pursuit of happiness. Even people who feel in the clear after having paid off their debts might **unexpectedly take on debt** to help support adult children or other family members, diminishing years of anticipated freedom.

Studies show that debt from credit cards, individual or bank loans, and unpaid medical expenses (referred to as types of unsecured debt) can be detrimental to physical and mental health.[5] Additionally,

- debt can limit the affordability of other goods and services needed for well-being, including health care activities;
- constant worry about paying off debt provokes high anxiety and depression;
- people who have long-term difficulty paying off debt are at most risk for negative health outcomes, though more recently accumulated debt was especially challenging for middle-aged individuals; and
- people with constant low debt were the least likely at age 50 to report body aches and stiffness that interfere with physical activity.

Debt can also be the result of other economic stressors—having to borrow money as a means to pay for surgery or car repair.

How Does Job Loss/Unemployment Influence Family Stress?

Sometimes the economy is conducive to high unemployment rates. Some industries diminish because of technological advances or outsourcing to other countries. Even highly educated heads of households with well-paying jobs can be laid off. For some there may be a silver lining to job loss—it can be an opportunity to reinvent oneself through education or training and establish a more satisfying career. What about those heads of households with major barriers toward reinventing themselves?

Regardless of circumstances, losing or not having a job creates significant pressure on families. Common stressors and outcomes associated with parental job loss/unemployment include the following:[6]

- Parents commonly feel distress, despair, anger, and sadness; a spouse and children often have similar feelings and worry about the parent. Unemployed parents who have a strong provider role identity (as is especially the case for fathers) may feel like failures and worthless to their families. (How does it feel to be a failure?)
- The unemployed parent's well-being appears to decline more than would be expected from the loss of income alone. Thus, other effects of a job loss, such as worrying about paying bills, losing employee benefits (including health insurance), and going through the job search process could have a cumulative, stressful effect. (What can be especially discouraging about looking for a job?)
- Unemployed parents have reported high levels of family conflict and negative parenting. However, some families appear able to take advantage of having more time together and emotionally supporting one another, improving their family relationships. (Which types of families might best be suited to do so?)

What Other Family Stressors Does the Economy Influence?

Most families probably seek a rewarding balance between their employment and family roles. **Work-family conflict** is a classic challenge for employed parents—though not always a detriment. Some family caregivers report that their job and family roles enhance each other, especially under certain conditions. Generally speaking, employed parents who report **more schedule flexibility and workplace autonomy**—especially mothers—are less likely to experience work-family conflict.

Professionals at the World Economic Forum speculated how millennial parents (those born between 1981 and 1996) will shape future workplaces by further blending work and family roles.[7] Specifically, they will insist on space for parenting while at work (e.g., on-site childcare, dedicated breast-feeding/pumping rooms), blend workplace and home-based technologies to facilitate work and family responsibilities (e.g., specialized calendaring apps), design flexible workspaces and scheduling (e.g., choose how long to work, in which location—including remotely), and prioritize parenting (e.g., a culture of ending meetings or shifts on time, adequate family benefits, wages conducive to raising a family). Though it appears that workplaces in the United States have overall trended in this direction, it remains to be seen how much employers can or will adapt to fully embrace such an aspiration.

Work-family conflict connotes that one realm makes the other realm more stressful. For example, some parents have strenuous, unfulfilling jobs that wear them down or foster negative feelings, **depleting** their abilities at home to be attentive and nurturing. Some parents have family responsibilities that take time and focus away from employment responsibilities, and that also **diminish** physical and emotional energy. Some parents "work from home" and struggle to keep these realms separate (e.g., young children, coworkers, and neighbors needing a favor may not differentiate the two realms). In short, workplace and family demands, coupled with economic shifts that increase the need to boost income, can produce major pressure on families; hardships and daily hassles can occur in the forms of reduced energy and focus to thrive in both realms and manage conflicting obligations (e.g., attending a meeting or a child's athletic event schedule at the same time).

Ensuring dependent family members are cared for can also be expensive, and each family arrangement has tradeoffs. Parents who are primarily at home caring for children save **costs associated with childcare and employment** (e.g., transportation, purchasing more meals and services) but also miss out on potential income. **Quality childcare** is indeed expensive: estimates vary by state and circumstances, but two-parent families on average pay the equivalent of about 10% of their income, and single parents about 34% of their income annually on childcare, which is in the range from about $19,000 in the South up to about $26,000 in the Northwest. Raising **children with special needs** can also be costly, including expenses for special schools and programs and possibly equipment (e.g., electric wheelchairs). Caring for **aging parents** often takes time away from earning and requires expenses that stretch the budget. One report indicated that over 20% of people caring for a family member or friend found it "somewhat" or "extremely" stressful on their finances.[8] Government assistance is a helpful resource for some families to offset childcare and other caregiving expenses, which should help minimize financial stressors.

Retirement can also be a financial stressor. Financial security during retirement requires good planning, financial literacy, and usually a history of substantial earnings. Having paid off a mortgage and facing fewer living expenses seems to be the ideal vision we have for middle-class retirement. Studies have shown that partial or full retirement can relieve symptoms of depression that come from work-family conflict.[9] However, **lingering debt and expenses** threaten the anticipated peace of mind. Some older family members postpone retirement when the economy slumps or to make up for earlier withdrawals from retirement accounts to cover unexpected costs (including medical bills). Health problems of the employee or the employee's family members can lead to early retirement, which can feel like a double financial burden. Of course, some families can't afford retirement and do their best just to pay rent.

Fortunately, pressures associated with retirement—or any family financial issue—need not damage family relationships. For example, analyses of national data indicated that couples who had retired within the prior 5 years, or who were old enough to retire but hadn't done so, were more likely to experience **marital conflict** when they had more negative emotions because of financial stress.[10] However, for couples who had already been retired for over 5 years, their negative emotions because of financial stress did not carry over into marital conflict. Consistent with what we know about family stress and coping, these couples had likely already adjusted well to retirement and found ways to cope that protected their relationship.

How Does Economic Inequality Contribute to Family Stress?

The concept of economic (or income or wealth) inequality is laden with ideological assumptions and controversy. Why do some families have more resources than others? What does it mean to have a "fair share" of a country's economic prosperity? What is the government's role in addressing gaps in family wealth? Furthermore, the term "economic inequality" may not mean the same thing to everyone.

First, try this little experiment. Seriously, give it a shot, you may surprise yourself. What do you think the average household income (combined income of earners) is for the poorest 20%

of the population in the United States in 2019 (we will use these numbers to avoid including the impact of the COVID-19 pandemic)? Write down or type a number. What do you think the average household income is for the wealthiest 20% of households? Now divide the larger income (top 20%) by the lower income (bottom 20%). *Don't* read further until you do it.

If, for example, the number you got was 10 (e.g., $200,000 divided by $20,000), then your interpretation would be that the ratio is 1:10, or that the average household income of the wealthiest 20% is 10 times more than the lowest 20%. **Before you look at the correct answer, what do you think the ratio should be?** The correct income numbers and ratio for 2019 are found at the bottom of Part A. Check them out *after* you give your best guesses.

How close were you to the actual average incomes and the ratio? Studies using this type of procedure using national data from online surveys have found that people generally overestimate both the highest income for the top 20% and the gap between the highest and lowest groups. For example, the average ratio in one study was 1:1,500. The same sample preferred an average of 1:50 ratio. Yes, you are reading these numbers correctly (and will see that they are far from reality). Preferring income differences suggests that people **expect unequal incomes** because of unequal effort or abilities, which is an assumption of a capitalistic or market-based economy. While both conservative and liberal survey respondents overestimated these numbers, liberal respondents overestimated them the most. These patterns are consistent with the moral foundations described in Chapter 2 regarding the foundation of **fairness versus cheating**.

Education is also a key ingredient in economic security (Figure 4.1). Poverty is about three times more common among people with less than a high school education than those who have a high school degree and about 100 times more common than those with a bachelor's degree. (*Yes, stay in school.*) **Married** individuals are more likely to have at least a bachelor's degree (42%) compared to unmarried (35%) and divorced individuals (29%). As is evident in the graph of 2020 U.S. Census data, **women** are somewhat more likely to have a bachelor's degree or higher except in the case of Asian

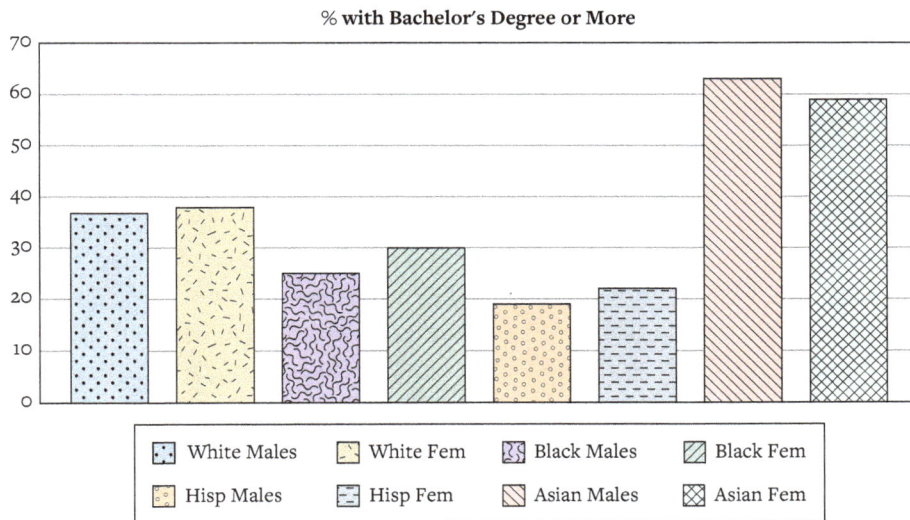

FIGURE 4.1 % with Bachelor's Degree or More

women.[11] Also evident are variations by **ethnicity**. Might there also be barriers to seeking and completing a college education that contributes to such income distributions?

Of course, effort and earnings do not perfectly match; some people are naturally more gifted as athletes, intellectuals, or artists. Some have disabilities that can hamper productivity. Some are clearly held back or advantaged because of discrimination or the circumstances they were born into. How precisely the combination of effort, opportunity, talent, discrimination, and economic institutional influences interact to produce gaps in household wealth is sufficiently unclear to keep philosophers and politicians busy. The bottom line for our purposes is that wealth gaps are stressors, but not only because of income itself.

Various psychological experiments and economic studies suggest that humans are highly comparison-oriented in nature—we feel good about ourselves when we believe we are doing as well or better than others. Living in the smallest house in a neighborhood feels worse than living in the largest house in another neighborhood, even if it were the exact same house in both scenarios. To some degree, wealth is a **relative perception** with real consequences. For example, consider the following:

- In areas of high-income gaps, people tend to trust each other less and report less happiness (especially lower earners).
- People tend to decrease productivity at work and experience lower job satisfaction when they know their pay is lower than their coworkers'.
- People who believe their circumstances are unfair are much more prone to feel negatively about themselves, which can be stressful.

Imagine the difference it would make for you if you believed your wages were lower because you choose not to work as many hours versus having lower wages because of your race. How would these beliefs affect your stress levels?

Some research has focused on what is referred to as **subjective social status** (**SSS**)—how high on the social ladder people believe they are regarding money, education, and having a respectable job.[12] SSS should reflect some sense of actual social status (e.g., education level and sufficiency of income for basic needs) and perceived relative status (e.g., assumptions about the circumstances of others throughout the country). SSS tends to correspond with negative mental health outcomes. Research of economically disadvantaged families revealed that unemployment and lower parental education levels corresponded with more parenting stress (but not parental depression), whereas lower SSS corresponded with higher depression (but not parenting stress).[13] SSS was only slightly correlated with the objective indicators of economic status (income and employment status), meaning that subjective ratings of having lower social status had only a little to do with actually having lower status. Feeling depressed added to parental stress and then to more child misbehavior. One might wonder: if these parents had less inflated assumptions about other families' wealth, would they have felt less depressed? What contributes to social comparison these days? Should that worry us?

A lack of economic resources undoubtedly puts families at risk for financial and other stressors and can threaten resiliency. Perceptions are important but so is **objective reality**. Yet, as we have seen, we tend to make judgments about ourselves based on our perceptions of others, which can be highly **inaccurate**. The meanings we form about our circumstances affect how we feel about our lives, which can be stressful in itself, regardless of our objective strengths and limitations.

How Do Families Adjust to Financial Stressors?

In the **FIM framework**, **adjustment coping** refers to using current resources in light of default interpretations of the stressor to address—in this case—economic pressure. More advantaged families can make fairly minor adjustments to ensure their financial demands don't strongly interfere with family functioning. That might be eating out less or choosing a cheaper vacation destination and duration when unexpected expenses arise. What other simple cost-cutting decisions can families make without creating major shifts in their routines? What other **resources** might be available to families who are generally financially stable? Disadvantaged families will likely have to do more than just adjust their lifestyles, as we will see in Part B.

Improve Your Learning

Without peeking, take a moment to review in your mind (or say out loud) the key concepts from this chapter (this is a proven learning technique). Then review the "Chapter Preview" section at the top and compare. Skim Part A of the chapter with extra attention to the **bolded words**. Skip to the end of the chapter to find more learning resources.

Answers to The Economic Inequality Experiment (Section II)

Here are the answers for the incomes in 2019 (to avoid including the impact of the COVID-19 pandemic): The lowest 20% of households averaged $14,589, and the highest 20% averaged $109,732, with a resulting ratio of about 1:7.5, or 7.5 times higher average income at the top compared to the bottom. Were you close?

Part B. Chronic Economic Hardship and Poverty Stressors

Living in a chronic state of financial uncertainty or deprivation makes families vulnerable to negative outcomes. Such families can also become overwhelmed by any of the economic shifts mentioned earlier. Personal characteristics and external contexts add to the diversity in which families perceive and experience economic hardship and poverty.

What Is Life Like for Families Experiencing Poverty?

Poverty statistics are typically based on family household income levels versus the required income needed to cover **basic needs**. Calculations adjust for the number of individuals in a household and the consumer price index that helps account for inflation and the costs of goods and services (e.g., food, medical care, and housing). They are not necessarily adjusted for cost of living differences in various regions. Some forms of government assistance are typically not counted in such numbers, such as public housing, food stamps, and Medicaid. According to the U.S. Census Bureau, the overall poverty rate in the United States in 2020 was 11.4% of U.S. households—about 37 million people, which represented a 1% increase from 2019, prior to which it had been declining.[14] While methods of poverty calculations are debated and include some subjectivity (e.g., what exactly are "basic needs" and what quality of goods is necessary to meet them?), what seems clear is that millions of families experience low-income-related hardships.

Growing up with chronic poverty or economic hardship is generally a strong predictor of various **negative outcomes** related to psychical health, mental and emotional health, academic performance, IQ scores, self-regulation ability, behavioral control, relationship functioning, parentification of children (children taking on parenting-type roles), and future economic standing. Domestic violence, substance problems, chronic stress, inadequate health care, divorce/an absent parent, and lower quality schools are thought to be important ways that bring about some of these negative outcomes. Several explanations for the impact of economic stressors on children help focus us on important processes disadvantaged families go through:

- Rand Conger and Glen Elder proposed a **family stress model** to account for why children suffer from economic problems.[15] Economic hardship puts high pressure on parents, which leads to excessive worry and discouragement that elevates **marital conflict** and **negative parenting behavior**, both of which create difficult challenges for the children. For example, parents with lower socioeconomic status display lower quality parental monitoring (e.g., knowing their adolescent's school performance and dating habits), which was linked to poorer adolescent self-control and greater adolescent substance usage.[16] The link between negative family interactions and poorer outcomes for children seems stronger for economically challenged families than wealthier families. Any thoughts as to why?
- Research is also consistent with what has been referred to as the **family investment model**—impoverished families have fewer resources to invest in their children (e.g., support for extracurricular activities, learning materials at home, prenatal and postnatal medical care, role modeling of healthy behavior, restrictive rules of media use, high-quality paid childcare, nutritious food), resulting in less optimal child development and well-being.[17]
- Economic pressure from poverty also appears to **directly** affect children (instead of just indirectly through their parents' behavior).[18] Specifically, poorer children worry about household financial circumstances, are excluded from social activities, have fewer friendships, and get bullied because they don't fit in (e.g., not adhering to popular clothing

styles and other social norms). Poorer adolescents have reported feeling more financial pressure or stress in the forms of missing out on activities, wearing old clothes or shoes that didn't fit well, pretending to family and friends to have their needs met, and not eating enough when hungry. These circumstances led to distress, which then contributed to parent-adolescent conflict related to money. However, when such child-reported financial pressure was accounted for in the analyses, the high-income parents tended to feel *more* distress from economic pressure than did lower-income parents. It could be that wealthier parents place more responsibility on their own shoulders to provide for their children, perhaps shoot for higher standards, and have fewer excuses when they fail.

Overall, low-income families are likely to struggle with meeting their needs, which becomes a major risk factor for parental and child health outcomes. Nevertheless, we shouldn't discount the **resilience** of lower-income families. Lower-income families can thrive and flourish because of effective coping and sometimes because of additional family, community, or government support. Poorer families who thrive may have **strengths and capacities** that some wealthier families lack because of differences in the obstacles they have learned to overcome.

What Key Stressors Are Associated With Poverty?

Families in poverty are at greater risk for having severe and enduring stress. Something to keep in mind, however, is that people **shift in and out of poverty**. According to U.S. Census data, between the years 2013 and 2016, about 35% of people in poverty were impoverished for 2 to 6 months and the percentages declined for each longer period of time, except for those who were in poverty for that whole time period or longer (see Figure 4.2).[19] In short, about 67% of people in poverty were out of poverty within a year. Time in poverty is an important factor in understanding the potential stress and coping mechanisms families experience. Additionally, many other families struggle with living on the **verge of poverty**.

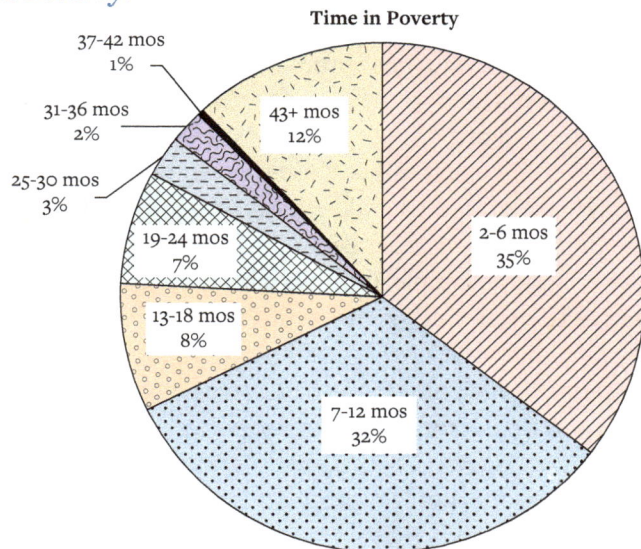

FIGURE 4.2 Time in Poverty

Generally speaking, **longer poverty durations** create more challenges and negative outcomes for families and children. A national study found that parents in shorter term poverty were able to demonstrate similarly high-quality parenting as those who had never experienced poverty, whereas chronically poor parents tended to demonstrate lower quality parenting.[20] However, children who first experienced poverty at a later age (between 4 and 9) had more behavioral and emotional problems than those who experienced it earlier. This could indicate that having to adjust to new financial difficulties can be more stressful in some ways than being familiar with poverty from the beginning.

How Do the Living Environments of Poor Families Contribute to Family Stress?

As you might suspect, poverty is not glamorous. Housing is typically of lesser quality and living conditions may be less comfortable and sanitary. Needed household repairs and upgrades may be neglected. The quality of products used by the family could be suboptimal. People who have money can more easily save money by purchasing **higher quality products**.[21] Cheaper products need to be repaired or replaced more often, which in the long term could end up costing more money. Similar to buying food in **bulk**—it is usually cheaper than buying the same amount of food on separate occasions. Wealthier people are also able to borrow money with **lower interest rates** because of higher down payments and establishing a strong credit history. In short, people can save money by paying more upfront, but one has to have sufficient funds in the first place to do so. At the same time, some expensive purchases are **costlier** to maintain and repair, so even moderate-to-high-income families are not immune to some of these stressors. Having a healthy savings account can bring peace of mind when things break down.

As mentioned in Chapter 3, neighborhoods are important contexts for daily living. Impoverished neighborhoods can put families at risk for various reasons. Living in disadvantaged neighborhoods often corresponds with higher depression rates and substance use.[22] Areas of concentrated poverty can lead to **physical neighborhood decay**, which tends to also link to more destructive behavior. Youth in disadvantaged neighborhoods who perceive that they have limited opportunities for future economic security can feel they have little to risk through delinquency and substance use. Overall, neighbors might close themselves off from one another and stay inside their residences.

However, as we would expect from our understanding of family stress theory, individual and family characteristics play important roles as potential **protective factors** from neighborhood poverty. For example, families with **higher incomes** in the neighborhood, or who perceive themselves to be **as well or better off than their neighbors**, are less likely to be negatively impacted by neighborhood poverty. Similarly, longitudinal research indicated that the low-income neighborhood of their childhood had lasting, negative mental effects for young adults, mostly explained by a cumulation of family stressors (e.g., divorce, abuse, deaths of loved ones) and neighborhood problems (e.g., crime, drug use, rundown buildings, noise).[23] Yet, for those whose parents had a **college education**, the neighborhood effects were *not* associated with poorer mental health in young adulthood. Why might education be related to such resiliency?

How Does Food Insecurity Contribute to Family Stress?

The U.S. Department of Agriculture defines *food security* as "access by all people at all times to enough food for an active, healthy life."[24] Food security also addresses the "quality, variety, or desirability of diet." Families experiencing **food insecurity** face stress associated with worry about having enough healthy food and with physical and mental symptoms of potential malnutrition and hunger—including poorer child developmental outcomes. Yet, obesity is also more common when families struggle with food insecurity for reasons that continue to be investigated, some of which seemingly have to do with preferences for high-energy foods that differ by social class, higher costs for healthy foods, potential differences in metabolism when food is perceived as scarce, and psychological responses to stress.

Lower and unstable income can put families at risk for food insecurity, especially in single-parent households with nonstandard work shifts or multiple jobs.[25] Family **attitudes and resources** also play an especially large role in the consumption of fruits and vegetables, such as being willing to adopt a healthy lifestyle, having better exercise habits, and having greater support from other family members. Some government programs are designed to help ensure disadvantaged families have access to healthy food, including Supplemental Nutrition Assistance Program; Special Supplemental Nutrition Program for Women, Infants, and Children; and reduced or free school lunches.

How Does Homelessness Contribute to Family Stress?

Let's take a moment to celebrate some **good news**. According to numbers by the U.S. Department of Housing and Urban Development,[26]

- only about 0.2% of the U.S. population is homeless on a given day (defined as lacking a "fixed, regular, and adequate nighttime residence");
- since 2007, the number of homeless families (defined as belonging to a household with at least one adult and one child) has decreased by 32%;
- 90% of homeless families sleep in homeless shelters (as opposed to sleeping on the streets)—unsheltered family homelessness has declined by 70% since 2007; and
- since 2007, people experiencing chronic homelessness (defined as a time span of at least 12 months) decreased by 8%.

Does that fit your perceptions of homelessness in the United States? Unfortunately, despite the positive trends, **over 171,000 families** experience homelessness on a given night. That constitutes about 30% of all homeless individuals. About 60% of individuals in homeless families are female, whereas 60% of all homeless individuals are male (who are also less likely to be sheltered than females). Though they make up less than 1% of all homeless individuals, over 3,500 homeless individuals on a given night are **children** under the age of 18 unaccompanied by an adult. Though having access to a shelter is a beneficial resource for families, **shelters** can be sources of stress associated with a lack of privacy and with rules and routines that disrupt children's familiar living patterns.

Like with poverty in general, families fluctuate in and out of homelessness.[27] About one quarter of homeless people live in **chronic homelessness**. This group disproportionately includes people who are a bit older with physical and mental disabilities and substance problems, and they are very difficult to employ. They are more likely to live in larger cities (40% live in California). Most homeless people are **transitory**—they may spend a few nights in a shelter as they transition into more stable housing after some kind of catastrophe. The rest are more **episodic**, meaning they are in and out of homelessness. They are typically younger individuals who have difficulty maintaining employment and may have problems with physical and mental health and substances.

Millions of people who may not fit the definition of homeless face **instability with housing**—they might stay with family and friends, rotating every few nights to avoid living on the streets or in shelters. Poverty increases the chances of eviction or loss of utilities because of a lack of payments. The stress of unstable housing can be emotionally draining and threaten overall family functioning.

How Does Class Discrimination Contribute to Family Stress?

Imagine you and your family own a small restaurant that attracts local families who enjoyed the safe, clean atmosphere. In walks a shoeless man and a male adolescent, both with unkempt hair and dirty and smelly clothes who grab a menu and sit down at one of the tables. Would you have any concerns? We don't hear as much about **class discrimination** (or discrimination against the poor), and we probably have no shortage of opinions on what would actually constitute such discrimination.

"Classism" and "povertyism" can be manifest through our attitudes toward others. Do we see poor (or even working-class) people as somehow inferior? Do we assume they deserve their circumstances or that they are a victim of their circumstances? Are they unfairly denied educational and recreational opportunities simply because they cannot afford them, or is that just the way life works? Many resources exist to help poor families have greater access to health, educational, and daily living resources, but sometimes people are **looked down upon** for using them. Poor families can have the added stress of being (or perceived to be) thought less of by others and feeling **excluded** from what the seeming majority of other families enjoy. They lack the resources that wealthy families have to ensure their children get the help they need to prepare for and be successful in pursuing **higher education**. Poorer families have less access to high-quality lawyers and other **services** that help wealthier families avoid harsher penalties for misconduct.

The clothes people wear, the accents or grammar they speak with, their interests, and even their names can be indicators of class that can trigger **prejudices** from others.[28] Victims of classism have reported more depression and overall negative mental health, sleep problems, risk-taking behaviors, and substance use. We tend to perceive people from lower classes as less competent—though warmer or friendlier than upper-class individuals. Teachers and peers may likewise be tempted to **expect less** from poorer children and treat them accordingly. Lower-class college students feel extra anxiety about possibly confirming low-expectation **stereotypes**, not fitting in, and being discriminated against. They also tend to be less socially integrated with other students.

Philosophical and political disagreements about universal economic rights aside, it appears clear that individuals from poorer families can easily be made to feel like **outsiders**. Even when they are given opportunities above what they can create for themselves, they might lack the history of socialization and other resources needed to navigate a path toward a middle-class or higher lifestyle. However, **upward mobility** is a real possibility, particularly in Western countries (though the United States is lower than most of Western Europe). Pew Economic Mobility Project data show that of those children born to the bottom 20% of household incomes, about two thirds move out of that bottom 20%, though only about 7.5% make it to the top 20% of earners (and about 11% of those born to the top 20% end up in the bottom 20%).[29] While the odds are tougher for poor families, some show great resilience toward improving the circumstances of the next generation through some combination of their own efforts and support from others.

How Do Families Adapt to Chronic Economic Stressors or Crises?

In the **FIM framework**, **adaptive coping** refers to using past and new resources in light of expanded interpretations of the stressor to address—in this case—being in a state of economic crisis. Various studies shed some additional light on the types of resources families in economic crisis might turn to:[30]

- Lower-income individuals with credit problems and who had card debt were more likely to file for bankruptcy or use payday loans to get by—short-term loans with extremely high interest rates (e.g., 400%). While bankruptcy policies can help struggling families eliminate much of their debt and get a fresh start (especially because of job loss, medical expenses, divorce, and unexpected expenses), the consequences of bankruptcy can be difficult to overcome, like having restrictions on future loans.
- On the positive side, families hit hard by an economic recession coped by using humor, unity, and blaming their hardships on the recession (instead of themselves). Financially strained families often mention that their strong family relationships help them get through the hard times.

Coping strategies poor families use to confront **food insecurity** include (1) strategic shopping (monitor prices, shop at multiple stores, purchase in bulk, use coupons, frequent discount stores, and rely on canned instead of fresh foods), (2) strategic meal preparation (use leftovers, have smaller serving sizes, skip meals, use large-pot meals to stretch ingredients, use spoiled food), (3) seeking assistance from friends and family (donations of food or money, sharing meals), and (4) using external resources (governmental food programs, food pantries, church charity, daycare, and school meals).[31] Do you see any downsides to any of these strategies?

Research consistently finds that having **married parents** is a large buffer for economic problems—such households are less likely to experience chronic poverty or homelessness, and the children are more likely to achieve higher education. Analyses like that of the Brookings Institute show that on average, **college education**, even a 2-year degree from a community college in many cases, dramatically increases the odds of becoming wealthier than the circumstances one was born into (i.e., **upward mobility**), particularly for impoverished families.[32]

The relevance of **perceptions** has been mentioned throughout the chapter, especially regarding the causes of income inequality and the subjective comparisons people make with one another. From the beginning, the theme of **control** has seemed relevant to the impact of poverty. Research has shown that most of the connection between one's income and well-being has been shown to depend on how much control people felt they had in their lives—people with higher income generally feel more in control and consequently have higher well-being.[33] Furthermore, the connection between income and well-being was stronger for people who cared more about having money, and people who equated money with success tended to have lower well-being. These findings suggest that **perceptions of control** and the **importance and meanings of money** could impact how someone is affected by their financial circumstances. Poorer people have been more likely than wealthy people to say that the **challenges in their lives give them meaning** and less likely to say the same about a career.[34]

Research has found that low-income fathers seem to shape their perceptions of *responsible fatherhood* by downplaying the role of providing money for daily care.[35] Instead, they focus on the importance of spending time with children, distancing from children if they thought it was in the child's best interest, acknowledging their paternity in public, and asking about the child's home life. These patterns imply that some disadvantaged fathers **construct meanings** from their experiences that help them feel successful instead of becoming discouraged and giving up completely.

How Do External Contexts Impact Families Facing Economic Stressors?

In Chapter 3 we focused on how social characteristics related to gender, sexuality, and ethnicity contribute to some diverse ways of experiencing family stressors. This chapter adds similar information related to social class. Prejudice and discrimination based on these characteristics can be major sources in the actual and perceived opportunities parents have to provide for their families. What was mentioned about minority stress is clearly relevant to economic stress, and worry and suspicion about getting a fair chance to earn a living add stress on top of the economic stressors themselves. Any kind of **real or perceived favoritism** can be discouraging for those who miss out—including members of advantaged groups who believe they were penalized for the sake of elevating someone from a disadvantaged background.

Financial Industry Regulation Authority Foundation research highlighted differences in finical stress and anxiety across households with various characteristics.[36] Key findings of this national sample of 19,108 adults illustrate some of our **external contexts in action:**

- Sixty percent reported being financially anxious and 50% financially stressed when thinking about or discussing their personal finances (even those who had higher than average income); 65% of **women** compared to 54% of **men** were financially anxious.
- Other adults who were more likely to be anxious or stressed were **younger**, had a **lower income**, had **less education**, were **less finically literate**, had **more children**, were **not married**, and were **unemployed**.
- Financial anxiety differed by **ethnicity**: 62% of Hispanic, 56% of Asian, 54% of White, and 51% of Black adults reported feeling financial anxiety.
- The biggest causes of financial anxiety and stress were low levels of **financial literacy** that led to poorer money management and less planning for the future.
- **Younger** adults (ages 21–34) reported the most financial stress and anxiety. Their financial concerns tended to be more abstract about their future educational and career paths and student loan debt rather than about their immediate circumstances.

When the analyses accounted for differences in age, gender, education, marital status, number of dependent children, income, employment status, and financial literacy, White adults were more financially anxious than Hispanic and Black adults, and more financially stressed than Black adults. In all groups, **women** were more anxious or stressed than men except for Black adults, which was the opposite. The study authors speculated that people of different ethnicities and genders have **differing expectations for themselves**, or perhaps different ways of coping with financial stressors that result in how they feel about their financial circumstances. Also, group differences in the variables that were accounted for in the analyses (e.g., education, marital status, employment status) seem to help explain why some groups of individuals might be more prone to feeling financial anxiety and stress.

What Does All This Mean for You?

Take a few moments to ponder:

- How have you been feeling while engaging with this information? Why?
- How much of this topic can you personally relate to?
- Did you grow up in a home that spoke openly about money management and problems?
- What other examples have come to mind that illustrate similar or diverse ways that families cope with economic stressors?
- What hope do families have for coping with chronic poverty? Can such families ever flourish?

Your insights can be valuable to your personal life, your family relationships, and your professional roles. Consider the elements of the **FIM framework** and other family stress concepts. As a person of influence, you can help guide people through the coping processes and ideally help foster a **flourishing** life. However, take care to avoid letting your personal interpretations push you toward **assuming** too much about somebody else's circumstances, perceptions, and motivations. Always be ready to address issues that might be hard for you to face because of your own history and be sure to **practice good self-care** (Chapter 2).

Opinions on how to solve poverty vary dramatically and go beyond the scope of this book. However, you can help others cope with economic stressors and perhaps avoid prolonged economic crisis—review some things we have learned so far to keep in mind when helping families with stressors in the "master table" (see Table 4.1 on the next page).

Some other considerations specific to helping families cope with economic stressors or foster resiliency have been suggested by various scholars:[37]

- **Normalize** economic struggles (help families realize they are not unique or alone in these kinds of problems, nor do these problems mean the family is broken or bad)
- **Empower** families to speak up for their needs
- Help families learn to identify and change any **problematic behavior** and improve their **problem-solving skills**

- Intervene within the **first year of life** for children born into poverty, focusing on parenting skills, couple relationship skills, and addressing financial concerns
- Encourage increased **parental involvement in children's education** to help them stay in school; encourage schools to be flexible with allowing children who move to attend the same school for continuity

TABLE 4.1 Master Table of Concepts for Helping Families With Stressors

Where	What	How
Chapter 1 Part A	Rules, roles, boundaries	Help families evaluate their patterns that contribute to creating stressors or difficulty in coping with stressors; explore more helpful patterns
Chapter 1	Resources, perceptions, coping, resilience	Help families explore their current resources and resources they need to cope with the stressors; explore perceptions and meanings of stressors and resources and help evaluate their usefulness or impact
Chapter 2 Part A	Family philosophy, external contexts, bias	When needed, encourage families to expand (alter) interpretations by exploring the influences on their perceptions; be aware of your own personal and professional biases
Chapter 2 Part B	Cognitive coping strategies	Help families explore the impact of negative coping (e.g., rumination, catastrophizing) and encourage replacement with positive coping (e.g., positive refocusing, acceptance, refocus on planning)
Chapter 2 Part B	Motivational interviewing (OARS components)	Use effective questioning and listening skills to help understand and empower families to cope and become more resilient
Chapter 2 Part B	Behavioral coping, informal and formal supports, family consolidation	Help families build and connect with support networks that provide social and physical resources to foster coping and resilience; encourage families to consolidate their resources and perceptions
Chapters 3 and 4	Diverse external contexts, minority stress, cultural competency	Be sensitive to diverse experiences based on gender, race, sexual orientation, location, immigrant status, minority status, and social class; use culturally competent procedures with families

Improve Your Learning

Without peeking, take a moment to review in your mind (or say out loud) the key concepts from this chapter (this is a proven learning technique). Then review the "Chapter Preview" section at the top and compare. Skim Part B of the chapter with extra attention to the **bolded words**.

Do You Want to Learn More?

We have only touched on a portion of information related to some elements of this topic. **What really sparked your interest? What do you wish was covered more thoroughly?** Consider taking some time to further deepen your understanding of personal and professional issues related to helping families cope with stressors. The following are a variety of resources that you might find helpful, and some references directly or indirectly referred to in this chapter. Your additional efforts will certainly pay off.

Videos

(Use links or do searches with the key words provided)
- Blending Work and Family: You Are Not Alone (16 mins). Dr. Bahira Sharif Trask. TEDx-WilmingtonWomen. https://www.youtube.com/watch?v=X1v2W7ZoLeQ
- Income Inequality Impairs the American Dream of Upward Mobility (1 hr 44 mins. debate). IntelligenceSquared Debates https://www.youtube.com/watch?v=3GHKp6tPsEY
- Poverty and (Economic) Inequality Defined, Explained and Compared in One Minute (2 mins). *One Minute Economics*. https://www.youtube.com/watch?v=rmF7uJaf1ho
- Growing Up Poor in America (53 mins). *Frontline* https://www.youtube.com/watch?v=qAxQltlGodA
- Poor Kids. *Frontline* (53 mins). https://www.youtube.com/watch?v=HQvetA1P4Yg
- Is American Dreaming? Understanding Social Mobility (4 mins). Brookings Institution. https://www.youtube.com/watch?v=t2XFh_tD2RA&t=103s
- We Won't Fix American Politics Until We Talk About Class (17 mins). Joan C. Williams. TEDxMileHigh. https://www.youtube.com/watch?v=v7I6D1i27Nw

Websites

- Economic Research Service, U.S. Department of Agriculture. (n.d.). Food security in the U.S. https://www.ers.usda.gov/topics/food-nutrition-assistance/food-security-in-the-u-s
- Fernando, J. (2021, October 29). Financial literacy. Investopedia. https://www.investopedia.com/terms/f/financial-literacy.asp
- Office of Publicity Development and Research, HUD USER. (n.d.). https://www.huduser.gov/portal/home.html
- U.S. Bureau of Labor Force. (2022, January 20). Labor force statistics from the current population survey. https://www.bls.gov/cps/cpsaat22.htm
- Unites States Census Bureau. (2021, April 21). Educational attainment in the United States: 2020. https://www.census.gov/data/tables/2020/demo/educational-attainment/cps-detailed-tables.html

Readings (Articles, Books, Book Chapters)

- Chzhen, Y., Howarth, C., & Main, G. (2021). Deprivation and intra-family conflict: Children as agents in the family stress model. *Journal of Marriage and Family.* https://doi.org/10.1111/jomf.12791
- Frech, A., Houle, J., & Tumin, D. (2021). Trajectories of unsecured debt and health at midlife. *Population Health, 15,* 100846. https://doi.org/10.1016/j.ssmph.2021.100846
- Friedline, T., Chen, Z., & Morrow, S. (2021). Families' financial stress & well-being: The importance of the economy and economic environments. *Journal of Family and Economic Issues, 42*(1), S34–S51. https://doi.org/10.1007/s10834-020-09694-9
- Hoffmann, S., Sander, L., Wachtler, B., Blume, M., Schneider, S., Herke, M., Pischke, C. R., Fialho, P. M., Schuettig, W., Tallarak, M., Lampert, T., & Spallek, J. (2022). Moderating or mediating effects of family characteristics on socioeconomic inequalities in child health in high-income countries—a scoping review. *BMC Public Health, 22,* 338. https://doi.org/10.1186/s12889-022-12603-4
- LeBaron, A. B., & Kelley, H. H. (2021). Financial socialization: A decade in review. *Journal of Family and Economic Issues, 42,* 195–206. https://doi.org/10.1007/s10834-020-09736-2
- Sano, Y., Mammen, S., & Houghten, M. (2021). Well-being and stability among low-income families: A 10-year review of research. *Journal of Family and Economic Issues, 42*(Suppl 1), 107–117. https://doi.org/10.1007/s10834-020-09715-7
- Starmans, C., Sheskin, M., & Bloom, P. (2017). Why people prefer unequal societies. *Nature of Human Behavior, 1,* 0082. https://doi.org/10.1038/s41562-017-0082

Notes

1 United States Census Bureau. (n.d.). Hinc-02. Age of householder-households, by total money income, type of household, race and Hispanic origin of householder. https://www.census.gov/data/tables/time-series/demo/income-poverty/cps-hinc/hinc-02.2019.html

2 LeBaron, A. B., Kelley, H. H. (2021). Financial socialization: A decade in review. *Journal of Family and Economic Issues, 42,* 195–206. https://doi.org/10.1007/s10834-020-09736-2

3 Pappas, S. (2022, February 21). Inflation could hit your mental health as much as your wallet, psychologists say. Live Science. https://www.livescience.com/inflation-mental-health-impact

4 Pierce, T., & Williams, A. (2021, April 28). Large number of Americans reported financial anxiety and stress even before the pandemic. Financial Industry Regulation Authority (FINRA) Foundation. https://www.finra.org/media-center/newsreleases/2021/large-number-americans-reported-financial-anxiety-and-stress-even

5 Frech, A., Houle, J., & Tumin, D. (2021). Trajectories of unsecured debt and health at midlife. *Population Health, 15,* 100846. https://doi.org/10.1016/j.ssmph.2021.100846.

6 McKee-Ryan, F., Song, Z., Wanberg, C. R., & Kinicki, A. J. (2005). Psychological and physical well-being during unemployment: A meta-analytic study. *Journal of Applied Psychology, 90*(1), 53–76. https://doi.org/10.1037/0021-9010.90.1.53; Schneider, W., Waldfogel, J., & Brooks-Gunn, J. (2017). The Great Recession and risk for child abuse and neglect. *Children and Youth Services Review, 72,* 71–81. https://doi.org/10.1016/j.childyouth.2016.10.016

7   Mickens-Dessaso, A. (2019, December 11). 4 ways millennial parents will shape the workplace of the future. World Economic Forum. https://www.weforum.org/agenda/2019/12/millennial-parents-will-shape-the-workplace-of-the-future

8   Tan, S., Kudaravalli, S., & Kietzman, K. (2021). Who is caring for the caregivers? The financial, physical, and mental health costs of caregiving in California. UCLA Center for Health Policy Research. https://healthpolicy.ucla.edu/publications/search/pages/detail.aspx?PubID=2252

9   Coursolle, K. M., Sweeney, M. M., Raymo, J. M., & Ho, J. (2010). The association between retirement and emotional well-being: Does prior work-family conflict matter? *Journal of Gerontology: Social Sciences*, 65(5), 609–620. https://doi.org/10.1093/geronb/gbp116

10 Dew, J., & Yorgason, J. (2010). Economic pressure and marital conflict in retirement-aged couples. *Journal of Family Issues, 31*(2), 164–188. https://doi.org/10.1177/0192513X09344168

11 Unites States Census Bureau (2021, April 21). Educational attainment in the United States: 2020. https://www.census.gov/data/tables/2020/demo/educational-attainment/cps-detailed-tables.html

12 Adler, N. E., Epel, E. S., Castellazzo, G., & Ickovics, J. R. (2000). Relationship of subjective and objective social status with psychological and physiological functioning: Preliminary data in healthy white women. *Health Psychology, 19,* 586–592. http://dx.doi.org/10.1037/0278-6133.19.6.586

13 Roy, A. L., Isaia, A., & Li-Grining, C. P. (2019). Making meaning from money: Subjective social status and young children's behavior problems. *Journal of Family Psychology, 33*(2), 240–245. http://dx.doi.org/10.1037/fam0000487

14 United States Census Bureau (2022, January). National poverty in America awareness month: January 2022. https://www.census.gov/newsroom/stories/poverty-awareness-month.html

15 Conger, R. D., & Elder, G. H. (1994). *Families in troubled times: Adapting to change in rural America.* Aldine de Gruyter.

16 Farley, J. P., & Kim-Spoon, J. (2017). Parenting and adolescent self-regulation mediate between family socio-economic status and adolescent adjustment. *The Journal of Early Adolescence, 37*(4), 502–524. https://doi.org/10.1177/0272431615611253

17 Hoffmann, S., Sander, L., Wachtler, B. *et al.* (2022). Moderating or mediating effects of family characteristics on socioeconomic inequalities in child health in high-income countries - a scoping review. *BMC Public Health, 22,* 338. https://doi.org/10.1186/s12889-022-12603-4

18 Chzhen, Y., Howarth, C., & Main, G. (2021). Deprivation and intra-family conflict: Children as agents in the family stress model. *Journal of Marriage and Family*. https://doi-org.proxy.bsu.edu/10.1111/jomf.12791

19 Mohanty, A. (2021, August 27). Dynamics of economic well-being: Poverty, 2013–2016. United States Census Bureau. https://www.census.gov/library/publications/2021/demo/p70br-172.html

20 National Institute of Child Health and Human Development Early Child Care Research Network. (2005). Duration and developmental timing of poverty and children's cognitive and social development from birth through third grade. *Child Development, 76*(4), 795–810. http://www.jstor.org/stable/3696729

21 Pratchett, T. (2003). *Men at arms.* HarperPrism.

22 Aneshensel C. S. (2009). Neighborhood as a social context of the stress process. In W. Avison, C. Aneshensel, S. Schieman, & Wheaton B. (Eds), *Advances in the conceptualization of the stress process* (pp. 35–52). *Springer.* https://doi.org/10.1007/978-1-4419-1021-9_3

23 Wheaton, B., & Clarke, P. (2003). Space meets time: Integrating temporal and contextual influences on mental health in early adulthood. *American Sociological Review, 68,* 680–706. https://www.jstor.org/stable/1519758

24 Economic Research Service, U.S. Department of Agriculture. (n.d.). Food security in the U.S. https://www.ers.usda.gov/topics/food-nutrition-assistance/food-security-in-the-u-s/

25 Sano, Y., Mammen, S., & Houghten, M. (2021). Well-being and stability among low-income families: A 10-year review of research. Journal of Family and Economic Issues, 42(Suppl 1), 107–117. https://doi-org.proxy.bsu.edu/10.1007/s10834-020-09715-7

26 Office of Publicity Development and Research, HUD user. (n.d.). https://www.huduser.gov/portal/home.html

27 Adavelli, M. (2020, August 4). Homelessness statistics in the US for 2021. PolicyAdvice. https://policyadvice.net/insurance/insights/homelessness-statistics; National Coalition for the Homeless. (n.d.). *Homelessness in America.* https://nationalhomeless.org/about-homelessness/

28 Rheinschmidt, M. L., & Mendoza-Denton, R. (2014). Social class and academic achievement in college: The interplay of rejection sensitivity and entity beliefs. *Journal of Personality and Social Psychology, 107*(1), 101–121. https://doi.org/10.1037/a0036553; Sartor, C. E., Haeny, A. M., Ahuja, M., & Bucholz, K. K. (2021). Social class discrimination as a predictor of first cigarette use and transition to nicotine use disorder in black and white youth. *Social Psychiatry and Psychiatric Epidemiology, 56*(6), 981–992. https://doi.org/10.1007/s00127-020-01984-9

29 Silver, L., Van Kessel, P., Huang, C., Clancy, L., & Gubbala, S. (2021, November 18). What makes life meaning-ful? Views from 17 advanced economies. Pew Research Center. https://www.pewresearch.org/global/2021/11/18/what-makes-life-meaningful-views-from-17-advanced-economies/?utm_source=pocket_mylist

30 Friedline, T., Chen, Z., & Morrow, S. (2021). Families' financial stress & well-being: The importance of the economy and economic environments. *Journal of Family and Economic Issues, 42*(1), S34–S51. https://doi.org/10.1007/s10834-020-09694-9

31 Jarrett, R. L., Bahar, O. S., & McPeherson, E. (2015). "Do what you gotta' do." In J. A. Arditti (Ed.), *Family problems: stress, risk, and resiliency* (pp. 101–116). Wiley.

32 Reeves, R. V., & Kraus, E. (2018, January 11). *Raj Chetty in 14 charts:* Big findings on opportunity and mobil-ity we should all know. Brookings. https://www.brookings.edu/blog/social-mobility-memos/2018/01/11/raj-chetty-in-14-charts-big-findings-on-opportunity-and-mobility-we-should-know/

33 Killingsworth, M. A. (2021). Experienced well-being rises with income, even above $75,000 per year. *PNAS, 118*(4), e2016976118. https://doi.org/10.1073/pnas.2016976118

34 Silver, L., van Kessel, P., Huang, C., Clancy, L., & Gubbala, S. (2021, November 18). What makes life meaningful? Views from 17 advanced economies. Pew Research Center's Global Attitudes Project. https://www.pewresearch.org/global/2021/11/18/what-makes-life-meaningful-views-from-17-advanced-economies

35 Myers, M.J.U. (2013). A big brother: new findings on how low income fathers define responsible fatherhood. *Journal of Family and Economic Issues, 34*(3), 253–264. https://ideas.repec.org/a/kap/jfamec/v34y2013i3p253-264.html

36 Pierce, T., & Williams, A. (2021, April 28). Large number of Americans reported financial anxiety and stress even before the pandemic. Financial Industry Regulation Authority (FINRA) Foundation. https://www.finra.org/media-center/newsreleases/2021/large-number-americans-reported-financial-anxiety-and-stress-even

37 Bae, D., & Wickrama, K.A.S. (2015). Family socioeconomic status and academic achievement among Korean ado-lescents: Linking mechanisms of family processes and adolescents' time use. *Journal of Early Adolescence, 35*(7), 1014–1038. https://doi.org/10.1177/0272431614549627; Edwards, J. B., Gomes, M., & Major, M. A. (2013). The charged economic environment: Its role in parental psychological distress and development of children, adolescents, and young adults. *Journal of Human Behavior in the Social Environment, 23*(2), 256–266. https://doi.org/10.1080/10911359.2013.747350; Ratcliffe, C., & McKernan, S. M. (2012, September 20). Child poverty and its lasting consequence. The Urban Institute. https://ssrn.com/abstract=2205388

Image Credits

Fig. 4.1: Source: Adapted from https://www.census.gov/data/tables/2020/demo/educational-attainment/cps-detailed-ta-bles.html.

Fig. 4.2: Source: Adapted from https://www.census.gov/library/publications/2021/demo/p70br-172.html.

CHAPTER 5

Fertility, Adoption, and Family Stress

In a given month of sexual activity without birth control, a woman has about a 30% chance of getting pregnant; that decreases to 20% for women aged 35 and 5% for women aged 40. A male partner over 40 also decreases the likelihood of pregnancy.[1]

Chapter Preview

- Various paths to parenthood differ, some of which are more controllable than others.
- Infertility can challenge a person's sense of masculinity or femininity.
- Infertility stressors put adults at risk for difficult outcomes, such as anxiety and depression.
- Family members, including spouses, can create pressure on those struggling with infertility.
- Infertility treatment is also a stressor and can trigger stigma associated with infertility.
- Miscarriages can cause significant grief for men and women and insecurity about their future families.
- Infertility treatments can lead to multiples (e.g., twins), which creates a variety of stressors for the whole family.
- The adoption process can be stressful for birth and adoptive parents.
- Children with a history of trauma or other disruptions put adoptive families at greater risk for stressors.
- Stressors can lead to adoptions being disrupted or discontinued.
- Transracial and international adoptions have some unique stressors related to ethnicity and/or culture.

What Is This Topic About?

Adjusting to parenthood can be one of life's greatest stressors. Parents also have to learn and change as their children age—it is constant adaptation. Parenthood can take its toll on marital relationships and on personal mental health, even when people enjoy being parents and believe it to be worth it. However, multiple paths to parenthood exist and others to unintended childlessness. Adults rarely anticipate having to use less conventional means of becoming parents and can feel inadequate for having to do so.

In this chapter, we focus on stressors related to family fertility, particularly when fertility doesn't go as planned. For some people that means struggling with **infertility**, sometimes for long periods of time. Some couples overcome barriers to conceiving their own biological child through medical assistance. However, **infertility treatments** can increase the likelihood of having **multiples** (e.g., twins, triplets), which can be intimidating. Couples can also pursue **adoption** as a unique means of becoming parents. Regardless of how people get there (or attempt to get there), various paths toward parenthood have both common and unique stressors that impact the process of becoming a parent and the experience of being a parent for many years, if not a lifetime.

What Are the Assumptions?

How important is blood? Not in the sense of blood keeping your organs alive but blood as a connection to other people—our **blood relatives**. We see some diversity in how families across cultures organize themselves based on their blood relations, and historical time and culture likely influence the emphasis we place on our bloodlines (e.g., think about the importance of having royal blood within a monarchy system—or for tabloid editors). A **kinship perspective** on parenting presumes that for evolutionary purposes, we are motivated to invest more in children who continue our bloodlines.[2] Much research suggests that indeed we do see this kind of favoritism. Yet, a **compensation perspective** suggests that those who become parents through the use of fertility treatments (including those that incorporate sperm and/or egg donations from nonrelatives) or adopting an unrelated child are highly motivated parents. Consequently, such parents might compensate for the bias toward blood relations and stigma against nonbiological children by investing even more in their non-blood-related children. Additionally (or alternatively), they might compensate by perceiving their children more positively than their behavior might merit. Some research appears to be consistent with this perspective as well.

On an individual level, some people are particularly focused on conceiving a biological child and have reluctance toward other options (if not fully opposed). Some are passionate about fostering or adopting needy children instead of conceiving their own. Cultural and religious perspectives can shape some of these decisions. Though political ideology itself doesn't seem to include clear, direct perspectives on the meanings of infertility or the value of adoption, they might inform some details about their specific elements. For example, **some conservative religions** have prohibitions toward certain fertility treatments, especially those that involve some kind of donor or surrogate. Regarding the meanings of parenthood, **liberals** seem more comfortable than conservatives viewing parenthood as a highly inclusive adult right of expression. Conservatives seem more comfortable than liberals in viewing parenthood as more of a societal obligation with emphasis on preserving the conventional mother-father dyad as a way to maintain social and economic stability for society.

As you **engage with** the rest of the chapter, remember the key elements of family stress theories (e.g., stressors, resources, perceptions, coping, and crisis) and consider the following:

- Why might men and women have different perspectives on infertility issues?
- Why might some couples with similar fertility challenges flourish while others are strained?
- How do the various pieces of information throughout the chapter fit together to help explain why each family might be affected differently by infertility or adoption challenges?
- What experiences are you aware of among people you know that help you relate to specific concepts?
- How might the ideological perspectives influence how people (including you) think about the different paths to parenthood?

Part A. Infertility-Related Stressors

What Is Stressful About Fertility Problems?

Assuming you ever endured the "birds and the bees" talk, or simply "the talk," were you told that intercourse often fails to lead to pregnancy even without the use of birth control? Were you told it can take months of frequent sex to successfully conceive? The American Society of Reproductive Medicine (ASRM) uses a very common definition of infertility as a failure to achieve a successful pregnancy after at least **12 months** of consistent, unprotected sexual intercourse. While the joke of "having fun while trying to get pregnant" seems cliché, those who have struggled with infertility seem unlikely to use the word "fun" to describe their experience (at least unironically). Stressors of fertility treatments and/or miscarriages can also contribute to an overall rocky path to parenthood.

How Can Infertility Contribute to Family Stress?

Infertility tends to generate various pressures and challenging consequences.[3] If you think about the **characteristics of stressors** (see Table 1.1 in Chapter 1), infertility is particularly stressful because it is usually unexcepted, is sometimes unexplainable, and can last for an unknown amount of time. People can have very specific plans about the number of children they want, when to have the first child, and the time gaps between multiple children. Some couples easily succeed in a having a child but are shocked when they struggle to have more. Fertility challenges can disrupt plans and threaten one's sense of **power and control** over one's life. A telling statement by a female study participant captures some of these sentiments: "I prepared my whole life for this moment, got married, bought a house, got good jobs, went to start a family and we couldn't."[4]

Infertility can take its toll on one's **mental health** and lead to negative self-perceptions. Anxiety and depression are common (though not necessarily extreme), as are feelings of self-doubt, guilt, embarrassment, shame, frustration, and sadness. Sometimes infertility is caused by other medical issues such as cancer treatments, leaving aspiring parents feeling extra angry and victimized. Of course, the more important parenthood is to someone, the more troubling infertility would feel. Why all these difficult feelings?

Furthermore, fertility has long been associated with **femininity** and **masculinity**, and having children has long been a societal expectation. Thus, fertility problems can feel embarrassing and lead to a sense of inadequacy. The inability to conceive a child is also often **perceived** as a loss that produces a grieving period for unfulfilled expectations and dreams. However, in contemporary times and in more individualistic countries, infertility might not be quite as **stigmatized**. People have increasingly felt freer to express disinterest in having children, and views on gender have broadened.

Women who have given up on trying to have a child can face challenges with **reshaping their identity**.[5] This can be a long process, especially when continually surrounded by reminders of the pain and loss, including the monthly menstrual cycle. Such women have described difficulty in overcoming feeling like they are incomplete, that life is meaningless, and that their dreams will go unfulfilled. They might know few if any women with the same experiences who can model how to flourish despite involuntary childlessness. Nevertheless, learning to prioritize present demands over future fantasies and choosing to find something else that gives one a goal and sense of purpose seem to help with moving on with optimism. Sometimes that involves reconnecting with prior passions and dreams that were put on hold or willingly sacrificed for potential parenthood.

How Can Infertility Stress Impact Family Relationships?

Couples are typically unprepared for infertility, and it could be the first (or early) major relational stressor partners face together. Infertility is generally a risk factor for a couple's relationship quality.[6] **Disagreement** about what each should be willing to do to conceive a child places extra pressure on the relationship. Some couples have an increase in **communication** problems and lack mutual emotional **support**. The sexual relationship can suffer when sex reminds couples of disappointment and insecurities related to infertility. It can also become so narrowly focused on pregnancy that it feels more like a **chore** on a to-do list. The spouse with the infertility problem might feel guilty about disrupting fertility plans or about the extra expenses of fertility treatments. Some worry about their spouse leaving them for someone else. Of course, like with any challenge, some couples are more **resilient** and grow together as they support one another and connect over a meaningful shared experience.

Other family members can also contribute to stress by voicing certain **expectations**. *When are you going to have children? I can't wait to be a grandparent! I know you are going to be such a great parent.* An only child might continually express the desire for a built-in playmate. Disappointing potential grandparents and aspiring siblings can be a weighty pressure on couples. Furthermore, well-intentioned family and friends might use hurtful words while attempting to be encouraging: *Maybe this means you just aren't ready to be a parent yet. You just need to relax and not worry about it; you are putting too much pressure on yourself.* They might also share questionable (at best) ideas they find on blogs or heard from a friend about tricks to getting pregnant. Being around other family members who are pregnant or have children can also be a painful **reminder** of fertility struggles, especially when others have unintended pregnancies or are perceived to be in less-than-ideal situations for raising children (e.g., a teen mother, financial insecurity). Individuals or couples might thus keep their distance to avoid painful interactions, creating more **social isolation** and loneliness.

How Can Infertility Treatments Influence Family Stress?

Science has helped couples overcome infertility through various assisted reproductive technologies (ART)—problem solved, right? While perhaps grateful for such assistance, couples can experience various pressures because of ART. By seeking treatment, the couple must **disclose** their possibly-perceived-to-be-embarrassing circumstances to somebody. Doing so can require that the couple more fully accepts the reality of their infertility. Couples must also decide whether to disclose their treatment to family and friends, some of whom may have negative perceptions or beliefs about "unnatural" means of conception. Infertility treatments signal that the couple struggles with infertility and thus trigger the potential **stigma** mentioned earlier. It appears that the stressors of fertility treatments can add to anxiety and depression carried over from experiencing infertility itself.

Treatments can also be invasive and uncomfortable and interfere with work and other obligations and schedules. Each failed attempt is disheartening and shatters raised hopes. The downside of having many treatment options available means couples must **decide when** to "give up" in light of the commitments and disappointments required with each treatment. Imagine the potential **regret** and guilt people might experience if they thought they stopped treatments too soon. *If I had just tried once more we might have a child.* And, in case you weren't aware, ART can be very expensive and is not necessarily covered by insurance. If you do a quick internet search on the price of in vitro fertilization (IVF), you will see numbers like $10,000, $15,000, $25,000, and higher—and this is just for one cycle of treatment (doing three cycles is pretty typical to achieve success, at least for younger women). Results are not guaranteed.

Even when fertility treatments bring relief and hope some pressure remains. Infertility-related stress can carry over into the pregnancy and beyond. Hits to self-esteem, consequences of social isolation, and changes to a couple's sexual relationship might endure. Interviews of childless couples in the late stages of pregnancy after IVF treatment revealed insightful perspectives on the pressures felt during such a pregnancy.[7]

- Couples tended to say little about their plans for the future. It appeared they were careful not to get their hopes too high until they actually had a healthy birth.
- Common concerns had to do with the baby's health—would it be healthy, would it inherit infertility, did doctors use the correct egg and sperm? Infants conceived through IVF are indeed at greater risk of being born prematurely and having low birth weight.
- Many suspected this would be the only child they could have (consider how that might influence the way they parent that child).
- Infertile men particularly struggled with guilt over all the extra treatments their wives had to endure.
- Women in particular reported that treatments disrupted their work schedules.
- The couples tended to be very committed to parenthood and tried to avoid complaining about the pregnancy experience because they were so grateful to be pregnant.

How Can Miscarriages Contribute to Family Stress?

Miscarriages—spontaneous pregnancy loss—happen within the first 20 weeks of pregnancy and appear to occur for up to half of all conceptions. People are often unaware of them, nor are they always an undesirable outcome. But for people who want to be pregnant, and for especially those who have struggled with infertility or multiple pregnancy losses, a miscarriage can be a major stressor. The ASRM labels two or more miscarriages as **recurrent pregnancy loss**. A series of miscarriages can create similar pressures and outcomes as the inability to conceive in the first place.

Couples who experience one or more miscarriages instead of a desired birth often experience stress in some form.[8] The loss associated with a miscarriage can feel just as devastating as the loss of a child at birth (we will explore the deaths of family members in Chapter 11 and elaborate on psychological processes that can also apply in the case of miscarriages). Anger, confusion, self-blame, loneliness, anxiety, and depression are common reactions. Feeling extra **vulnerable**, some women perceive health-care personnel as lacking sympathy and sometimes perceive that friends and family don't take the loss seriously enough. Women who lack the opportunity to fully express themselves to supportive listeners are more likely to struggle with their mental health.

Miscarriages can also bring concerns over the ability to have a successful pregnancy in the future, though a single miscarriage is unlikely to signal fertility problems. Stressful uncertainty can abound through the time periods between (1) the miscarriage and the next attempt at conception, (2) attempting conception and a positive pregnancy test, and (3) becoming pregnant and confirming that the pregnancy is healthy and stable. Couples sometimes avoid getting their hopes up about the future or telling others about the pregnancy until later than they prefer, which is yet another form of pressure.

How Can Giving Birth to Multiples Contribute to Family Stress?

One outcome of ART is conceiving/birthing multiples—twins, triplets, and so on. (particularly through IFV). According to the Centers for Disease Control, births of multiples have grown exponentially alongside the expanded use of ART.[9] More than a third of twins and three quarters of higher order multiple (i.e., triplets or more) in the United States are due to some form of fertility assistance. Thus, having multiples is highly associated with infertility treatment, which links back to potential **stigma** and insecurities about infertility.

Couples might struggle to decide whether to tell others that the multiples were the result of treatment, and they can be sensitive about the topic when strangers bring it up (which appears to be a fairly common experience). Discussing treatment can also trigger painful memories for those who endured great **hardship** and discouragement. Not disclosing, especially to friends and family, can also feel disingenuous and enhance feelings of isolation. Some women even believe that they deserved less sympathy and support than others who have multiples more naturally; choosing to use fertility treatments meant to them that they had essentially asked for multiples to happen, so they shouldn't complain.[10] Is that a good thing?

Having multiples brings other types of pressures, including concerns about the infants' health and future. Multiples are at **higher risk** for prematurity, low birth weight, developmental delays, disabilities such as cerebral palsy, and lack of school readiness.[11] They are also more likely to suffer a **perinatal death** (i.e., toward the end of the pregnancy or within the first seven days of birth). Mothers are at higher risk for birth complications (including more cesarean births) and symptoms during and after birth and exhaustion once caring for the babies at home. Parenting stress, anxiety, and depression (including postpartum depression) are generally higher for men and women raising multiples, and sometimes parents are less responsive and stimulating toward the children. When parents of multiples seek advice from parents of singletons (most parents) or even experts they will realize that much of the parenting advice available doesn't apply to handling multiple same-aged children. The table in Figure 5.1 includes additional data from a large study in Great Brittan.[12]

Percentage of Mothers Raising

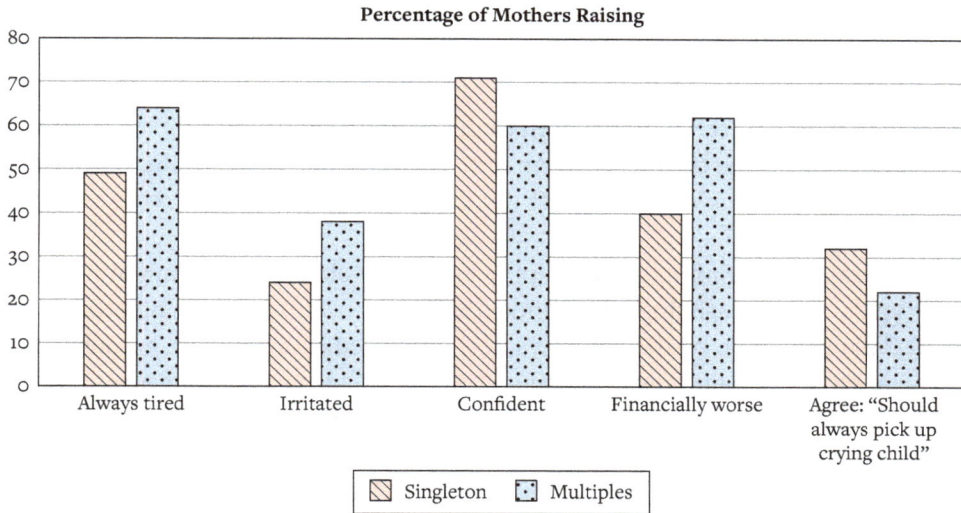

FIGURE 5.1 Percentage of Mothers Raising Singleton and Multiples

A perusal of parenting websites offers insights on other possible pressures when raising multiples that could be categorized as follows:[13]

- **Juggling:** Multiples often means juggling several tasks at once, like feeding one baby while needing to burp another, chasing toddlers running in various directions, helping with different homework at the same time, dividing attention among children who demand it, trying to find time to sleep when multiple infants have different sleeping patterns, and attending to the needs of other people in the family (e.g., other children, spouse, aging parents) while maintaining healthy relationships with them.
- **Expenses:** While some resources can be shared across children, multiples create more expenses. Even couples who have already accumulated resources from prior children will need duplicities (e.g., cribs, car seats, high chairs) or replacements (e.g., upgrade to a double stroller). Some parents struggle to finance bigger expenses, like an expensive school trip or two sets of dance lessons, and opt-out. They might feel guilty that their children are "punished" just because they were born at the same time. Mothers of multiples are typically slower to return to work (if applicable), which can also impact economic circumstances.
- **Managing comparisons:** Two or more children of the same age are easy to compare, which can contribute to more sibling competition and friction. Their identities can

become overly simplified because people label them in contrast to one another—*he is the funny one and his twin is the shy one*. Multiples can be extra sensitive to perceived fairness and equal treatment—parents can't get away with attributing differential treatment to age differences like they might with other children. Identicals are likely especially touchy about being compared and might put extra pressure on themselves to portray uniqueness and divergent interests.

- **Fostering individuality:** Multiples often have a joint identity—*Where are "the twins"*? The need to feel like and be treated as an individual could be threatened when parents struggle to have one-on-one time with each child and choose to jointly acknowledge their milestones (e.g., same birthdays, same first day of school, same graduation). At the same time, one of the multiples can feel left out if both/all aren't invited to the same sleepover or birthday party.
- **Sibling challenges:** Siblings of multiples, especially older siblings, might play a larger-than-typical role in assisting with childcare, for better or worse. A singleton sibling might also feel ganged up on by the multiples, feel unneeded as a playmate because the multiples have each other, and resent getting less attention than what multiples tend to attract inside and outside the home. Some siblings, though, might enjoy less attention and more independence.

On the bright side, for those who struggle with infertility, getting two (or more) with one pregnancy saves time, **resources**, pregnancy pains, and emotional energy. The children have playmates of their age who can keep each other occupied and give parents a break. Multiples can support one another in unfamiliar surroundings, like going to preschool or a community event for the first time (though they might lean on each other so much that they don't make many other friends or feel lost without each other). Some fathers, who might otherwise be more peripheral when caring for an infant, can be thrust into feeding and diaper-changing rotations that help them bond with their children.

How Do External Contexts Impact Families With Infertility Stressors?

Women tend to report more anxiety and depression from infertility than men.[14] Some of that difference could be due to fertility treatments. Even when a man is infertile, a woman likely takes special medications and gets poked and prodded. Women also seem more prone to feeling inadequate and embarrassed when they struggle with fertility. **Gender** biases in society can contribute to stronger stigmas for childless **women**, especially in some **cultures**. For example, interviews of women in Nigeria revealed significant maltreatment of infertile women by husbands, family, and community members.[15] Those women with higher education and who married later in life were often blamed for infertility because they didn't marry sooner. Some women felt pressured to get a divorce so their husbands could remarry and try again.

Yet, **men** tend to feel pressure to "fix" problems for their partners, and infertility and miscarriages can bring a strong sense of helplessness, guilt, and self-blame.[16] Men grieve because of miscarriages and can feel overwhelmed and isolated, but they are often looked upon to manage daily life so a woman has a break to mourn. Men can feel pressure to hide their emotions, sometimes as a way to appear sufficiently strong to comfort a grieving partner and sometimes because people think they have less reason to grieve than a woman. At the same time, if he comes off as too unemotional, he is at risk of being perceived as uncaring. Men can also be sensitive to having a wife inseminated with another man's sperm, triggering insecurities and possible resentment.

Black and Hispanic women tend to wait longer to seek out infertility treatment, perhaps because of differing perceptions or meanings within cultural groups, less trust in the mainstream medical system, and economic or availability barriers. In a study of women seeking treatment in the Midwestern United States, racial **minority** women tended to have greater concerns about feeling like a failure (especially Black women), experiencing social stigma (especially Asian women), disappointing a spouse (especially Black women), friends and family finding out about the treatment (especially Asian women), having a miscarriage (especially Hispanic women), having twins (especially Black women), and having triplets or greater (especially Hispanic women).[17] While income differences were accounted for in the ethnic group comparisons, women with overall lower household **income** tended to have greater concerns about friends or family finding out, high financial costs, and treatment complications.

Same-sex couples seeking treatment might face some unique stressors, especially in places where there is a stigma against lesbian, gay, and bisexual orientations or same-sex parenting. Gender, culture, and sexual identity appear to intersect in ways that can influence different types of pressures and experiences. For example, a study in Sweden indicated that lesbian couples who became parents after receiving infertility treatment reported feeling more competent, less socially isolated, and less restricted in other areas of their lives (by having a baby) than heterosexual couples receiving the same treatments.[18]

Improve Your Learning

Without peeking, take a moment to review in your mind (or say out loud) the key concepts from this chapter (this is a proven learning technique). Then review the "Chapter Preview" section at the top and compare. Skim Part A of the chapter with extra attention to the **bolded words**. Skip to the end of the chapter to find more learning resources.

Part B. Adoption Stressors

When infertility treatments don't work out, some couples turn to adoption. Of course, people adopt for other reasons, but it is commonly linked to infertility. Stressors of infertility and miscarriages are part of the context in which many infertile couples approach adoption, so such stressors could have **carryover effects** during and after the adoption process. Similarly, adopted children have a history that can impact their experiences with their new adoptive families.

How Does Adoption Influence Family Stress?

The adoption process depends on many different factors including state and country laws and type of adoption (e.g., from foster care, international).[19] The process requires adoptive parents to make high-stakes decisions and experience various other pressures, such as the following:

- They must determine how **selective** to be about the child they are willing to adopt, including race, gender, age, and country of origin. The narrower the criteria, the longer it can take for a match (adoptions typically take several months to over a year to complete).
- They must decide whether to do a **private agency adoption** (agencies provide many services and tend to charge between $15,000 to $30,000), **independent adoption** (hire a lawyer who can sometimes simplify and speed up the process but tends to charge more—between $25,000 to $50,000), or a **foster care adoption** (through government-subsidized agencies with minimal costs, perhaps $2,000 to $3,000). Other expenses can also apply, particularly when travel is involved with visiting prospective birth families, or fees associated with international adoptions.
- They also decide (and potentially negotiate) how much contact adoptive children should have with their birth families. **Open adoptions** appear to be the norm, and they give birth parents the ability to continue a relationship with their children (some are semi-open adoptions in which photos and updates are shared with biological parents).
- They must be willing to open up their homes, lifestyles, and personal histories to scrutiny and evaluation to **qualify** to adopt a child.

While adoptive parents take on the stressors of any parent, they also experience "**adoption strains.**"[20] Classic pressures and fears somewhat unique (or intensified) to adoptive parents include bonding with an unrelated child, becoming an instant parent (especially to noninfants), raising children with greater risks for mental health or developmental issues, fearing the possibility of having to return the child to a birth parent (see the following discussion), a child potentially preferring to go back to a biological or foster parent, and deciding when and how to disclose the fact (and other details) that the child was adopted. As with any stressor, the resources and perceptions of the adoptive parents should contribute to how they are affected by these adoption strains. For example, wealthier households and greater parental readiness for adoption tend to predict healthier family outcomes. And child characteristics also influence outcomes—older children tend to be a greater source of distress, particularly those with a long, traumatic past.

Of course, it can also be highly stressful to willingly (or at least willingly enough) **place a child for adoption**. Perceiving one's child to have been adopted into a better situation can be a source of peace, however. Though giving up a child can ease certain pressures, other pressures can take their place, particularly psychological and emotional in nature. For example, individuals or couples might face anger or rejection from other family members who disagree with the decision. They might endlessly worry about the child's welfare or constantly regret that things didn't work out differently. Perhaps they wonder if their children could ever understand why they were given up and if they hate them. Biological parents can typically **change their minds** and have their children returned to them within a certain number of days. The timing and procedures vary by state, but it appears that 30 days is a common length. Imagine how painfully slow those 30 days must seem to go by for all involved. Of course, children can be forcefully removed from their homes because of abuse or neglect and eventually go through the adoption process against the will of former parents, which could certainly be distressing.

How Do Adopted Children Influence Family Stress?

Typically, at least half of adoptions are of children from the **foster care** system. Many foster children experience some form of **maltreatment or trauma** (see Chapter 7). Some were exposed to addictive substances while in the womb. Foster care itself can be challenging, especially when children are moved around to multiple placements. Most adopted foster children have been in foster care for over two years (only about 7% are adopted within two years of entering the system).[21] Thus, adopting foster children potentially invites stressors of the children's **internalizing** (e.g., anxiety, depression, fear) and **externalizing** (e.g., acting out, disruption, delinquency) behaviors rooted in their past challenges. The adopted children could appear detached and have difficulty emotionally connecting with the parents. They might struggle in forming other social relationships and with paying attention at school. The **coping strategies** they learned in their past can be disturbing to others—hoarding food, stealing things or sneaking around, turning off their emotions, or using aggression. They might even try to sabotage their circumstances hoping to be returned to birth or foster parents. Indeed, a relative few adoptive parents do admit that they would not have accepted the child had they known the child's full history, especially when the child had an attachment disorder.[22]

On the other hand, the adoptive parents have had their backgrounds checked, homes screened, and income and health analyzed. They generally have completed specific training and have access to support resources from adoption services. They also tend to be older than other first-time parents, better established in their home and work lives, and are highly motivated to be parents.[23] One might expect that on average, adoptive parents are especially capable of handling difficult parenting situations. Will such attributes compensate for adoption strains and a history of maltreatment?

Adopted children tend to show decreases in **anxiety** and **depression** over time, though some challenging behavior can increase as children adjust to later life stages and transitions or distinct home environments.[24] Studies that compare adopted children to children raised by their biological parents generally find that when there are differences (perhaps in a minority of cases), adopted children are more likely to have health issues (e.g., asthma), learning disabilities and delays, and behavioral problems. Parent-adolescent relationships can be less warm and more conflicted. In families that include an adopted child and biological child of about the same age, parents rated the adopted children more negatively than the biological children (on average); these adopted children were also rated more negatively than adopted children in families that had adopted a pair of children the same age. It is possible that the combination of an adoptive and biological sibling of about the same age creates some unique types of stress or conflict, or an opportunity for unhelpful comparisons.

The risk for **generally poorer outcomes** of adopted children is possibly attributable to both preadoption and postadoption experiences.[25] Once adopted,

- children might be teased or bullied at school because of their distinct family circumstances;
- their attributes can differ dramatically from other family members in ways that make them feel like oddballs;
- they might become fixated on who their birth families are and why they were given up for adoption; or
- as alluded to in the assumptions section, nonbiological children might not solicit the same amount of responsiveness from parents—possibly because their features don't trigger the same natural reactions as blood relatives.

Difficult children can also challenge the quality of **parent-child relationships** which could contribute to ongoing suboptimal parental responsivity and support. While it is likely that most adopted children function at high levels, especially those without a highly traumatic history, families with adopted children typically have some unique stressors that can require committed, intentional parenting.

How Can Adoption Stressors Impact Other Family Relationships?

Around 70% of adoptions are by married couples (another 3% by unmarried couples), and like with other new parents, adopting a child is generally linked to lessening marital satisfaction.[26] Spouses who already struggle with depression at the time of adoption tend to have greater marital problems over time. Spouses who have already experienced a failed adoption or who have struggled with infertility (without treatment) also appear to struggle more with maintaining marital positivity after adoption. Sometimes foster parents desire to adopt their foster child but have to wait months or over a year for a judge to terminate birth parents' rights, followed by months of a possible appeal process, only to end up having the foster child returned to biological parents. Imagine learning to love a child to the point of desiring adoption but also knowing that if the child's biological parents "get their act together," the child will go back home—and it could take a year or longer to know if that will happen. Having a supportive partner is often a key resource to managing the various transitions to parenthood, and couples who work harder at being supportive and strengthening the marriage *before* the adoption experience less of a relationship satisfaction decline.

How might other children in the home be affected by an adopted sibling? As with any family, the addition of a child changes family needs and disrupts family patterns (which by definition is a stressor). Family **rules, roles, and boundaries** will need adjusting. Some children abruptly take on the role of an older or younger sibling. Consider how an older child might differently view the addition of a sibling through adoption versus the typical reproductive process. Birth order can change quickly when older children are adopted. Suddenly the oldest child becomes a younger child, or two children of the same age simulate some dynamics of raising twins. In general, siblings are sensitive to fairness and favoritism in the household, and an adopted child might require extra attention. Sibling competition for parental attention might intensify. Having a mix of biological and adopted children can be an enriching experience for all involved, but the family **patterns and transitions** are a little different or happen at a different pace for adoptive families, creating unique pressures for every family member.

What Happens When the Adoption Doesn't Work Out?

Some adoptions are **disrupted** before being legally finalized (i.e., the child is already placed in the adoptive home but something goes wrong). This happens in about 10% to 25% of cases.[27] Sometimes it occurs because the adoptive parents are unable to afford specialized treatment for an adopted child's health problems and having a child enter the foster care system gives access to government-funded resources. After a time, children commonly return to their adoptive homes. Fortunately, only a small portion of children adopted from foster care reenter foster care, somewhere between 5% and 20%; from about 1% to 10% of adoptions permanently end.

Adoption **discontinuity** can happen *after* an adoption is legalized—the child spends some time in the foster care system or the adoption ends before the child becomes an adult. Risk factors for the occurrence of discontinuity include the following:

- Adopting an older child, especially a teenager
- Having been in multiple foster care placements
- Child behavioral challenges and difficulty with forming attachments
- Adoptive parents with a lower commitment to caregiving
- Adoptive parents with unrealistic expectations about adoption
- Being unmarried adoptive parents
- Being unrelated to the adopted child (especially when compared to grandparents or uncles/aunts)
- Having had inadequate postadoption services, training, and support
- Having insufficient knowledge of the child's background circumstances
- Having been pressured to take on more difficult cases than the parents can handle
- Perceptions of inadequate subsidy (government funding) to meet expenses

The disruption of children's placement is stressful. Children get attached and adjusted to a certain environment and are then moved to another environment, adding to uncertainty and to difficulty connecting with and trusting others (see Chapter 7).

How Do External Contexts Impact Families With Adoption Stressors?

Adopted **boys** appear to struggle more than adopted **girls**.[28] Boys in general, from very early on, struggle with more externalizing and aggressive behavior and impulse control. It appears that some combination of natural temperament crossed with environmental factors contributes to such a disparity. Boys entering school for the first time also seem to exhibit more behavioral problems that can inhibit building good relationships with teachers and peers and overall functioning in the classroom environment. Boys at risk because of early trauma, separation, or poor prenatal care might have these tendencies amplified and be especially challenging for foster and adoptive parents to raise.

The age of adopted children also seems to make a difference in individual and family outcomes, though connections are complex. Logically, younger children tend to have spent less time in potentially challenging living conditions and to have experienced placement disruptions. They might also have more formative years ahead of them in which to adapt to and benefit from better circumstances. Research tends to indicate that indeed being adopted at an older age (e.g., after age 4 or 6) is a greater risk for psychological problems, externalizing behavior, and school problems.[29] Older children are also more **aware** of what it means to be adopted and can experience more confusion and uncertainty, and grieve past losses (even when they like their current circumstances). Thus, as children adopted at a young age mature and increase their awareness of their less-normative circumstances, they likely face some stressors similar to those of children adopted when they were older.

Same-sex couples are much more likely to be raising a foster or adopted child, perhaps up to seven times more likely than male-female couples.[30] Though adoption by same-sex couples is legal in every state in the United States, some social **stigma** persists. We would expect that some of the **minority stressors** discussed in Chapter 3 would also apply to this situation. While much less is known about same-sex adoptive parents, studies seem to show very similar stressors and outcomes for couples regardless of the gender combination—though women in both same-sex and male-female couples have reported greater decreases in couple relationship quality (compared to reports by men) after adoption.[31]

Transracial adoption (adopting a child of a different race than one's own) has become more common over the last decade. National data shed some light on this adoption trend.[32] About 28% of all adoptions are transracial. Around 51% of children of color are adopted into a family with a White mother, and around 45% of White adoptive parents adopt a child of color. The pie charts in Figure 5.2 show the racial demographics of children who were in kindergarten and their adoptive

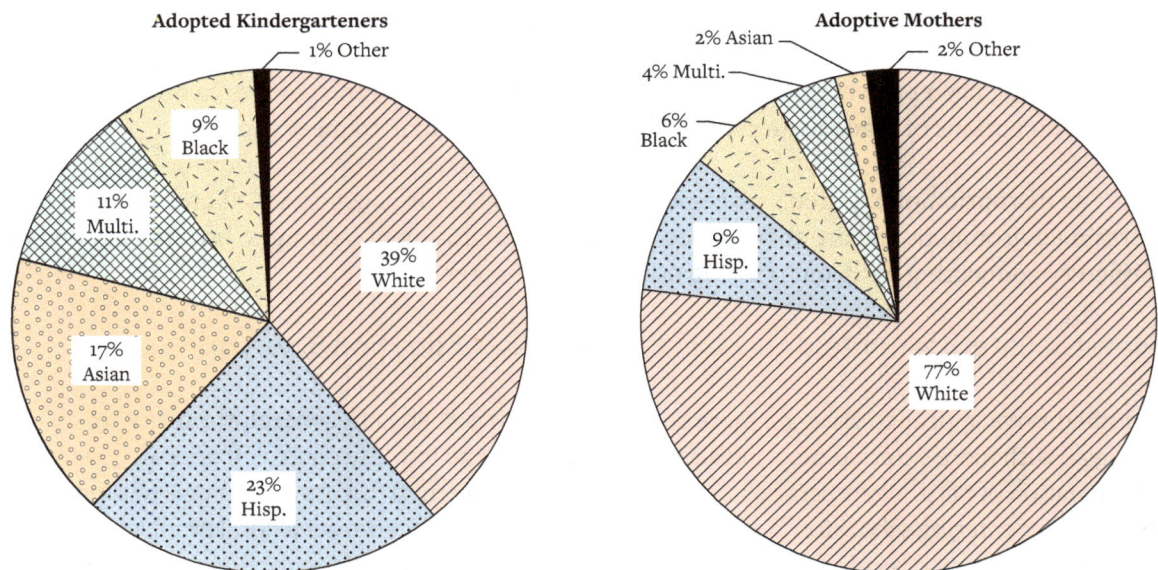

FIGURE 5.2 Adopted Kindergarteners and Adoptive Mothers

mothers. Though such estimates can fluctuate, we can generally conclude that the most common form of transracial adoption is a White parent raising a child of color.

Adopting a child of a different race can be a pressure-filled situation. People have mixed views, and some have strong opinions about matching children with parents of the same race, even though it is illegal to prevent an adoption based just on race. Hence, families with transracial adoptions could face social **backlash**, potentially from multiple directions (i.e., from people of the same race as the parents and from people of the same race as the children). Regardless of the racial combination, the adoptive parents have pressure to help their children develop a healthy sense of **ethnic identity** and to prepare to navigate a life the parents might have difficulty relating to. How are they to know what is important to teach? How much credibility do they have to talk about a certain racial heritage or about being victimized by racism?

Interviews with adopted children and researchers illustrate some of the stress commonly experienced by families that include children of color with adoptive White parents.[33] Such parents tend to worry about how well their children will fit in with other children in the neighborhood and school. Nevertheless, some of the parents avoided moving to more ethnically diverse areas because they believed the schools were better and neighborhoods were safer where they already lived. However, some children of color receive **undesired attention** from others, some of whom are fascinated by their different types of hair or eye shape. They can also be pestered by questions about being adopted. Children who complain to their parents about such things sometimes feel invalidated by their parents' efforts to downplay the attention as innocent curiosity. These reactions contribute to **perceptions** that their parents just can't relate to racial minority issues or are simply uncomfortable talking about race—so children might stop bringing it up. Some children feel hurt when White parents interpret high-profile events related to race differently than a majority of the child's ethnic group or disallow the children to participate in protest rallies or marches. The overall effect of such potential **mismatches** inside and outside the family can lead to feelings of isolation.

Adoptive parents might believe they expose their children to important cultural connections but their efforts might be too superficial, like merely eating at certain restaurants or attending a cultural festival (though some visit the child's birth country or befriend others from that country).[34] Furthermore, as part of a White family, the children might be treated as if they are White in some contexts (e.g., in the family's social groups), which could contribute to feeling unprepared when treated more like a racial minority in others. They can also feel **stigmatized** or rejected by some who share their ethnicity because of being raised in a White context. Adoptive parents typically seem concerned with connecting their children to their ethnic heritage, but doing so likely requires pressures on time, effort, and creativity.

International adoptions have the potential for some of the same concerns as transracial adoptions. However, some cultural or environmental differences could be even more dramatic than those between subcultures in the United States. In some cases, children are adopted from particularly difficult living conditions that contribute to health problems with intestinal parasites, lead toxicity, anemia, and tuberculosis.[35] Orphanages or similar institutions are common in some countries, and children in such settings could have additional challenges associated with suboptimal living conditions and a potential lack of individual attention. Children adopted from various countries by U.S. families tend to have more problems with attention and other cognitive deficits when they have lived in an institution for more than 4 months. Older children, regardless of how long they lived in an institution, are especially prone to have these challenges along with more internalization and externalization problems in general.

What Does All This Mean for You?

Your insights can be valuable to your personal life, your family relationships, and your professional roles. Take a few moments to ponder:

- How have you been feeling while engaging with this information? Why?
- How much of this topic can you personally relate to?
- What opinions do you have about infertility or infertility treatment that might differ from other peoples' opinions?
- How do you think you would feel toward an adopted child compared to a biological child of your own?
- What other examples have come to mind that illustrate similar or diverse ways that families cope with fertility-related stressors?

Reminders for Helpers

As a person of influence, you can help guide people through the coping processes and ideally help foster a **flourishing** life. However, take care to avoid letting your personal **interpretations** push you toward assuming too much about somebody else's circumstances, perceptions, and motivations. Always be ready to address issues that might be hard for you to face because of your own history.

Draw upon the elements of the **FSS integrated model of family stress and crisis framework** and other family stress concepts. Remember, **coping** refers to an action or response based on available or new resources and perceptions related to stressors. Families have either successfully **managed** a stressor's pressure through **adjustment coping** or reached crisis in which **adaptive coping** is needed to reestablish some level of **general family functioning**. Resources and **perceptions** are key concepts to focus on when confronting family stress. **Review the master table** in Chapter 4 as a guide for exploring the following ideas on how to help families with stressors.

What Are Some Ways to Encourage Effective Family Coping?

Drawing primarily from citations and insights noted in the chapter thus far, we will explore **suggested resources and noteworthy perceptions** that can contribute to successful coping and more optimal family functioning.

How Can You Help With Fertility-Related Stressors?

A general theme for the situations explored in this chapter is ensuring that couples **understand what they are getting** into when they consider infertility treatments, prepare to have multiples, or begin the adoption process. Fertility stressors are easier to cope with when couples have realistic expectations, know how to deal with disappointment, are prepared for possible stigmas associated with their paths to parenthood (or with having a large family), and develop skills that facilitate **cooperative** and **supportive behavior** in their relationship. They also benefit by having plenty of **social support** from others who can help them in various ways. Support groups of parents in similar situations are helpful sources of practical information and encouragement. Family members and friends can also show support by

- listening to expressions of painful feelings and frustration over infertility or miscarriages so that the couple has more than just each other to complain to (but the couple should be communicating with each other more than with other people);
- comforting and encouraging at times of loss, self-doubt, and apathy;
- assisting with the challenges of juggling multiples with other daily tasks;
- filling in for parents who need a break;
- helping **normalize** a family's circumstances and the value of each child: that being conceived through ART doesn't make someone less of a person, that having miscarriages doesn't mean someone did anything wrong, that looking identical to a sibling doesn't mean one isn't an individual, and that adopted children are as valuable and loved as biologically related children; and
- being alert to siblings who may feel neglected because of increased attention to other needy children and freeing up time for parents to have one-on-one time with each child.

One of adopted children's greatest needs is to have **trusting relationships** with others, especially if they have experienced abuse or neglect or have been in multiple placements. Children and parents might need help realizing that building trust can take a long time and that setbacks are likely and normal. Parental consistency and patience are important for cultivating trust. Anticipating children's emotional and behavioral challenges can help parents avoid some anxiety and worry, especially when they understand that a child's way of **coping** may have little to do with how the child feels about the parents. As you have learned, sometimes coping that helps someone survive or endure a traumatic situation forms habits that create problems in more stable circumstances. Children also need permission to express their feelings, even when they are hard to hear, but they can be assisted through **emotion coaching** as noted previously as a technique for helping maltreated children.

Parents who adopt children from different ethnic cultures and/or internationally might need help preparing children for possible prejudice and connecting with their culture of origin. Parents learning to comfortably talk about race and racial conflict (and differing **perceptions** of relevant issues) can help children feel comfortable sharing their related experiences and concerns. Adoptive parents in general differ in their **perceptions** of whether their families are just like everybody else's families or they have uniquely difficult challenges, and multiracial adopted families might especially be perceived as the latter.[36] Those who believe their families to have uniquely different challenges tend to talk openly about the adoption and its challenges, though they also potentially overattribute family problems to their adoption strains. However, those who have more strains might also be more likely to view their families as especially different from other families. Regardless, the **meanings** that families make out of their circumstances could contribute to overly negative perspectives on adoption (or on race) and are worth analyzing.

Finally, **couples** enduring infertility, miscarriages, raising multiples, and adjusting to adoption face stressors that can lead more **vulnerable** couples toward a less satisfying relationship. Conversely, some couples embrace that pressure to energize or fortify their relationship. A unique application of **integrative behavioral couples therapy** toward assisting infertile couples illustrates some potentially helpful goals that we might generalize toward helping families cope with the stressors discussed in this chapter: **empathic joining around the problem** (each partner focusing on the other's pain and efforts), **unified detachment** (partners see the problem as something outside of themselves instead of blaming each other), **tolerance building** (learning to accept and value different coping styles in a partner), and **self-care** (fortifying each partner so each can handle undesirable reactions from or differences in one another).[37] Encouraging couples to work together while making decisions and managing their circumstances, be sensitive to each individual's experience, and develop effective coping skills to preserve and strengthen their relationship can help facilitate a strong foundation for families dealing with fertility stressors.

Improve Your Learning

Without peeking, take a moment to review in your mind (or say out loud) the key concepts from this chapter (this is a proven learning technique). Then review the "Chapter Preview" section at the top and compare. Skim Part B of the chapter with extra attention to the **bolded words**.

Do You Want to Learn More?

We have only touched on a portion of information related to some elements of this topic. **What really sparked your interest? What do you wish was covered more thoroughly?** Consider taking some time to further deepen your understanding of personal and professional issues related to helping families cope with stressors. The following are a variety of resources that you might find helpful and some references directly or indirectly referred to in this chapter. Keep your mind fertile by adopting a healthy sense of curiosity and love of learning.

Videos

(Use links or do searches with the key words provided)
- Infertility Counselor Peggy Daglian: How Infertility Affects Couples and Families (5 mins). Santa Monica Fertility. https://www.youtube.com/watch?v=YA7kcUhgnw8
- This Is What Infertility Really Looks Like (11 mins). Shara Hutchinson, TEDxColumbusWomen. https://www.youtube.com/watch?v=QdzG_k5YeDU

- We Survived With Infertility, and Now We Have Quadruplets (8 mins). BuzzFeedVido. https://www.youtube.com/watch?v=YlYNvJXZfCQ
- What It's Like Having Triplets (24 mins). Birth Days, Real Families. https://www.youtube.com/watch?v=mrXT0JGv9NE
- Why Adoption Is Traumatizing Even at Birth (8 mins). Elizabeth Kromhout. https://www.youtube.com/watch?v=3zvsLtZYUk4
- Adopting a Child of a Different Race? Let's Talk (19 mins). Susan Devan Harness, TEDxMileHigh. https://www.youtube.com/watch?v=uORk3TGSCl4
- How My Adoption Helped Me to Become the Best Version of Myself (7mins). Alyssa Belcher, TEDxYouth@Dayton. https://www.youtube.com/watch?v=_Krf9K5UyqE
- Adoptees Speak (21 mins). Pactadopt. https://www.youtube.com/watch?v=Dw5-Vd9tlmY
- Parents Open Up About Their Experience Adopting Teenagers (6.5 mins). *Today*. https://www.youtube.com/watch?v=gN--er0kyeo

Websites

- American Society for Reproductive Medicine. https://www.asrm.org/
- Centers for Disease Control. https://www.cdc.gov/art/index.html
- Children's Bureau, Administration for Children & Families. https://www.acf.hhs.gov/cb/focus-areas/adoption
- Fierro, P. (2021, August 1). The hardest things about raising twins. Verywellfamily. https://www.verywellfamily.com/hardest-things-about-having-twins-2447101
- North American Council for Adoptable Children. https://nacac.org/
- Raising Multiples. https://www.raisingmultiples.org/

Readings (Articles, Books, Book Chapters)

- Hatzipanagos, R. (2021, December 13). "I know my parents love me, but they don't love my people": Adoptees of color with White parents struggle to talk with their families about race. *The Washington Post*. https://www.washingtonpost.com/nation/interactive/2021/transracial-adoption-racial-reckoning/
- Segal, N. L., Li, N. P., Graham, J. L., & Miller, S. A. (2015). Do parents favor their adoptive or biological children? Predictions from kin selection and compensatory models. *Evolution and Human Behavior, 36*(5), 379–388. https://doi.org/10.1016/j.evolhumbehav.2015.03.001

Notes

1   Jean Haliles for Women's Health. (n.d.). Eight facts you may not know about fertility. https://www.jeanhailes.org.au/news/eight-facts-you-may-not-know-about-fertility

2   Segal, N. L., Li, N. P., Graham, J. L., & Miller, S. A. (2015). Do parents favor their adoptive or biological children? Predictions from kin selection and compensatory models. *Evolution and Human Behavior, 36*(5), 379–388. https://doi.org/10.1016/j.evolhumbehav.2015.03.001

3   Greil, A. L., Slauson-Blevins, K. S., Lowry, M. H., & McQuillan, J. (2020). Concerns about treatment for infertility in a probability-based sample of US women. *Journal of Reproductive and Infant Psychology, 38*(1), 16–24. https://doi.org/10.1080/02646838.2019.1587395; Kaur, N., & Ricciardelli, R. (2017). "I asked for it": How women experience stigma in their transition from being infertile to being mothers of multiples through assisted reproductive technologies. *Journal of the Motherhood Initiative for Research and Community Involvement, 8*(1–2), 232-248. https://jarm.journals.yorku.ca/index.php/jarm/article/view/40459; National Council on Family Relations. (n.d.). *Family focus.* https://www.ncfr.org/ncfr-report/focus; Péloquin, K., & Lafontaine, M. (2010). What are the correlates of infertility-related clinical anxiety? A literature review and the presentation of a conceptual model. *Marriage & Family Review, 46,* 580–620. https://doi.org/10.1080/01494929.2010.543042; Wichman, C. L., Ehlers, S. L., Wichman, S. E., Weaver, A. L., & Coddington, C. (2011). Comparison of multiple psychological distress measures between men and women preparing for in vitro fertilization. *Fertility and Sterility, 95*(2), 717–721. https://doi.org/10.1016/j.fertnstert.2010.09.043

4   Kaur, N., & Ricciardelli, R. (2017). "I asked for it": How women experience stigma in their transition from being infertile to being mothers of multiples through assisted reproductive technologies. *Journal of the Motherhood Initiative for Research and Community Involvement, 8*(1–2), 232-248. https://jarm.journals.yorku.ca/index.php/jarm/article/view/40459

5   Fieldsend, M., & Smith, J. A. (2020). 'Either stay grieving, or deal with it': The psychological impact of involuntary childlessness for women living in midlife. *Hum Reproduction, 35*(4), 876–885. https://doi.org./10.1093/humrep/deaa033

6   Chaves, C., Canavarro, M. C., & Moura-Ramos, M. (2019). The role of dyadic coping on the marital and emotional adjustment of couples with infertility. *Family Process, 58*(2), 509–523. https://doi.org/10.1111/famp.12364; Pasch, L. A., & Sullivan, K. T. (2017). Stress and coping in couples facing infertility. *Current Opinion in Psychology, 13,* 131–135. http://dx.doi.org/10.1016/j.copsyc.2016.07.004; Onat, G., & Kizilkaya Beji, N. (2012). Marital relationship and quality of life among couples with infertility. *Sexuality and Disability, 30,* 39–52. https://doi.org/10.1007/s11195-011-9233-5

7   National Council on Family Relations. (n.d.). Family focus. https://www.ncfr.org/ncfr-report/focus

8   Andersson, I., Nilsson, S., & Adolfsson, A. (2012). How women who have experienced one or more miscarriages manage their feelings and emotions when they become pregnant again—a qualitative interview study. *Scandinavian Journal of Caring Sciences, 26*(2), 262–270. https://doi.org/10.1111/j.1471-6712.2011.00927.x; Bellhouse, C., Temple-Smith, M. J., & Bilardi, J. E. (2018). "It's just one of those things people don't seem to talk about …" women's experiences of social support following miscarriage: A qualitative study. *BMC Women's Health, 18*(1), N.PAG. https://doi.org/10.1186/s12905-018-0672-3; Nelson, S., Robbins, M., Andrews, S., & Sweeny, K. (2017). Disrupted transition to parenthood: Gender moderates the association between miscarriage and uncertainty about conception. *Sex Roles, 76*(5–6), 380–392. https://doi-org/10.1007/s11199-015-0564-z

9   Centers for Disease Control. (2016, April 1). *ART and multiple births.* https://www.cdc.gov/art/key-findings/multiple-births.html

10 Kaur, N., & Ricciardelli, R. (2017). "I asked for it": How women experience stigma in their transition from being infertile to being mothers of multiples through assisted reproductive technologies. *Journal of the Motherhood Initiative for Research and Community Involvement, 8*(1–2), 232-248. https://jarm.journals.yorku.ca/index.php/jarm/article/view/40459

11 Kehoe, A., Dempster, M., McManus, J., & Lewis, S. (2016). Stress and coping in parents of newly born twins. *Journal of Psychosomatic Obstetrics & Gynecology, 37*(3), 110–118. https://doi.org/10.1080/0167482X.2016.1175427; McKay, S. (2010, March). The effects of twins and multiple births on families and their living standards. Twins & Multiple Births Association (TAMBA); Twins Research Australia (TRA). (2019, April). Multiple perspectives: What support do multiple birth families need to live happy and healthy lives. https://www.twins.org.au/images/PDFs/Multiple_Perspectives_Discussion_Paper_Final.pdf

12 McKay, S. (2010, March). The effects of twins and multiple births on families and their living standards. Twins & Multiple Births Association (TAMBA). https://twinstrust.org/

13 Fierro, P. (2021, August 1). The hardest things about raising twins. Verywellfamily. https://www.verywellfamily.com/hardest-things-about-having-twins-2447101; Geddes, J. K. (2017, June 19). 17 reasons why raising twins is easier than you think: Raising twins may mean double the work, but they also offer twice the joy. Care.com. https://www.care.com/c/17-reasons-why-raising-twins-is-easier-than-y/

14 Wichman, C. L., Ehlers, S. L., Wichman, S. E., Weaver, A. L., & Coddington, C. (2011). Comparison of multiple psychological distress measures between men and women preparing for in vitro fertilization. *Fertility and Sterility, 95*(2), 717–721. https://doi.org/10.1016/j.fertnstert.2010.09.043

15 Naab, F., Lawali, Y., & Donkor, E. S. (2019). "My mother in-law forced my husband to divorce me": Experiences of women with infertility in Zamfara State of Nigeria. *PLoS ONE, 14*(12). https://doi.org/10.1371/journal.pone.0225149

16 Casey, P., Jadva, V., Blake, L., & Golombok, S. (2013). Families created by donor insemination: Father-child relationships at age 7. *Journal of Marriage and Family, 75*, 858–870. https://doi.org/10.1111/jomf.12043; Chaves, C., Canavarro, M. C., & Moura-Ramos, M. (2019). The role of dyadic coping on the marital and emotional adjustment of couples with infertility. *Family Process, 58*(2), 509–523. https://doi.org/10.1111/famp.12364; National Council on Family Relations. (n.d.). Family focus. https://www.ncfr.org/ncfr-report/focus

17 Missmer, S. A., Seifer, D. B., & Jain, T. (2011). Cultural factors contributing to health care disparities among patients with infertility in Midwestern United States. *Fertility and Sterility, 95*(6), 1943–1949. https://doi.org/10.1016/j.fertnstert.2011.02.039

18 Borneskog, C., Lampic, C., Sydsjö, G., Bladh, M., & Skoog Svanberg, A. (2014). How do lesbian couples compare with heterosexual in vitro fertilization and spontaneously pregnant couples when it comes to parenting stress? *Acta Pædiatrica, 103*, 537–545. https://doi.org/10.1111/apa.12568

19 Adoption Network. (n.d.). Home page. https://adoptionnetwork.com; adoption.com. (n.d.). *Home page.* https://adoption.com

20 Bird, G. W., Peterson, R., & Miller, S. H. (2002). Factors associated with distress among support-seeking adoptive parents. *Family Relations: An Interdisciplinary Journal of Applied Family Studies, 51*(3), 215–220. https://doi.org/10.1111/j.1741-3729.2002.00215.x; Neil, E. (2009). Post-adoption contact and openness in adoptive parents' minds: Consequences for children's development. *British Journal of Social Work, 39*(1), 5–23. https://doi.org/10.1093/bjsw/bcm087; Nadeem, E., Waterman, J., Foster, J., Paczkowski, E., Belin, T. R., & Miranda, J. (2016). Long-term effects of pre-placement risk factors on children's psychological symptoms and parenting stress among families adopting children from foster care. *Journal of Emotional and Behavioral Disorders, 25*(2), 67–81. https://doi.org/10.1177/1063426615621050

21 Children's Bureau. (2018, July 11). Adoption data 2016. https://www.acf.hhs.gov/cb/data/adoption-data-2016

22 Agnich, L. E., Schueths, A. M., James, T. D., & Kilbert, J. (2016). The effects of adoption openness and types on the mental health, delinquency, and family relationships of adopted youth. *Sociological Spectrum, 36*(5), 321–336. https://doi.org/10.1080/02732173.2016.1198950

23 South, S. C., Lim, E., Jarnecke, A. M., & Foli, K. J. (2019). Relationship quality from pre- to postplacement in adoptive couples. *Journal of Family Psychology, 33*(1), 64–76. http://dx.doi.org/10.1037/fam0000456

24 Nadeem, E., Waterman, J., Foster, J., Paczkowski, E., Belin, T. R., & Miranda, J. (2016). Long-term effects of pre-placement risk factors on children's psychological symptoms and parenting stress among families adopting children from foster care. *Journal of Emotional and Behavioral Disorders, 25*(2), 67–81. https://doi.org/10.1177/1063426615621050; Agnich, L. E., Schueths, A. M., James, T. D., & Kilbert, J. (2016). The effects of adoption openness and types on the mental health, delinquency, and family relationships of adopted youth. *Sociological Spectrum, 36*(5), 321–336. https://doi.org/10.1080/02732173.2016.1198950; Segal, N. L., Li, N. P., Graham, J. L., & Miller, S. A. (2015). Do parents favor their adoptive or biological children? Predictions from kin selection and compensatory models. *Evolution and Human Behavior, 36*(5), 379–388. https://doi.org/10.1016/j.evolhumbehav.2015.03.001

25 Segal, N. L., Li, N. P., Graham, J. L., & Miller, S. A. (2015). Do parents favor their adoptive or biological children? Predictions from kin selection and compensatory models. *Evolution and Human Behavior, 36*(5), 379–388. https://doi.org/10.1016/j.evolhumbehav.2015.03.001; Gunnar, M. R., van Dulmen, M. H. M., & The International Adoption Project Team. (2007). Behavior problems in postinstitutionalized internationally adopted children. *Development and Psychopathology, 19*(1), 129–148. https://doi.org/10.1017/S0954579407070071

26 Children's Bureau. (2018, July 11). Adoption data 2016. https://www.acf.hhs.gov/cb/data/adoption-data-2016; Goldberg, A. E., Smith, J. Z., & Kashy, D. A. (2010). Pre-adoptive factors predicting lesbian, gay, and heterosexual couples' relationship quality across the transition to adoptive parenthood. *Journal of Family Psychology, 24*(3), 221–232. https://doi.org/10.1037/a0019615; South, S. C., Lim, E., Jarnecke, A. M., & Foli, K. J. (2019). Relationship quality from pre- to postplacement in adoptive couples. *Journal of Family Psychology, 33*(1), 64–76. http://dx.doi.org/10.1037/fam0000456

27 Child Welfare Information Gateway. (2021). Discontinuity and disruption in adoptions and guardianships. U.S. Department of Health and Human Services, Administration for Children and Families, Children's Bureau. https://www.childwelfare.gov/ pubs/s-discon

28 Agnich, L. E., Schueths, A. M., James, T. D., & Kilbert, J. (2016). The effects of adoption openness and types on the mental health, delinquency, and family relationships of adopted youth. *Sociological Spectrum, 36*(5), 321–336. https://doi.org/10.1080/02732173.2016.1198950; Gunnar, M. R., van Dulmen, M. H. M., & The International Adoption Project Team. (2007). Behavior problems in postinstitutionalized internationally adopted children. *Development and Psychopathology, 19*(1), 129–148. https://doi.org/10.1017/S0954579407070071; Freeman, D., & Freeman, J. (2017, November 19). Are boys genetically predisposed to behavioural problems? *OUPblog*. https://blog.oup.com/2017/11/boys-genetically-predisposed-to-behavioural-problems/; Owens, J. (2016). Early childhood behavior problems and the gender gap in educational attainment in the United States. *Sociological Education, 89*(3), 236–258. https://doi.org/10.1177/0038040716650926

29 Nadeem, E., Waterman, J., Foster, J., Paczkowski, E., Belin, T. R., & Miranda, J. (2016). Long-term effects of pre-placement risk factors on children's psychological symptoms and parenting stress among families adopting children from foster care. *Journal of Emotional and Behavioral Disorders, 25*(2), 67–81. https://doi.org/10.1177/1063426615621050; McConnachie, A. L., Ayed, N., Foley, S., Lamb, M. E., Jadva, V., Tasker, F., & Golombok, S. (2021). Adoptive gay father families: A longitudinal study of children's adjustment at early adolescence. *Child Development, 92*(1), 425–443. https://doi.org/10.1111/cdev.13442

30 UCLA School of Law Williams Institute. (2020, October 27). Same-sex parents are 7 times more likely to raise adopted and foster children. https://williamsinstitute.law.ucla.edu/press/lgbt-parenting-media-alert/

31 McConnachie, A. L., Ayed, N., Foley, S., Lamb, M. E., Jadva, V., Tasker, F., & Golombok, S. (2021). Adoptive gay father families: A longitudinal study of children's adjustment at early adolescence. *Child Development, 92*(1), 425–443. https://doi.org/10.1111/cdev.13442; Goldberg, A. E., Smith, J. Z., & Kashy, D. A. (2010). Pre-adoptive factors predicting lesbian, gay, and heterosexual couples' relationship quality across the transition to adoptive parenthood. *Journal of Family Psychology, 24*(3), 221–232. https://doi.org/10.1037/a0019615

32 Allon, K., Gosciak, J., & Spielfogel, J. (2020, November). The multiethnic placement act 25 years later: Trends in adoption and transracial adoption. Office of the Assistant Secretary for Planning and Evaluation. https://aspe.hhs.gov/pdf-report/mepa-transracial-adoption; Zill, N. (2017, August 8). *The changing face of adoption in the United States*. Institute for Family Studies https://ifstudies.org/blog/the-changing-face-of-adoption-in-the-united-states

33 Hatzipanagos, R. (2021, December 13). "I know my parents love me, but they don't love my people": Adoptees of color with White parents struggle to talk with their families about race. *The Washington Post*. https://www.washingtonpost.com/nation/interactive/2021/transracial-adoption-racial-reckoning/; National Council on Family Relations. (n.d.). Family focus. https://www.ncfr.org/ncfr-report/focus

34 Friedlander, M. L., Larney, L. C., Skau, M., Hotaling, M., Cutting, M. L., & Schwam, M. (2000). Bicultural identification: Experiences of internationally adopted children and their parents. *Journal of Counseling Psychology, 47*(2), 187–198. https://doi.org/10.1037//0022-0167.47.2.187

35 Jacobs, E., Miller, L. C., & Tirella, L. G. (2010). Developmental and behavioral performance of internationally adopted preschoolers: A pilot study. *Child Psychiatry & Human Development, 41*(1), 15–29. https://doi.org/10.1007/s10578-009-0149-6; Gunnar, M. R., van Dulmen, M. H. M., & The International Adoption Project Team. (2007). Behavior problems in postinstitutionalized internationally adopted children. *Development and Psychopathology, 19*(1), 129–148. https://doi.org/10.1017/S0954579407070071

36 Palacios, J., & Sánchez-Sandoval, Y. (2006). Stress in parents of adopted children. *International Journal of Behavioral Development, 30*(6), 481–487. https://doi.org/10.1177%2F0165025406071492

37 Pasch, L. A., & Sullivan, K. T. (2017). Stress and coping in couples facing infertility. *Current Opinion in Psychology, 13*, 131–135. http://dx.doi.org/10.1016/j.copsyc.2016.07.004

Image Credits

Fig. 5.1: Source: Adapted from Stephen McKay, "The Effects of Twins and Multiple Births on Families and Their Living Standards," 2010.

Fig. 5.2a: Source: Adapted from https://ifstudies.org/blog/the-changing-face-of-adoption-in-the-united-states.

Fig. 5.2b: Source: Adapted from https://aspe.hhs.gov/reports/multiethnic-placement-act-transracial-adoption-25-years-later.

CHAPTER 6

Intergenerational Challenges, Polarization, and Family Stress

An estimated 68 million people in the United States are currently estranged (cutoff) from a family member.[1]

Chapter Preview

- Generation gaps can be conducive to disagreement and power struggles.
- The perceived value of family unity is culturally and ideologically influenced.
- Political and religious polarization in families can inhibit communication, limit time together, and contribute to hurt feelings that threaten family cohesion.
- Acculturation differences across generations can lead to disagreement and stress.
- Generational knowledge and preferences related to technology and social media contribute to concerns and disagreements that can damage relationships.
- Family estrangement is a fairly common reaction to intergenerational polarization.
- Multigenerational households (three or more generations) can help families manage economic conditions and have mixed consequences.
- Grandparents raising grandchildren typically experience pressures that can strain the resources of these unexpected parental figures.
- Grandchildren raised by grandparents tend to be at higher risk for negative outcomes at least in part because of problems related to their parents.
- Helping families enhance their social and emotional resources and evaluate their assumptions can be helpful in promoting effective coping with intergenerational stressors.

What Is This Topic About?

Parents and their children typically have a sizable age gap—around 15 to 40 years, though that gap can be smaller or larger because of adoption and stepfamily formation. Rapid social change accentuates **generation gaps** in families—social norms, customs, and fads can differ for a parent's generation and a child's generation, even more so for a grandparent and grandchild. This gap can be a source of stressors regarding how family members relate to one another, including the potential for disagreements about social issues, changes in socially acceptable lifestyle options, religious beliefs or affiliations, acculturation, and technology-related abilities and preferences. Sometimes **intergenerational conflict** leads to family estrangement, creating more stress in the process. However, resilient families are able to maximize the benefits of intergenerational differences and minimize polarization that tends to promote damaging outcomes.

    Power differentials between the generations can contribute to intergenerational conflict. Young children especially depend on their parents for survival and overall well-being. Parents tend to exert their power over children by using their resources of superior size, knowledge, and bank accounts. Growing children tend to exert their independence by resisting parental power and finding their own ways to gain power—like embarrassing a parent in public or wearing down a parent to get what they want. Adolescents and young adults push back against parental power as they prepare for independence—particularly in individualistic cultures that predominate the United States. Parental attempts to influence their children of any age can be perceived as a declaration of power regardless of the intentions. As mentioned in Chapter 2, **reactance** is a bias (or tendency) to resist perceived attempts to limit our freedom even when the request/demand is in our best interest. Parents and children alike are tempted by reactance. Overall, intergenerational relationships are inherently conducive to disagreement and conflict because of generation gaps and power struggles. Navigating such interaction brings along various kinds of family stressors.

What Are the Assumptions?

How important is family unity? Do the benefits of unity (support, comfort, collaboration) outweigh the costs of unity (rigidity, pressure to conform, stifling personal expression)? Families vary in their degrees of **collectivism** (or **familism**) versus **individualism**, especially when comparing families across different cultures. Whether we view one tendency as better than the other depends in part on our own cultural and ideological perspectives. How much tolerance families have for intergenerational differences and conflict, how stressful such conflict is for a family, and how families cope with conflict are influenced by family members' assumptions about unity, loyalty, authority, and power. For our purposes, **family unity** refers to a strong sense of conformity among members who put the stability of the family unit and relationships above individual expression.

    Compared to a liberal viewpoint, a conservative viewpoint tends to value more highly the moral foundations of **authority**, **loyalty**, and **sanctity**. Authority and loyalty could contribute to a push for unity and respect for parents' wishes for the sake of family stability. Sanctity could be seen in expectations for children to minimize activities perceived as wasteful, immoral, or degrading.

Family conflicts and power struggles likely emerge when children seek greater individuality that contradicts the **family philosophy** and prefer activities that the parents view negatively. A liberal viewpoint tends to be less constraining to **social change** and **individual expression** and might promote less concern over intergenerational differences. Such openness could make it more difficult at times when parents feel the need to exercise authority to restrict their children's worrisome values and activities.

Some intergenerational political disagreement is to be expected given that, generally speaking, polls show that younger people are more liberal than older people.[2] As we explore in this chapter, parents and children with different political or religious beliefs can become polarized and distant regardless of who leans ideologically one way or the other. As you **engage with** the rest of the chapter, remember the key elements of family stress theories (e.g., stressors, resources, perceptions, coping, and crisis) and consider the following:

- How can families effectively juggle the need for cooperation and the honoring of independence?
- Why might some families with similar intergenerational differences flourish while others are strained?
- How do the various pieces of information throughout the chapter fit together to help explain why each family might be affected differently by intergenerational challenges?
- What experiences have you had or observed that help you relate to specific concepts?
- How might the ideological perspectives influence how people (including you) think about potential causes of and solutions to families' intergenerational struggles?

Part A. Intergenerational Stressors

What Are the Sources of Intergenerational Stressors?

Have you ever had an argument with a parent or grandparent about a political policy or candidate? Have you ever cringed because of the word choices of a family member of a different generation? Most people probably desire a basic level of family harmony and look toward the home as a respite from external conflicts and competition, but what happens when that isn't the case? Some homes are the prime source of contention in people's lives, which not only adds stress but also denies family members a supportive resource to help cope with stressors. Even relatively mild disagreements can disrupt togetherness and feelings of acceptance, especially chronic disagreements that are **perceived** in ways that threaten **trust**.

How Does Viewpoint Polarization Influence Intergenerational Stress?

Parents and children can have strong, differing, and even polarizing viewpoints about politics and religion. Such disagreement is not necessarily a consequence of generation gaps—couples can certainly disagree on their viewpoints. However, growing up in distinct generations creates the opportunity for cultural and social norms of each generation to contribute to varying perspectives of a parent and child, especially regarding **social or political issues**. Of course, parents heavily influence their children's perspectives, but it is not unusual for their opinions to diverge. For example, research has shown that only about 65%–68% of adult children correctly perceived their parents' political party affiliation, and about 28%–34% had chosen to *not* adopt the same political party as their parents.[3] Adult children were more likely to have adopted their parents' views when they had frequently heard parents talk about politics in the past, felt more current parental social support, and had two parents agree politically with one another. Any thoughts on why? How accurate do you think your perceptions are of family members' political views?

In Chapter 2, we explored some of the political polarization that occurs in the United States. Commentary about the extreme or unprecedented nature of this polarization abounds. Several factors play into political polarization and its consequences when it seeps into families.[4] These days, people appear to integrate an increasingly high level of importance of their political affiliation into their overall **identity**. The rise in more politically specialized media outlets makes it easier to find the news we like to hear (or think we should be supporting), and the growth of social media contributes to the pressures we feel to signal our beliefs in certain ways. Our **biases** and our natural need to reserve cognitive effort (think of it like energy) tend to push us toward preferring perspectives that already match our own—they are easier to integrate and relate to.

Favoring like-mindedness means we also tend to miss out on hearing other perspectives and understanding the rationales behind them. We can become less and less tolerant of diverse viewpoints. It appears that the more extreme voices within political groups or movements effectively pressure toward conforming with polarizing views. With viewpoint polarization, we tend to **perceive** people with differing viewpoints as less intelligent, brainwashed, or even enemies of our political group, as if it were a team competition. Many observers express concern that failing to learn respectful disagreement and to explore diverse viewpoints can have detrimental consequences for a democratic society.

Some good news is that recent data from the American National Elections Study indicated that only about 16% of adults reported that political differences hurt family relationships "moderately" to "a great deal" (though another 18% said it hurt "a little").[5] The downside is that that translates to millions of families with stressful political disagreements (or who at least feel harmed by such disagreement). Intergenerational political disagreement can contribute to family stress in many ways. For example, consider the following:[6]

- **Family conversations**: Some family members feel less able to openly share their political beliefs and experience a lesser sense of belonging. Families may completely avoid certain topics, which could feel constraining or inauthentic. After the highly polarizing 2016 U.S. election, nearly 40% of families reported avoiding political conversation during the holidays. Children in families that struggle to talk about politics without getting hostile might learn to hide their perspectives and feel alone. Watching television shows or movies together that include subtle (or not so subtle) political commentary might also become too uncomfortable, which further threatens closeness.
- **Visiting for the holidays**: Families can feel tremendous pressure to keep the peace during holidays. Compared to 2015, those who traveled to spend Thanksgiving with

family in 2016 stayed for less time (30–50 minutes) when visiting family members from the opposite political party. The more hours of political ads aired in the region where the travelers lived, the shorter their visit lasted (e.g., about 69 minutes shorter in Orlando, Florida which was inundated with about 26,000 political ads).

- **Choosing a mate, becoming an in-law:** Parents are showing less tolerance for their children dating or marrying someone who has a different political orientation. Accordingly, spouses appear to be more similar in their politics than they are in their physical attributes and personalities, mostly due to choosing mates with similar beliefs rather than becoming more similar over time. Such similarity could be a sign of family pressure and internalized political polarization.

- **Hurtful opinions:** Hearing a family member's political beliefs that are perceived to be bigoted or narrow-minded can feel hurtful, especially when we have strong feelings about the topic. It might even feel confusing or embarrassing to be related to someone with a certain viewpoint. Some perspectives can feel like a personal attack or rejection, like holding certain views about lifestyle choices or identity declarations that apply to our own sense of self. It can also hurt when a family member assumes the worst about our motives behind our beliefs—*don't they know me enough to believe my intentions are good?*

- **Estrangement:** As will be explored next, family members distance themselves from each other, sometimes fully and permanently, over political disagreements. This seems especially likely to happen when a mismatch in beliefs focuses on the identity or lifestyle of a parent or child.

Religious differences are not unusual in intergenerational relationships. About half of people in the United States change religion at least once at some point. American Enterprise Institute data indicate that about 24% of young adults who were raised in a religion are no longer religiously affiliated (compared to only 14% of adults aged 50–64).[7] Young adults particularly are less certain about religious beliefs and are also increasing the frequency of interfaith marriages, creating more potential for intergenerational conflict among in-laws. Religious disagreements in a family can be at least as polarizing as political disagreements. Family conversations, hurtful opinions, and the other stressful circumstances mentioned earlier can play out very similarly with religious polarization, and sometimes religious and political disagreements overlap. Can you think of any types of pressure that are unique to religious-based conflict?

For religiously devout family members, having another family member leave the faith can bring up concerns about the child's, parent's, or future generations' **salvation** (or their destination in the next life). Parents especially might feel like **failures** when a child abandons or rejects their faith. Children might feel bad about **disappointing** their parents and could even face parental **rejection**. Joining another religious denomination, especially one that starkly contrasts with the rest of the family's denomination, could introduce **contradictory rituals and beliefs** that feel threatening to family unity and traditions. As with politics, some families find it impossible to talk about religion without creating major conflict and hurt feelings. Hostility from family members about religious differences or changes of affiliation—including becoming religious or nonreligious—can make any exchange highly stressful. As explored in Chapter 3, political and religious perspectives can contribute to the **concealment** of one's sexual or religious identity, which then creates its own types of pressure. Disclosing such identities also places stress on families to decide how to talk about polarizing issues and how to treat one another.

How Does Acculturation Contribute to Intergenerational Stress?

Immigrant parents face stressors based on the extent to which their children **acculturate** into mainstream society (see Chapter 3), which is also a source of intergenerational disagreement and conflict. For immigrant families, the parents' life experiences could be dramatically different than their children's, having been raised in two different generations *and* cultures. The values and beliefs of their cultural heritage might not mesh well with those of their new home. Greater levels of acculturalization for the children can also lead to dating and marrying outside of one's culture, a major source of disagreement and conflict for some families. Similar to political and religious intergenerational differences, disagreements about whether children should retain certain elements of their heritage can cause conflict and stress.

Studies show that larger acculturation gaps between parents and children generally lead to **less family cohesion**.[8] For example, Vietnamese parents who more strongly identified with their cultural heritage were more disgruntled about their children who only weakly identified with their heritage. Parents sometimes encourage their children to speak their native language to keep them connected with their past, as illustrated by studies of Turkish and Japanese immigrants. However, some children fear speaking their **native language** outside the home because of discrimination; such hesitance seemingly then contributed to the lessening of family cohesion. Though not immigrants, Native American families can experience similar pressures and disagreements about acculturating into mainstream society. At the same time, families of various cultures have reported perceived **advantages** of children's acculturation. For example, parents feel better about their children's ability to succeed in the broader society and help the family as a whole gain a greater understanding of societal conventions and expectations.

How Does Technology Use Contribute to Intergenerational Stress?

Have you ever been frustrated with an older relative having trouble using a computer or smartphone? Have you ever felt judged by an older family member for your social media use? With generation gaps come different experiences and meanings of technology use that can lead to disagreement and to barriers toward family cohesion (see also Chapter 10 on addictions and compulsions).

Intergenerational differences in technology use can lead to significant pressure on a family.[9] In the case of raising young children, parents are prone to be the culprit of letting technology interfere with family togetherness. Technology use can even disrupt the **bonding process** with young children by distracting from active parenting. Children of any age can perceive that they compete for attention with their parents' smartphone and social media feed, causing stress about the level of care they receive and resentment that their parents love technological gardens more than them. Many parents, however, report that technology helps them be better parents, particularly as it assists with monitoring their children and finding parenting resources and support.

While parents can be just as into technology as their older children, the rising generation is likely more heavily influenced by the latest technological and social media trends and advancements. Many advancements are subtle and may do little to trigger generation gap stressors, but major technological shifts can make parents feel out of touch with the times. For example, parents unfamiliar with email, texting, and social media platforms when such activities first became popular could struggle with relating to their children's relevant habits. Such unfamiliarity breeds **fear and concern**, which at times might be justified, that fosters disagreement and power struggles. Regardless of familiarity, parents can have concerns about the sexual and violent content their children are exposed to online or in video games or the amount of screen time compared to time exploring the outdoors, being physically active, and having face-to-face social contact.

New technologies pressure families to revisit their rules, roles, and boundaries that help **regulate the usage** of such technology, requiring time, effort, and some research. Parents face challenging decisions of how much to honor children's privacy and autonomy versus closely **monitoring** their technology and social media use, knowing that children have less experience and reasoning capacity to consistently form sensible judgments for their own well-being. When parents cross the line—from the child's standpoint—children can feel betrayed, not trusted, and resentful, and work harder to deceive their parents. A stressful dilemma, isn't it?

Children's reliance on technological gadgets for leisure gives parents an easy target for **leverage**. Regulating such leisure time as a means of punishing and rewarding children's behavior puts technology at the forefront of family contention, especially when parents themselves demonstrate heavy use of similar gadgetry. Conflict can also ensue when parents and children share devices and parents ask (or demand) to take their turn. Conversely, technology can bring families together as they negotiate its use, create shared leisure experiences, and use it to increase their communication.

Why Does Polarization in Families Create Stress?

Family polarization can be perceived as a threat that activates our attachment systems.[10] If you have studied child development, you are probably familiar with the concept of **attachment**. You might recall that early childhood attachment to caregivers helps children feel safe exploring their environment. Children look to the attachment figure for reassurance as a way to regulate emotions. Attachment processes continue throughout childhood and adulthood—we all turn to loved ones for social support and reassurance. Feeling psychologically and emotionally safe becomes more difficult when our attachment figures are perceived as unreliable or rejecting, leading to greater anxiety or depression. Family togetherness and closeness, which are valuable **protective factors** for all family members, are more difficult to maintain in the face of polarization.

Imagine that the person a child or young adult would turn to in times of anxiety believes their worldview is "crazy," "stupid," "immoral," or "meaningless." Similarly, imagine the youth believes the parent's views are "hateful," "clueless," "evil," or "obsolete." Polarization threatens the ability to foster **empathy and respect** that reinforce secure attachments, especially when parents and children feel they are on different sides of a social battlefront. Who will they turn to instead? Consider that a family gathering around the lone radio or television set has gradually been replaced by most family members viewing their own preferred media and news in the palms of their hands wherever they choose to be. How can that play into polarization? Research shows that people who consume high amounts of partisan media appear to be less polarized by it when they also have political discussions with others who have different views.[11] That might be good information for parents to keep in mind.

How Can Intergenerational Stress Contribute to Estrangement?

In some cases, intergenerational conflict and polarization lead to estrangement—cutting communication or ties with a family member. **Family estrangement** has various causes, consequences, and cures.[12] Estrangement might be more common than one might think. A national study of adults in the United States found that about 27% of adults reported a current family estrangement, 24% of which was with a parent, 14% with a child, 30% with a sibling, and 32% with extended family members, including grandparents (see the pie chart in Figure 6.1). It appears that the likelihood of family estrangement differs little if any by gender, race, marital status, region, or education level. Based on projections of this data, it could be that around 68 million people are currently (not to mention any past instances) estranged from family. How do you feel about that?

Percent Estranged with a Family Member

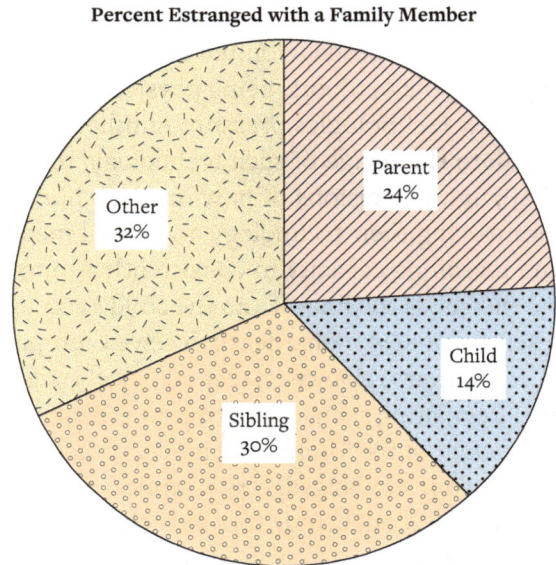

FIGURE 6.1   Percent Estranged With a Family Member

Estrangement is not an inevitable outcome of major intergenerational conflict—two families might have similar problems, but for various reasons, one family ends in estrangement while the other avoids doing so. If we think about estrangement as a form of **family crisis**, referring to the **FSS integrated model (FIM) of family stress and crisis framework** will remind us that resources and perceptions help explain why and how estrangement can be avoided. Furthermore, **family philosophy** and **external contexts** should influence decisions about estrangement. For example, family values about loyalty, self-sacrifice, and open communication could act as protective or risk factors when a family member considers cutting connections—assuming that such values have been internalized. Family philosophy and **general family functioning** could contribute to how members perceive and take offense to one another, and whether things escalate to a boiling point. How might external contexts contribute to decisions about estrangement?

While estrangement is not new, modern estrangements seem to be more uniquely characterized as a means toward **personal growth**. Contemporary trends in focusing on mental health and personal well-being mixed with highly individualistic cultural norms have arguably made estrangement more **socially acceptable**. Estrangement levels are likely to persist if not grow as more individuals are able or encouraged to rely less on family and place greater emphasis on personal happiness and growth than on family obligations and responsibility.[13] Have you observed a strong societal message of not letting anyone—including family—"hold you back"? What do you think about that message?

It appears that most intergenerational estrangements are **initiated by the adult child/grandchild.** Most of those adult children report that it was the best option for their own household, though some report remorse over their children missing out on a relationship with grandparents. Common problems that lead family members to consider cutting off a family relationship include the following:

- Experiencing abusive parenting (physical, emotional, verbal)
- Parental favoritism toward one child over another
- Efforts to control older or adult children (e.g., exerting undesired levels of influence over one's choices about friendships, employment, timing of marriage)
- Conflict related to money (wills, inheritance, favoritism in spending)
- Value differences often related to sexual identity, politics, religion, "alternative" lifestyles
- Choice of adult child's mate or spouse, in-law problems
- Consequences of a divorce such as pressure to take sides, being unhappy with division of emotional or financial resources between households, or displeasure about a parent's remarriage or stepfamily members
- Concern about exposing grandchildren to grandparents' views and word choices

Estrangement itself is a stressor. It can cause stress by limiting the benefits that come from a cohesive family—a sense of belonging, social and other forms of support, and companionship. Also, consider when only one married parent cuts off a child but the other parent disagrees. Spouses in such cases likely feel **pressure** to side with one of the estranged loved ones or to somehow fix the estranged relationship. The estranged parent and child might each resent that spouse/other parent for maintaining a close relationship with both parties. Losses owing to estrangement can be especially profound and stressful in times when family is critically important to lean on (e.g., quarantine during a pandemic) or in moments that trigger happy memories of being together (e.g., holidays). Some families do **reconcile**, however, which can be a major source of pride and confidence for those who worked through that crisis.

How Do External Contexts Impact Families With Intergenerational Stressors?

Some examples of external contexts in the form of ethnic culture and social norms of political polarization have already been mentioned in this chapter. Individual and external contexts can contribute to intergenerational stressors in various other ways.[14] For example, Asian cultures tend to highly value **parental authority and control**. Research has indicated that Asian immigrant parents in the United States are especially likely to closely monitor their children's social media histories (e.g., Facebook logs). This monitoring style contributes to frequent parent-child disagreements and shame and anxiety for children when their activities have been discovered. Sexualized social media or virtual communication is particularly taboo. Children who are highly

acculturated into a society that would view such parental behavior as overly intrusive would be especially likely to resist parental control and thus contribute to more family conflict.

Muslim families in the United States are especially likely to have **strict religious laws and customs** that shape their daily rituals and behavioral expectations. These daily rituals and behaviors can accentuate differences in mixed-religious families and therefore contribute to more frequent family disagreements and conflict. Generational acculturation could also breed more stress and conflict if children adopt more mainstream habits and values contrary to strict religious expectations.

Some lesbian, gay, bisexual, and transgender (LGBT) parents rely heavily on social media to increase awareness of their barriers, advocate for their rights, and connect with a larger LGBT community. A **visible social media presence** could bring unwanted attention to a child who is embarrassed or unaccepting of a parent's sexual or gender identity, or who is bullied because of it. This issue can thus trigger multiple types of intergenerational friction and stress in the home that some other types of parents wouldn't need to worry about.

> **Improve Your Learning**
>
> Without peeking, take a moment to review in your mind (or say out loud) the key concepts from this chapter (this is a proven learning technique). Then review the "Chapter Preview" section at the top and compare. Skim Part A of the chapter with extra attention to the **bolded words**. Skip to the end of the chapter to find more learning resources.

Part B. Multigenerational Household Stressors

Generation gaps are obviously larger between grandparents and grandchildren. Much of the content in Part A applies to families when three or more generations live together. In fact, there are at least three different generation gaps in such households—grandparent to adult child, grandparent to grandchild, and adult child to grandchild (own child). Thus, opportunities for the intergenerational disagreements mentioned earlier seem more abundant. However, other unique stressors emerge when grandparents are involved with daily family patterns. Can you think of any?

What Are Common Stressors for Multigenerational Households?

Households that contain three or more generations of family members are typically referred to as **multigenerational households**. U.S. Census data indicate the presence of nearly five million multigenerational households.[15] A large national report by Generations United provides numerous estimates and firsthand accounts about multigenerational households that can help explain a broader context of why such families are common and the nature of likely family stressors.[16] Though this was a national survey, it was a nonrandom online survey, so the findings may not accurately represent the full diversity of multigenerational households.

The overall **economic climate** was the most common reason mentioned for living in a multigenerational household. Though the pandemic played a part in that climate (see Chapter 12), finances are typically a major motivator for multigenerational household living. Other major reasons included elder care, childcare, job loss, health-care costs, cultural/family norms, high tuition costs or student debt, divorce, and home foreclosure. Multigenerational households seem to be on the rise given that many young adults continue or return to live with their parents after college (especially during a bad economy), with people waiting longer than in the past to marry, and with more people living to advanced ages who might need family care.

Multigenerational living seems to have **mixed consequences** for families. About 75% of the sample said that the arrangement causes stress from time to time, though about 76% stated that overall it had a positive effect on their mental or physical health, and 79% thought it helped bond family members. Given what we know about stressors, it shouldn't be surprising that some families cope better with these circumstances than others. Common sources of stress include the following:

- Managing caregiving responsibilities for elder- and/or childcare
- Navigating multiple schedules
- Lack of privacy and personal space
- Conflicting tastes in music, decorative styles, and entertainment
- Maintaining family routines
- Managing finances

Common **benefits** to multigenerational households included having a constant support system, less worry about the well-being of an aging parent living alone, frequent conversations with extended family members, and less social isolation. Families who were most positive about the arrangement tended to have homes with more bedrooms and bathrooms, spaces for both privacy and for being together, modifications or additions to their homes, and designated time for kitchen use. About 28% of the sample planned to **discontinue** the living arrangement in the future.

Overall, multigenerational households add **complexity** to family roles, rules, and boundaries. How do you think such complexity can help or hurt a family? If managed well, multigenerational households can add to family resilience and protective factors through **resources** of support and cooperation among individuals with a greater variety of knowledge and experiences. Children likely have more adults in their corner to support and encourage them. If managed poorly, intergenerational friction because of conflicting preferences and worldviews, along with potential spatial constraints, can reduce resiliency and increase risk factors.

What Are Stressors for Grandparents Who Raise Their Grandchildren?

Most of the approximately seven million grandparents living with at least one grandchild have no or only partial responsibility for helping raise grandchildren. Let's refer to them as **noncustodial grandparents** (**NC-GPs**). As will be explored in Chapter 9, many such grandparents live with their adult children and grandchildren to receive caregiving support. However, nearly 2.5 million grandparents living in their own homes are raising over 4.7 million grandchildren—let's call them

custodial grandparents (C-GPs). In many cases, the children's parents also live in that same home (at least temporarily).

The table in Figure 6.2 shows numbers from the 2020 U.S. Census Bureau, indicating how the 7.6 million children living in a home with at least one grandparent (either as NC-GP or as C-GPs) are distributed among various types of **family configurations.**[17] For example, in the first column, you see that most of the households in which two NC-GPs lives also have both parents in the home, the next most common being a mother only in the home. What do you notice about single fathers overall? How about single (or widowed) grandfathers? Even if all three generations are not living in the home at the same time, we will consider C-GP households as multigenerational because in most cases, the middle generation has at least a **psychological presence** in the household if not a physical one at least occasionally. Such households are sometimes referred to as **skipped-generation** families.

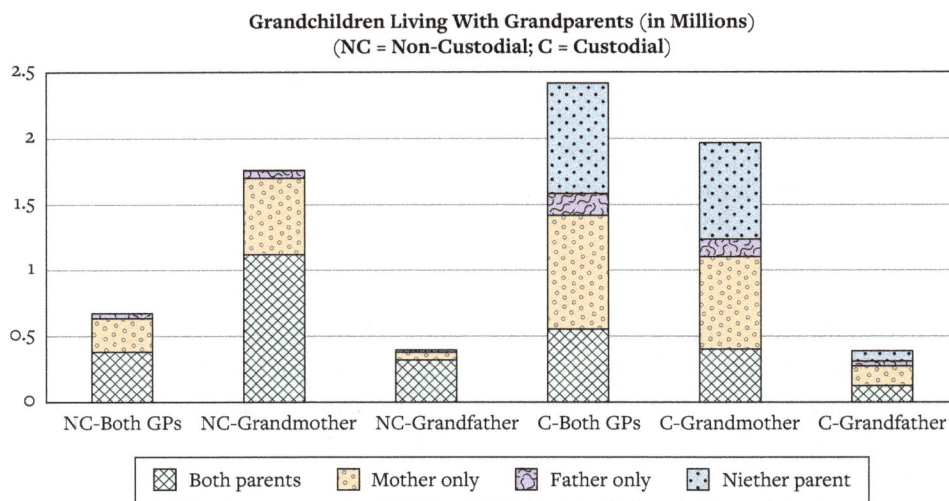

Grandchildren Living With Grandparents (in Millions)
(NC = Non-Custodial; C = Custodial)

Legend: Both parents | Mother only | Father only | Niether parent

FIGURE 6.2 Grandchildren Living With Grandparents

C-GPs don't always have official custody of the grandchildren they raise, and sometimes only raise them for a short time. For example, in recent years, about 18% of C-GPs raise a grandchild for less than a year, and only about 44% raise one for over 5 years. Estimates suggest that about 25% of C-GPs are Black, which is higher than would be expected based just on the population distributions in the United States (12.4% Black). As noted in Chapter 3, **minority stressors** associated with teen and single-mother parenthood and economic challenges likely contribute to more grandmothers stepping in to care for grandchildren, and doing so could be part of cultural expectations. Why else might grandparents raise their grandchildren? Why might it be stressful?

Parental **substance use problems** account for about 40% of grandchildren being raised by grandparents. Parental **abuse, neglect, or abandonment** account for about another 30%. Other reasons relate to teen parenthood; parental imprisonment, military deployment, or death; and family economic hardship. Grandparents often serve as family foster parents for children who are removed from their homes by Child Protective Services—most often for neglect (frequently related to substance problems; see Chapter 7). Doing so can help children feel more comfortable living with someone they likely know, and it can help prevent siblings from being divided across multiple households if foster families can only take one child. Grandparents raising grandchildren save taxpayers more than $6 billion annually by preventing the grandchildren from being in foster care. However, grandparents are not always eager and prepared to take on such responsibilities.

Common pressures among C-GPs include the following:[18]

- **Adjusting expectations**: C-GPs typically hadn't expected to be raising their grandchildren. Long-anticipated vacation and travel plans, or simply having time to rest, might be put on hold. Some grandparents feel obligated to step in and take custody of grandchildren even if it isn't their true preference to do so; they might feel trapped, unable to refuse. Some are motivated to ensure their grandchildren avoid the foster care system. They could struggle with feelings of guilt and shame about their perceived contributions to their adult children's decisions or circumstances that put the grandchildren at risk in the first place.
- **Struggling with adult children**: Imagine discovering that your adult child uses and deals illegal drugs, has been arrested, and is likely to be imprisoned for years. Even if the news is expected, these types of circumstances can be emotionally and psychologically draining. Aging parents likely face disappointment, surprise, and anxiety about the welfare of their adult children who lose custody of their children. As seen in Figure 6.2, parents are often living with the C-GPs, so their interaction could also be a source of tension, especially if the adult parents don't meet their parents' expectations. Grandparents can also feel burdened by questions of how much they are enabling the problematic behavior of their adult children. *Should I continue to let my child live here for free? Should I report legal violations to the police?*
- **Parent problems**: The adult children as parents can raise hope in their children's expectations for better parental involvement or sooner reunification that they are able or even intend to deliver. The grandparents then have the role of helping soothe disappointments and perhaps take on the role of the "bad guy" who has a more realistic understanding of what the children should hope for. When parent-child interactions are problematic the C-GPs might find themselves mediating the relationship and having to protect the grandchildren. As with any children, disappointed grandchildren are prone to act out in ways that bring stress to the environment. Sometimes the presence of their parents triggers traumatic memories that cause emotional and psychological responses that can disturb eating and sleeping patterns. Children voicing the desire to be in their previous home with parents could hold anger and resentment toward their parents and/or grandparents, neither of which is something most grandparents likely find appealing.
- **Financial circumstances**: About 20% of C-GPs live in poverty, and 1.3 million C-GPs actively earn wages to care for their grandchildren. Retired grandparents typically live on

a fixed income that may be insufficient for additional members of the household. C-GPs are affected by the same downward swings in the economy that might have contributed to the grandchildren having been removed from their homes. As noted, C-GPs don't always have legal custody or authority over their grandchildren—the arrangement may be informal. This can limit their eligibility for some of the financial resources to help with raising grandchildren.

- **Support issues**: C-GPs can lack important support from a variety of sources. Some have mentioned feeling stigmatized or judged by social service providers. The time and attention required to raise grandchildren take away time from C-GPs' social lives that they could be spending with similar-aged people, and they might have few peers who can empathize with their situation. Some C-GPs feel judged by their peers for having raised "troubled" children and for now having to take on their grandchildren. Their other adult children might resent the resources their parents devote to their sibling (the adult parent of a custodial grandchild) or pressure their parents to avoid being "taken advantage of" buy the sibling. Consider the grandparents who live in a retirement community that disallows younger family members from living there. *Now what do we do, move?*

- **Grandchildren challenges**: Raising children requires some stamina. Grandparents inhibited by health issues could struggle to actively engage their grandchildren, especially younger children who thrive off of active play. As noted in Part A, generation gaps can be conducive to various forms of disagreement and polarization. Children who have been removed from their parents are likely to have experienced some form of trauma—or at least suboptimal parenting—and therefore predisposed to experiencing behavioral and emotional challenges that can exhaust any parental figure. Traumatized grandchildren can struggle to let their guard down to bond with and trust their grandparents. They can also bring with them health problems that tax grandparents' resources. Furthermore, grandparents might lack knowledge about updated understandings of optimal child development and parenting practices, let alone how to parent a traumatized child. They might also have to navigate an unfamiliar school system.

Overall, research suggests that grandchildren raised by grandparents are at elevated risk for problems with behavior, emotional regulation, paying attention, and academic performance. As noted, their experience with their parents could be a main contributing factor to these outcomes. C-GPs also tend to be at elevated risk for psychical and psychological consequences. Nevertheless, as you well know by now, people can be **resilient** and stressors can lead to **positive consequences**. For example, C-GPs can find satisfaction in helping continue routines and cherished family traditions for their grandchildren, in sparing children anxiety from having to live with strangers, and in bonding with young family members. This can be a second chance at parenting—a chance to learn from some regrets the first time around, to feel more alive, and to feel important. C-GPs who are married, highly educated, and surrounded by social support have a better chance for resiliency and family flourishing, especially if they are able to **focus on** the potential benefits of their circumstances.

How Do External Contexts Impact Multigenerational Stressors?

So far you will have noted some reference to contextual factors related to multigenerational stress, including some **gender** differences in who makes up the households that contain grandparents (see Figure 6.2). C-GPs are much more likely to have a daughter living with them than a son, and custodial single grandfathers are relatively rare. Grandchildren with C-GPs are thus less likely to have daily interaction with their fathers, and many will also have no interaction with a grandfather. Some children without a male influence in their lives feel deprived of a desired relationship and perhaps certain experiences, especially when they already had a connection with their fathers. Boys tend to struggle more than girls in single-mother homes, which can be a sign of their extra vulnerability when lacking a same-sex parental figure. Of course, some of these grandparent households could receive visits from uncles or family friends who contribute as male influences.

You might also remember that a disproportionate number of C-GPs are Black and some of the contributing factors to those numbers. Interestingly, a study found that when comparing the well-being of grandmothers across different **ethnicities** and circumstances, Black grandmothers who were C-GPs had higher well-being than NC-GPs who assisted their adult children with parenting.[19] The opposite trend was found for Hispanic grandmothers. White noncustodial and custodial grandmothers had about the same level of well-being as one another, though custodial grandmothers had more positive *and* negative emotional reactions. The researchers suggested that a longer, more normalized tradition of Black grandparents raising grandchildren contributed to a lesser burden of custody. Additionally, while Latino and White custodial grandmothers had more conflict with their adult children than did their noncustodial counterparts, Black grandmothers had the same amount of conflict regardless of whether they were NC-GPs or C-GPs and less conflict overall with their adult children. This study illustrates how **culture and circumstances can interact** to create unique family dynamics.

As mentioned in Part A, intergenerational Native American families can face challenges with confronting **acculturation** into mainstream culture. Grandparent-grandchild relationships tend to be a common form of strengthening the rising generation, helping to minimize risks of youth's substance problems and trauma related to minority stressors. Hence, Native American families seem to struggle less with generation gap stressors and draw great strength from multigenerational closeness. Have you benefited from a close relationship with a grandparent?

Finally, **social class differences** are likely to appear when considering the types of grandparenting scenarios. C-GPs are less likely to live in middle-class homes and neighborhoods than NC-GPs. The grandchildren in wealthier circumstances are likely exposed to different and more stable parenting and to intergenerational values and standards than those from poorer custodial circumstances. That is not to say that one type of circumstance inherently comes with a superior set of values, just that the children from the circumstances might learn **different life lessons** and **acquire different coping strategies**. A C-GP might be a strong model of sacrifice, loyalty, and perseverance; an NC-GP might be a strong model of cooperation, interdependence, and supplementary support.

What Does All This Mean for You?

Your insights can be valuable to your personal life, your family relationships, and your professional roles. Take a few moments to ponder the following:

- How have you been feeling while engaging with this information? Why?
- How much of this topic can you personally relate to?
- Did you grow up in a home with polarization owing to generation gaps? What was it like?
- How can families avoid estrangement? What is worth sacrificing to do so?
- What other examples have come to mind that illustrate similar or diverse ways that families cope with intergenerational/multigenerational stressors?

Reminders for Helpers

As a person of influence, you can help guide people through the coping processes and ideally help foster a **flourishing** life. However, take care to avoid letting your personal **interpretations** push you toward assuming too much about somebody else's circumstances, perceptions, and motivations. Always be ready to address issues that might be hard for you to face because of your own history.

Draw upon the elements of the **FIM framework** and other family stress concepts. Remember, **coping** refers to an action or response based on available or new resources and perceptions related to stressors. Families have either successfully **managed** a stressor's pressure through **adjustment coping** or reached crisis in which **adaptive coping** is needed to reestablish some level of **general family functioning**. **Resources** and **perceptions** are key concepts to focus on when confronting family stress. **Review the master table** in Chapter 4 as a guide for exploring the following ideas on how to help families with stressors.

What Are Some Ways to Encourage Effective Family Coping?

Drawing from the aforementioned scholars, with some additional insights based on other scholars noted next, we will explore **suggested resources and noteworthy perceptions** that can contribute to successful coping and more optimal family functioning.

How Can You Help With Generation Gap Stressors?

Having family members adopt political or religious views and practices that are contrary to one's own can feel like a major betrayal. Finding ways to reconcile a need to accept a loved one while not accepting the person's beliefs can be difficult and require major shifts in mindset and relationship interaction. However, viewpoint polarization is often fueled by **unhelpful perceptions and misunderstandings** that could be avoided or changed. For example, seeing members of political parties or people with certain viewpoints as inherently inferior or evil puts us at risk of creating enemies in our own families. Overly relying on biased or deceptive sources often lead to misconceptions of a particular political position or religious doctrine. It is easy to assume that the meaning an issue has for us must be the opposite meaning for someone who disagrees.[20] Furthermore, we can draw questionable assumptions about other people who disagree with us. For example, take a close look at a comment by an adult who had a recurring disagreement with her mother:

> "I got nowhere with her and just don't have the same level of respect for her at this time. However, if one day she starts digesting other media and information sources and breaks the spell she's under, I could absolutely have a relationship with her again."

Can you think of any possible biased perceptions within that statement? Here is another one from a frustrated woman who disagrees with her father. What possible biases or assumptions might exist here?

> "We weren't fully aligned before, but his political beliefs have become more fanatic, obsessive, and emboldened. ... I didn't bother trying to change his mind—to have a conversation, the other person has to be willing to listen, and he's not. To avoid him influencing my son, I've limited their contact."

Regardless of the topic, or the accuracy of the perceptions, assumptions about others' motives and thinking can interfere with finding common ground or harmony. Apparent polarization in both of the aforementioned cases led to damaged relationships. When we perceive differing views as threats, we easily fall into a **self-preservation mode**, protecting ourselves from possible rejection and feelings of inferiority and from threats to our comfortable ways of thinking; we are then more prone to attack the threat's source, even if it is family.

Families with strong **relational resources** of trust and bonding are likely more resilient when facing potential viewpoint polarization. Being able to monitor and manage **cognitive coping strategies and emotional reactions** can help people short-circuit a polarizing interaction. Establishing clear and helpful goals for potentially polarizing conversations can help avoid negative outcomes. For example, the goals to change someone's mind or to be validated or respected because of full agreement could be less useful and more volatile than just seeking to understand someone's perspective or to find some common ground. Helping people **evaluate their goals** for such conversations and their motivations behind the goals could help them determine how to approach differing viewpoints in a family. Such a process could require deep **self-reflection and emotional transparency**; this can be difficult for individuals to do when they feel vulnerable and insecure about their identities and the commitment levels of their relationships.

Families can develop other resources related to personal and family characteristics. For example, research has found **intellectual humility** to be helpful for people with religious disagreements.[21] Intellectual humility consists of understanding one's own limits to their knowledge, having an openness to new ideas, presenting one's ideas in a nonarrogant and nonoffensive way, and avoiding taking offense to alternative viewpoints. Research shows that conversations between people of different faiths who had mutual intellectual humility ended with greater closeness and trust. Similarly, establishing **mutual curiosity** likely helps depolarize disagreements by honoring knowledge gained from others. Learning to listen to understand instead of listening for "flawed logic" to attack can also be a helpful resource. Helping families foster these types of characteristics in individual members, family rules, and family philosophy could help prevent major relationship problems and promote healing when polarization gets out of control.

As noted in Part A, polarization might threaten the safety and reassurance we thrive on through **attachment** to family members. They have found success in their clinical practices by helping disconnected families prioritize their **role identities** in the family. Specifically, family members should think about what it means to be a daughter, brother, parent, and so on, particularly regarding loyalty and support even in times of difficulty. Family roles can also include assuming the best about each other's motives and thoughtful consideration that goes into controversial viewpoints. Hearing each other **articulate their acceptance and love** of one another, regardless of beliefs, can strengthen that attachment bond and help avoid escalation. Families may need to agree on some rules and boundaries regarding if and when to discuss potentially volatile issues, be they political, religious, or acculturation related. At the same time, learning to discuss volatile issues in a nonthreatening manner can be a valuable skill if families can pull it off. A tricky balance.

Polarization related to **acculturation** can likewise be reduced by following the aforementioned ideas. Additionally, intergenerational differences in acculturation itself are not necessarily a problem unless they lead to distress and conflict.[22] Interventions that target acculturation-based stress tend to focus on families seeing benefits in their **bicultural identities**—or in other words, abilities to navigate two different cultures. Helping increase parental **empathy** toward the needs and desires of their children, and emphasizing intergenerational open communication are also useful. Similarly, parents who struggle to relate to their children's technology use can reduce conflict when they better understand their children's **motivations and needs** for using technology. One developmental psychologist suggests that parents focus less intently on simply the *amount* of time children use their gadgets and focus more on (1) the content they are exposed to, (2) the context in which they use their devices (where, why, how), and (3) connections (how technology helps or hinders their relationships).[23] Encouraging parents to think deeper about technology use might challenge some assumptions that lead to conflict.

Finally, what if a family has already experienced estrangement—how can they reconcile? First, family members might need help determining whether **reconciliation** is safe and advisable, which could require intense **self-reflection**. They might need to evaluate the potential consequences of reentering into a relationship, particularly when family members are at higher risk for unhealthy levels of emotional dependency or physical danger. Assuming reconciliation is beneficial, self-reflection can also help us discover how we contributed to the estrangement and what we might need to do differently from now on. Families who are able to successfully reconcile **change their focus** from the past to the present.[24] They are able to give up the need to have others agree with their interpretation of events and look at the state of the current relationship and find ways to improve it. Reconciliation was also more likely when families could **revise their expectations** of one another and give up the need to try to force someone to change their lifestyle. However, such families were also able to **establish clear rules and boundaries** for future interaction and lines that could not be crossed for the relationship to continue. Families might need assistance facilitating such a process and may need help seeing the benefits of considering increasing their humility, forgiveness, and patience with one another.

How Can You Help With Multigenerational Stressors?

Common stressors for multigenerational households generally pertain to pressure or conflict due to managing schedules and routines, space or privacy, and financial struggles. While those whose housing accommodated spatial needs for larger and intergenerational households, many families are unable to produce such a resource—especially if financial struggles were a key motivation for their living arrangement. Thus, perceptions and resources related more to **attitudes** and **relational abilities** could be of primary concern for coping. Research suggests that focusing on **mutual respect** among the generations helps prevent generational conflict.[25] While respecting older generations might be more built into some cultures and family philosophies, showing respect toward a younger generation's perspectives and needs could require more deliberate efforts. Such respect can also help **diffuse potential power struggles** that lead to conflict. Younger generations may need to work on being slower to assume that guidance from above is intentionally dominating or controlling, while older generations may need to work on sharing their guidance in a way that is less likely to trigger sensitivity to perceived dominance.

Custodial grandparents (C-GPs) likely need help with building up their physical, psychological, and emotional resources to enable positive care of grandchildren. They might need help creating a **social network** with other C-GPs who can provide social support and advice. An important skill-based resource is knowing how to **advocate** for their family's needs in educational, legal, and social services contexts. C-GPs might need guidance establishing household rules, roles, and boundaries that involve at least three generations of family members, including adult children who often struggle with substance use or who have a history of neglecting their own children. However, some programs that focus on skills and knowledge have helped C-GPs improve their parenting skills and relationships with grandchildren but also increased their levels of parenting stress, financial stress, and depression.[26] The new knowledge might sensitize C-GPs to the various demands and expectations they should be living up to, creating more distress. Perhaps additional support resources and guidance with perceptions could help them feel less overwhelmed.

In that knowledge itself likely doesn't solve everything, ensuring C-GPs engage in **self-care** also helps them maintain a capacity to nurture their grandchildren. As mentioned, C-GPs might need encouragement to adjust their **expectations** about their purposes and responsibilities and to find ways to think about such changes as opportunities to use their wisdom and experience to bless the lives of their grandchildren and to form a unique bond with them. Finally, C-GPs (or any parent) could benefit by practicing **self-compassion**, especially when they feel guilt for their children's problematic behaviors. Learning self-compassion is like having a close friend help you feel better about yourself, point out the limits of your power to control other people's choices or burdens, and encourage patience with yourself as you, like everyone else, are just learning how to navigate situations nobody has trained for. This type of cognitive coping can lessen discouragement and perhaps resentment toward adult children who choose a different path than their parents had in mind for them.

Improve Your Learning

Without peeking, take a moment to review in your mind (or say out loud) the key concepts from this chapter (this is a proven learning technique). Then review the "Chapter Preview" section at the top and compare. Skim Part B of the chapter with extra attention to the **bolded words**.

Do You Want to Learn More?

We have only touched on a portion of information related to some elements of this topic. **What really sparked your interest? What do you wish was covered more thoroughly?** Consider taking some time to further deepen your understanding of personal and professional issues related to helping families cope with stressors. The following are a variety of resources that you might find helpful, and some references directly or indirectly referred to in this chapter. Impress the older and younger generations with how much you have learned.

Videos

(Use links or do searches with the key words provided)
- Helping Loved Ones Divided by Politics (65 mins). Braver Angels. https://youtu.be/YwGpv3ZTqpQ
- Finding Happiness: How Forgiving My Mother Radically Changed My Life (12 mins). Sonia Weyers, TEDxFHNW. https://www.youtube.com/watch?v=3I4R_em_6wE
- Between Two Cultures (8 mins). Smrithi Ram, TEDxUCincinnati. https://www.youtube.com/watch?v=qv_UfDBNWI8&t=312s
- The Problem With Parents, Kids, and Social Media (3 mins). *The Atlantic*. https://www.youtube.com/watch?v=RAFSrGX0mxk
- The Superpower of Intergenerational Living (13 mins). Derenda Schubert, TEDxMt-Hood. https://www.youtube.com/watch?v=xb0fzZJuOoU
- Multigenerational Homes Are on the Rise, Offering a Sense of Community (4 mins). *Sunday TODAY*. https://www.youtube.com/watch?v=6dtYa6mzPow
- Raising Children for a Second Time, 'Grandfamilies' Struggle During the Pandemic (7 mins). *PBS NewsHour*. https://www.youtube.com/watch?v=CInufouwJQE
- Video: Grandparents Raising Grandchildren (5 mins). *SiouxCity Journal*. https://www.youtube.com/watch?v=cqAy9905dio
- When Family Bonds Are Broken (8 mins). *CBS Sunday Morning*. https://www.youtube.com/watch?v=zVN1BiB_-O0

Websites

- Braver Angels. https://braverangels.org/
- U.S. Census Bureau. (n.d.). American community survey. https://data.census.gov/cedsci/table?q=multigenerational&tid=ACSDT1Y2019.B11017
- Generations United. (2021). Family matters: Multigenerational living is on the rise and here to stay. https://www.gu.org/resources/multigenerational-families/
- U.S. Census Bureau. (2021, November 29). America's families and living arrangements: 2021. https://www.census.gov/data/tables/2021/demo/families/cps-2021.html
- Pillemer, K., (2021, December 20). Family rifts affect millions of Americans—research shows possible paths from estrangement toward reconciliation. *The Conversation.* https://theconversation.com/family-rifts-affect-millions-of-americans-research-shows-possible-paths-from-estrangement-toward-reconciliation-165781

Readings (Articles, Books, Book Chapters)

- Beyens, I., & Beullens, K. (2017). Parent-child conflict about children's tablet use: The role of parental mediation. *New Media & Society, 19*(12), 2075–2093. https://doi.org/10.1177/1461444816655099
- Chen, M. K., & Rohla, R. (2017). Politics gets personal: Effects of political partisanship and advertising on family ties. *Science, 360,* 1020–1024. https://doi.org/10.1126/science.aaq1433
- Coleman, J. (2021). *The rules of estrangement: Why adult children cut ties and how to heal the conflict.* Harmony.
- Dolbin-MacNab, M. L., Rosberto, K. A., & Finney, J. W. (2013). Formal social support: Promoting resilience in grandparents parenting grandchildren. In B. Hayslip & G. Smith (Eds.), *Resilient grandparent caregivers: A strengths-based perspective* (pp. 134–151). Routledge.
- Kildare, C. A., & Middlemiss, W. (2017). Impact of parents' mobile device use on parent-child interaction: A literature review. *Computers in Human Behavior, 75,* 579–593. https://doi.org/10.1016/j.chb.2017.06.003
- Rodriguez, D., Hook, J. N., Farrell, J. E., Mosher, D. K., Zhang, H., Van Tongeren, D. R., Davis, D. E., Aten, J. D., & Hill, P. C. (2019). Religious intellectual humility, attitude change, and closeness following religious disagreement. *The Journal of Positive Psychology, 14*(2), 133–140. https://doi.org/10.1080/17439760.2017.1388429

Notes

1   Pillemer, K. (2021, December 20). Family rifts affect millions of Americans—research shows possible paths from estrangement toward reconciliation. *The Conversation.* https://theconversation.com/family-rifts-affect-millions-of-americans-research-shows-possible-paths-from-estrangement-toward-reconciliation-165781

2   Parker, K., & Igielnik, R. (2020, May 14). On the cusp of adulthood and facing an uncertain future: What we know about gen Z so far. Pew Research Center's Social & Demographic Trends Project. https://www.pewresearch.org/social-trends/2020/05/14/on-the-cusp-of-adulthood-and-facing-an-uncertain-future-what-we-know-about-gen-z-so-far-2/

3   Ojeda, C., & Hatemi, P. K. (2015). Accounting for the child in the transmission of party identification. *American Sociological Review, 80*(6), 1150–1174. https://doi-org.proxy.bsu.edu/10.1177/0003122415606101

4   Chen, M. K., & Rohla, R. (2017). Politics gets personal: Effects of political partisanship and advertising on family ties. *Science, 360*, 1020–1024. https://doi.org/10.1126/science.aaq1433; Kim, Y. (2015). Does disagreement mitigate polarization? How selective exposure and disagreement affect political polarization. *Journalism & Mass Communication Quarterly, 92*(4), 915–937. https://doi.org/10.1177/1077699015596328

5   Abrams, S. J. (2021, September 20). Are American families really being torn apart by politics? Institute for Family Studies. https://ifstudies.org/blog/are-american-families-really-being-torn-apart-by-politics

6   Chen, M. K., & Rohla, R. (2017). Politics gets personal: Effects of political partisanship and advertising on family ties. *Science, 360*, 1020–1024.

7   Cox, D. A. (2019, December 11). The decline of religion in American family life: Findings from the November 2019 American perspectives survey. American Enterprise Institute. https://www.aei.org/research-products/report/the-decline-of-religion-in-american-family-life/

8   Bezcioglu-Goktolga, I., & Yagmur, K. (2018). Home language policy of second-generation Turkish families in the Netherlands. *Journal of Multilingual and Multicultural Development, 39*(1), 44–59. https://doi.org/10.1080/01434632.2017.1310216; Ho, J., & Birman, D. (2010). Acculturation gaps in Vietnamese immigrant families: Impact on family relationships. *International Journal of Intercultural Relations, 34*(1), 22. https://doi.org/10.1016/j.ijintrel.2009.10.002; Myhra, L. L., & Wieling, E. (2014). Psychological trauma among American Indian families: A two-generation study. *Journal of Loss & Trauma, 19*(4), 289–313. https://doi.org/10.1080/15325024.2013.771561

9   Beyens, I., & Beullens, K. (2017). Parent–child conflict about children's tablet use: The role of parental mediation. *New Media & Society, 19*(12), 2075–2093. https://doi.org/10.1177/1461444816655099; Kildare, C. A., & Middlemiss, W. (2017). Impact of parents' mobile device use on parent-child interaction: A literature review. *Computers in Human Behavior, 75*, 579–593; Shah, R., Chauhan, N., Gupta, A. K., & Sen, M. S. (2016). Adolescent-parent conflict in the age of social media: Case reports from India. *Asian Journal of Psychiatry, 23*, 24–26. https://doi.org/10.1016/j.ajp.2016.07.002

10   National Council on Family Relations. (n.d.). Family focus. https://www.ncfr.org/ncfr-report/focus

11   Kim, Y. (2015). Does disagreement mitigate polarization? How selective exposure and disagreement affect political polarization. *Journalism & Mass Communication Quarterly, 92*(4), 915–937. https://doi.org/10.1177/1077699015596328

12   Coleman, J. (2021). *The rules of estrangement: Why adult children cut ties and how to heal the conflict.* Harmony; Pillemer, K., (2021, December 20). Family rifts affect millions of Americans—research shows possible paths from estrangement toward reconciliation. *The Conversation.* https://theconversation.com/family-rifts-affect-millions-of-americans-research-shows-possible-paths-from-estrangement-toward-reconciliation-165781

13   Coleman, J. (2021). *The rules of estrangement: Why adult children cut ties and how to heal the conflict.* Harmony

14   Alghafli, Z., Hatch, T., & Marks, L. (2014). Religion and relationships in Muslim families: A qualitative examination of devout married Muslim couples. *Religions (Basel, Switzerland), 5*(3), 814–833. https://doi.org/10.3390/rel5030814; Blackwell, L., Hardy, J., Ammari, T., Veinot, T., Lampe, C., & Schoenebeck, S. (2016, May). LGBT parents and social media: Advocacy, privacy, and disclosure during shifting social movements. In *Proceedings of the 2016 CHI conference on human factors in computing systems* (pp. 610–622); Shah, R., Chauhan, N., Gupta, A. K., & Sen, M. S. (2016). Adolescent-parent conflict in the age of social media: Case reports from India. *Asian Journal of Psychiatry, 23*, 24–26. https://doi.org/10.1016/j.ajp.2016.07.002.

15   U.S. Census Bureau. (2021, November 29). America's families and living arrangements: 2021. https://www.census.gov/data/tables/2021/demo/families/cps-2021.html; U.S. Census Bureau. (n.d.). *American community survey.* https://data.census.gov/cedsci/table?q=multigenerational&tid=ACSDT1Y2019.B11017

16   Generations United. (2021). Family matters: Multigenerational living is on the rise and here to stay. https://www.gu.org/resources/multigenerational-families/

17 U.S. Census Bureau. (2021, November 29). America's families and living arrangements: 2021. https://www.census. gov/data/tables/2021/demo/families/cps-2021.html;

18 Dolbin-MacNab, M. L., & Keiley, M. K., (2006). A systematic examination of grandparents' emotional closeness with their custodial grandchildren. *Research in Human Development, 3,* 59–71. https://doi.org/10.1207/s15427617rhd0301_6; Dolbin-MacNab, M. L., Rosberto, K. A., & Finney, J. W. (2013). Formal social support: Promoting resilience in grandparents parenting grandchildren. In B. Hayslip & G. Smith (Eds.), *Resilient grandparent caregivers: A strengths-based perspective* (pp. 134–151). Routledge; Shakya, H. B., Usita, P. M., Eisenberg, C., Weston, J., & Liles, S. (2012). Family well-being concerns of grandparents in skipped generation families. *Journal of Gerontological Social Work,* 55(1), 39–54. https://doi-org/10.1080/01634372.2011.620072.; Gaille, B. (n.d.). 23 statistics on grandparents raising grandchildren. *Father Matters.* https://fathermatters.org/23-statistics-on-grandparents-raising-grandchildren/

19 Goodman, C., & Silverstein, M. (2002). Grandmothers raising grandchildren: Family structure and well-being in culturally diverse families. *The Gerontologist, 42*(5), 676–689. https://doi-org/10.1093/geront/42.5.676

20 Hickok, H. (2021, November 24). When family politics change, every conversation feels like battle. *Glamour.* https:// www.glamour.com/story/when-family-politics-change-how-to-cope

21 Rodriguez, D., Hook, J. N., Farrell, J. E., Mosher, D. K., Zhang, H., Van Tongeren, D. R., Davis, D. E., Aten, J. D., & Hill, P. C. (2019). Religious intellectual humility, attitude change, and closeness following religious disagreement. *The Journal of Positive Psychology, 14*(2), 133–140. https://doi.org/10.1080/17439760.2017.1388429

22 National Council on Family Relations. (n.d.). Family focus. https://www.ncfr.org/ncfr-report/focus

23 Abdullah, M. (2021, July 1). How to reset your family's screen time after the pandemic. *Greater Good Magazine.* https://greatergood.berkeley.edu/article/item/how_to_reset_your_familys_screen_time_after_the_pandemic?

24 Pillemer, K. (2021, December 20). Family rifts affect millions of Americans—research shows possible paths from estrangement toward reconciliation. *The Conversation.* https://theconversation.com/family-rifts-affect-millions-of-americans-research-shows-possible-paths-from-estrangement-toward-reconciliation-165781

25 Merriweather, L., & Morgan, A. (2015). Two cultures collide: Bridging the generation gap in a non-traditional mentorship. *The Qualitative Report, 18,* 1–16. https://doi.org/10.46743/2160-3715/2013.1558

26 Dolbin-MacNab, M. L., Rosberto, K. A., & Finney, J. W. (2013). Formal social support: Promoting resilience in grandparents parenting grandchildren. In B. Hayslip & G. Smith (Eds.), *Resilient grandparent caregivers: A strengths-based perspective* (pp. 134–151). Routledge.

Image Credits

Fig. 6.1: Source: Adapted from Karl Pillemer, "Fault Lines: Fractured Families and How to Mend Them," 2021.

Fig. 6.2a: Source: Adapted from https://www.census.gov/data/tables/2021/demo/families/cps-2021.html.

Fig. 6.2b: Source: Adapted from https://data.census.gov/cedsci/table?q=multigenerational&tid=ACSDT1Y2019.B11017.

CHAPTER 7

Intimate Partner Abuse, Child Maltreatment, and Family Stress

W hen looking at the current location of foster children on a given day, about 4,500 foster children have run away and are missing from their foster care placement.[1]

Chapter Preview

- Family violence and stress can have a bidirectional relationship.
- Abuse in families typically involves one-sided domination, sometimes related to gender.
- Most intimate partner violence is situational and mutual.
- Intimate partner abuse creates a variety of concerns and questions for victims to confront, all of which can create stress.
- Men can also be abused by a female partner, and abusers who wish to change face several stressors themselves.
- Children who witness intimate partner abuse often suffer from anxiety and fear and are subject to poorer parenting and a diminished parent-child relationship.
- Parental neglect is the most common source of child maltreatment stress.
- Abused children can suffer from trauma that they express through emotional or behavioral problems that create stress for themselves and others.
- Child sexual abuse is commonly associated with stress related to secrecy and shame.
- Children can also be traumatized by an older/more powerful sibling or by witnessing parental abuse of a sibling.
- Family and neighborhood factors can interact to increase risks for child maltreatment.

What Is This Topic About?

How is it that the people we love the most can also hurt us the most? Doesn't that seem counter to what people want from a family? Richard Gelles, a prominent scholar of family violence, concluded that "virtually every type and form of family and intimate relationship has the potential of being violent."[2] Think about that for a moment. In this chapter, we focus mostly on family conflict that rises to the level of **abuse or maltreatment**, including physical, sexual, emotional, psychosocial, or verbal. In the case of raising children, various forms of **neglect** also constitute maltreatment. Why would it feel different when someone in your family purposely hurts you compared to harm caused by an acquaintance or stranger?

This chapter mostly highlights **stress that results** from various types of family abuse and maltreatment, while some elements of scope, causes, and other consequences are provided to contextualize the topic. Parts of this chapter might resonate with your personal experience and could trigger painful thoughts and feelings. The fact that you are reading this shows **you have already shown great resilience** in your life, and it is normal to continue to struggle with the effects of abuse. Use proper self-care as needed, consider meeting with a professional if you generally feel overwhelmed, and monitor yourself as you push through reading at your own pace. Addressing and **making meaning** out of your experiences help build resilience, but be sure you have others who **support** you when it is difficult, and it may be wise to take things slow.

What Are the Assumptions?

In Chapter 1, we briefly discussed **reciprocal or bidirectional influences** between stress and family problems, which can also apply to stress and violence (or any type of abuse or maltreatment). From a **family stress perspective**, we would suspect that stressors can trigger violence depending on (1) family vulnerabilities and level of functioning, (2) how family members cope with the stressors in light of their resources and perceptions, and (3) how family philosophy and individual and external contexts influence risk factors and coping. With the right (or wrong) combination of those factors, stress becomes a **risk factor** for violence—but not necessarily a *cause* of violence. Some people are quick to become violent while others in similar circumstances or stress levels completely avoid doing so—people make choices about violence. Violence that threatens a family's ability to meet all its member's needs pressures the family to make changes to ensure needs are met. Violence can also be a **type of resource for coping with stressors**. It might be an attempt to control a situation or person or a way to vent overwhelming feelings by those who lack healthy emotional regulation and expression. Size and strength are also resources used to intimidate or control a family member. Violence can be a sign that a family has reached **crisis** because the family is not coping with stressors in ways that maintain a healthy level of **family functioning**.

Feminist and conflict theories highlight the role of **power** in family violence. Family violence (particularly between heterosexual partners) is understood as a manifestation of social roles, cultural expectations, and societal structures that elevate men over women. **Competition for**

limited resources (e.g., decision-making power, attention, status, comfort) between societal subgroups also happens in the home between adult partners, siblings, and a parent and child. Assumptions about what it means to be a spouse or parent can also influence tolerance for violence (e.g., whether marriage gives one the right to force sex upon a spouse and how much lenience parents should have in the way they punish their children). Liberal politics tends to align with feminism, so liberals are more prone than conservatives to view family violence through that lens. As you will see, however, various forms or incidents of family violence can have diverse motivations and meanings.

As noted in Chapter 2, liberals also generally value **care** above other moral foundations, which would seem to motivate avoiding intimate violence. Conservatives tend to place more emphasis on **loyalty** and **respecting authority** than do liberals, which could be reflected in different parenting approaches. For example, traditionally, conservatives have shown more approval of spanking than have liberals (though Black parents, who tend to have more liberal politics, also tend to be more approving of spanking), which could be a means toward enforcing obedience and respect to ultimately maintain family and societal stability. Whether spanking is considered a form of abuse is a matter of debate, but it seems logical that someone who refuses to spank or strike a child avoids the prospect of "losing control" during spanking. Similarly, if one's conservatism is tightly linked to religious or cultural views that justify men enforcing wives' or children's submission, families could be at higher risk for violence (though some religiously conservative groups strongly emphasize treating wives and children with the utmost care).

Ideology can also inform how we think about abuse **victims**. Politically liberal voices especially seem to condemn apparent "victim blaming." Well-intended responses to violence can infer that the victim in some way deserved the violence. *What did you do to make him angry? I can't believe you haven't left her yet!* At the same time, clinicians also mention the importance of **empowering** victims to take actions that free them from abuse. Some attempts to avoid victim blaming arguably reinforce the powerlessness of victims, telling victims that they must be saved by someone else. Yet, this line of thinking might lead some to conclude that by not making immediate, drastic changes, victims are somehow choosing to be part of the problem. People often reveal differing perspectives and interpretations of victim blaming or empowerment through the types of interventions and policies they propose.

As you **engage with** the rest of the chapter, remember the key elements of family stress theories (e.g., stressors, resources, perceptions, coping, and crisis) and consider the following:

- How do violence and abuse create stress that can change the patterns of family functioning (rules, roles, boundaries)?
- What hope do families have to flourish if they have already experienced stress from abuse?
- How do the various pieces of information throughout the chapter fit together to help explain why each family might respond differently to threats or signs of abuse?
- What experiences have you had or observed that help you relate to specific concepts?
- How might the ideological perspectives influence how people (including you) think about potential causes of and solutions to family violence and other maltreatment?

Part A. Intimate Partner Abuse Stressors

What Is Stressful About Intimate Partner Abuse?

That might seem like a dumb question—*of course it is stressful to be abused!* Let's assume, however, that not all forms of violence or abuse create the same pressures and that not all victims experience stress the same way. Let's see what kind of nuance we can capture that helps us better appreciate life through the eyes of someone being abused by an intimate partner. That should help us in our attempts to support and guide others who have shared such experiences. Though so far the chapter has emphasized violence, you will soon see why this section refers more to abuse. But first, let's talk about the potential for family violence.

Perhaps you have heard it said that someone had "reached their boiling point." Did you know that different liquids have different boiling points (i.e., the temperature required before they boil)? Did you know that water can boil at different temperatures depending on the altitude? Before you get worked up about a possible chemistry lesson (I'm saying that to myself as much as anyone), just consider the idea that as water molecules heat up they increase in pressure until they turn into bubbles that pop into the air as vapor. Boiling occurs once the water molecule pressure equals the level of pressure in the surroundings (i.e., atmospheric pressure, like the thickness or thinness of the air). What does this have to do with abuse?

Whether everyone can reach a boiling point (become abusive) when under enough pressure is hard to know, but people do seem to have different boiling points. **Personalities and brain physiology** could differ like liquids differ—some liquids need less heat to boil. Pressure in our surroundings could represent our different **social contexts**. Notice that some people can keep their calm at work or in other public spaces but at home lash out with harmful words or actions. Perhaps the atmospheric pressure outside the home requires more heat before the boiling point is reached. At home, where bosses, coworkers, police, and random onlookers with cameras are unable to observe us, we feel less motivated to "keep it together." Furthermore, those who know us best seem able to turn up the heat and raise our temperature.

What Is Intimate Partner Abuse?

Imagine a couple who reunites at home after a long, stressful day and starts to bicker. Little complaints escalate into louder accusations that eventually turn into a mutual shoving match. Maybe slaps or scratches or even punches are exchanged before partners back off, cool down, and ultimately apologize for letting things "get out of hand." Nobody is seriously hurt. This kind of exchange is the most common form of **intimate partner violence** (**IPV**). Men and women are equally likely to engage in it. Michael Johnson has famously coined this type of violence as **situational couple violence** (**SCV**).[3] In contrast, what you might see in movies is a male partner or husband dominating his wife, using strength and violence to intimidate and control her, leaving her bloodied and bruised, and reminding her that he as a man is entitled to her submission. Johnson called this scenario **intimate terrorism** (**IT**). Gender need not have to be a defining characteristic of IT—women engage in it against men, and it occurs within same-sex couples—but cultural norms and internalized beliefs that excuse male domination can enable IT, and women are more often the victims and tend to experience more severe harm.

Like with IT, the concept of **intimate partner abuse** (**IPA**) suggests a continued, more one-sided harmful pattern that victimizes a romantic partner. IPA could be physical, sexual, verbal, emotional, and psychological in nature, often including a combination of these forms. Abuse is usually about **controlling** another person, though it can also be an outlet for **one's frustration or anger** redirected at someone more vulnerable (e.g., a partner or child compared to a boss). Some abusers seemingly regret the abuse but have difficulty with **impulse control** when it matters; **chronic substance problems** can also contribute to lowering inhibitions that would otherwise deter abusive behavior. While SCV and other mutually aggressive behavior (e.g., verbal sparring) are often problematic and cause stress, such stress tends to be milder and can be addressed by helping couples find better ways to communicate their frustrations and to calm themselves. IPA, however, is usually a larger threat to one's safety, sense of identity, and overall well-being, hence the emphasis for Part A of this chapter.

How Does IPA Influence Family Stress?

Being abused by someone who committed to love and care for you creates some unique psychological and emotional challenges. *This isn't supposed to happen. Am I a bad spouse? Am I keeping up my end of the deal?* Trying to make sense of something that feels so violating is a form of **pressure**. Accepting the reality of having an abusive intimate partner might be so painful that our minds form thoughts and interpretations that help us minimize or deny the abuse. That can lead to self-blame or to tolerating the abuse as "normal" behavior. Why might some people be especially prone to deny this reality? What might they have experienced in their past to make it easier to blame themselves and excuse the abuse?

While some victims struggle less with recognizing abuse, all victims face the **pressure** of deciding what to do about it. Table 7.1 includes some examples of questions a victim might consider and pressure that might occur based on possible answers (keeping in mind that the answers are based on perceptions and might not be accurate predictions). Try to add at least one more potential stressful outcome for each of the "yes" and "no" columns for every question—there are plenty of other possibilities. Some of the questions are interrelated.

TABLE 7.1 Decisions Faced When Experiencing Abuse

Questions	Stress If "Yes"	Stress If "No"
Is this behavior normal for couples?	I have to learn to live with it.	I am upset with my inability to choose a good partner.
Do I fight back?	Violence could escalate and I could be more seriously injured.	I feel more helpless.
Did I cause this to happen?	I feel like a bad spouse.	I may not be able to see it coming next time.

Questions	Stress If "Yes"	Stress If "No"
Will this likely happen again?	I will have to endure more pain.	Uncertainty about my ability to really trust him again.
Was he under the influence of a substance?	I have to decide if the abuse will go away if he gets his substance issue under control.	It is harder to make excuses for his behavior.
Do I tell a friend or family member?	I will feel embarrassed and ashamed.	I will feel alone.
Do I call the police?	If the police aren't able to do anything (especially If not physically assaulted) then it will just get him angrier.	I might feel like I allowed it to happen.
Am I in legal trouble because I fought back?	I worry about being in trouble if I report this.	I need to be sure I am believed that I only used self-defense.
Do we still love each other?	I need to find a way to make this work.	I might struggle to understand how I made such a big mistake so I don't do it again.
Are the children at risk?	I need to decide if the risk is greater than the risk of being without the other parent.	I need to be really sure that they actually aren't at risk.
Will I ever find someone who will treat me better?	I would worry about how this would affect the children, especially if I don't have full custody.	I might have to just hope for the best for our situation.
Will it get more dangerous if I try to leave?	I don't know if I can protect myself.	I have to decide if this situation is tolerable.
Do I leave?	I might not find a safe place where I can't be found.	I must find ways to prevent this from happening again.

From the outside, sometimes the **victim's perspective** seems irrational. Consider though that an abusive partner might not be constantly abusive—in fact, abuse could be fairly infrequent. Abusers might have many attractive qualities and can show genuine remorse for the abuse. They might be victims of abuse themselves and thus engender sympathy—*If he could just get that aspect under control things would be great. If I can just stop triggering his pain everything will be fine.* These factors can contribute to abuse lasting longer—it is much easier to leave "a monster" than someone who seems to be 95% good. None of this diminishes the fact that IPA of any frequency is damaging and inexcusable, just that things often look different from inside the home, so to speak.

How might the table of questions look different in the case of a **woman abusing a man**? Men are not always bigger and stronger than their female partners (or as willing to strike with an object), but society at large tends to question the **legitimacy** of male victimhood. Male victims are less likely than women to be believed or receive sympathy and are more likely to be mocked.

And if men do defend themselves, they risk injuring a female abuser, which could be something they simply don't want to do or that could have negative social and legal consequences. While men may worry less than women about their economic survival if they were to leave an abusive situation, they might fear losing **custody** of their children because of not being taken seriously and perceived or real legal biases in favor of mothers.

Regardless of gender, abuse victims don't always know what they should do about their situation. As mentioned in Chapter 1, **ambiguous** circumstances are particularly stressful, and obtaining clarity (if possible) requires additional effort and other resources. Other possible **hardships** that result from IPA include the following:

- Physical pain and impairment
- Anxiety over threats of abuse and about making decisions with potentially major consequences (see Table 7.1)
- Depression and even suicidality related to feelings of hopelessness and worthlessness
- Feeling powerless to affect one's life or to make a change
- Fear and possible guilt related to other family members' safety and welfare
- Possible shame for embarrassing or dishonoring family or defying cultural expectations
- Isolation from others as a means of being controlled by the abuser or as a result of not disclosing the abuse to others
- Sexually transmitted infections or unwanted pregnancy
- Diminished ability to trust and connect with others (including in future romantic/sexual relationships)
- Diminished satisfaction and increased friction within the couple relationship
- Using maladaptive coping strategies (e.g., misusing substances, venting anger by hurting others, self-harm)
- Post-traumatic stress disorder (PTSD)

After traumatic events, including IPA, having **PTSD** typically means that disturbing feelings and thoughts tied to the event persist for an extended time. Symptoms can include nightmares or flashbacks, difficult emotional reactions (e.g., fear, anger, sadness), and feeling disconnected from other people. Such responses can be triggered by encountering things that remind one of the traumatic event. As you would expect, PTSD is stressful for family relationships. Can you think of any examples of what that might include?

What About Pressure for Abusive Partners?

Seldom do we encounter much information about pressure *for* the abuser that *results from* the abuse. It is understandable that we would have more sympathy for victims than abusers. Assuming the abuser shows interest in making changes, having awareness of the stress such an abuser faces because of the abuse might be insightful and help encourage change. The intent here is not to justify any kind of abuse, just to understand stressors for all family members involved with abuse. Carrie Askin, codirector of a program for abusive partners (Courdea), suggested eight things an abusive partner (in this case a man) would need to do to change and restore family relationships, which can give us clues about the pressures and distress such an abuser would face.[4] Some of these changes could include altering beliefs, attitudes, and behaviors one had learned many years ago.

1. **He'll need to sit with his guilt and stop focusing his blame on others** (think about what it means to take the blame for hurting someone you assumingly love).
2. **He'll have to expand his understanding of what is abusive** (this could involve major self-reflection and a willingness to change his worldview about healthy behavior—then perhaps feeling worse as he better recognizes the harm he caused).
3. **He'll have to learn to tolerate emotional injury** (this could require changes in how he normally reacts to feeling hurt—instead of lashing out, he has to find ways to control himself).
4. **He'll need to identify and share his feelings** (he may be unaccustomed to doing this in a healthy way and might even feel stigmatized by sharing feelings; he will have to learn to cope with the guilt he feels).
5. **He'll need to practice humility** (this could require him to feel vulnerable and resist the urge to aggressively defend himself).
6. **He'll have to develop deeper empathy** (sometimes people struggle to see past their own concerns and understand where someone else is coming from; empathy might feel like a form of weakness).
7. **He'll need to be accountable for real change** (making needed changes is likely more difficult than lashing out with abusive behavior, but he has to find the strength to do it).
8. **He'll need to be patient and accept uncertainty** (doing the work of making changes won't guarantee that the relationship will be restored, and that can be discouraging).

How Does IPA Influence Children's Stress?

As you likely suspect, growing up in a home with IPA is far from optimal for children. Such abuse becomes a source of stress for the entire household—or multiple households if children rotate where they live. Stress is created through witnessing the abuse and, in some cases, having the abuse spill over into other relationships.

What Pressures Come From Witnessing IPA?

Research has shed light on some of the specific processes and outcomes related to a child witnessing IPA.[5] Children sometimes directly see or hear the abuse as it is happening, or they learn of it by observing wounds or upset demeanors or hearing reports from others. Merely **knowing** about the abuse can be stressful.

A child's age and level of exposure to IPA could affect how children are impacted by IPA, but overall such children are prone to feeling anxious or depressed (**internalizing problems**) about their safety. They might blame themselves when the abuse seems to stem from disagreements about parenting. When their need for a safe, secure, and loving environment is threatened, children might lean more on themselves and turn their fears inward, elevating risks for depression. They might act out (**externalizing problems**) as they struggle to process their fears, to draw attention to their own needs, or even to distract the parents from "fighting." Children who witness IPA thus experience **extra pressure** to be on guard for their own safety and to possibly help soothe the physical or emotional wounds of a demoralized parent. Perhaps as an attempted means of coping with these additional pressures, substance use problems are more common among children who witness abuse in the home.

Abused parents might also be less able to care for the needs of children and can be harsher and colder in how they parent. The child then suffers from poorer parenting, which can add stress to one or both parents in this situation. **Parent-child relationship quality** can also suffer, adding to children's anxiety and their risk for poorer child outcomes, be they cognitive, emotional, social, or academic. Suspecting that a child is witnessing IPA is sufficient reason to contact **Child Protective Services** or the police and could be a requirement that you do so (consult the laws of your state).

How Can IPA Stress Spill Over Into Other Relationships?

You might wonder if a parent who abuses a child's other parent will also abuse the child. Abuse estimates are complicated, especially since so much abuse is likely unreported and definitions of violence and abuse vary. Studies also differ in the populations they draw from, making generalizing difficult. You might also wonder if children who witness IPA or experience abuse will eventually abuse a partner or child. If you are really into pondering, you might also wonder if children who witness or experience abuse become victims of IPA as an adult. The quick answer to all these questions is "not necessarily." Experts tend to agree that **abuse spills over** in a sizable minority of cases, but in more cases than would have occurred if abuse hadn't happened.[6] Children from abusive homes appear at higher risk for perpetrating or receiving aggressive and abusive behavior, possibly because of the following:

- Poor role modeling from parents
- The effects of trauma on their own abilities to self-regulate or form healthy attachments
- The roles they played in the home (they may only know how to navigate certain types of family patterns that shaped their identities)
- A continued presence of environmental risk factors (e.g., poverty stressors or substance problems)
- Shared genes with abusers that contributed in some way to the abuse
- Some kind of combination of the above

How Do External Contexts Impact IPA Stressors?

As mentioned, **gender** is a recurring theme when focusing on IPA, especially when related to issues of male power or sexual abuse. **Ethnicity** is less clear. Data from the National Intimate Partner and Sexual Violence Survey (2010) indicated some differences by ethnicity in percentages of women who had ever experienced physical violence from an intimate partner:[7] White, 31.7%;

Black, 40.9%; Hispanic, 35.2%; and Native American, 45.9%. Rates for male victims also differed: White, 28.1; Black, 36.8; Hispanic, 26.5; and Native American, 45.3. Differences among groups related to poverty or minority stress possibly account for such variation, and these numbers do not distinguish between types of violence or other forms of potentially abusive behavior that might also differ in unique ways across groups.

IPA appears more prevalent in places that perceive women as inferior to or property of men, or in which women should sacrifice their own well-being to appease a man's desires. Some countries view behavior that happens in the home to be highly **private**—a perspective that can help hide and maintain abusive relationships. Some countries underappreciate the negative impacts of **alcoholism** on families and are less likely to address it as a risk factor for family violence. More **collectivist** cultures tend to deal with family abuse by emphasizing ways to improve and maintain family relationships while more **individualistic** cultures prioritize separating abuse victims from their abusers. Thus, particular cultural values and practices of some immigrants to the United States could contribute to different perspectives on family violence among cultural groups.

Family violence also appears to be somewhat more prevalent among people living in **poverty** or from lower **social classes**. However, some argue that wealthier people are better able to hide family violence, and we should be cautious about presuming that abuse is infrequent in higher social classes. We hear much about sexual assault and date rape on **college campuses**, which is somewhat related to social class. When investigating contextual factors that correspond with (but not cause) sexual assault on campus, studies find higher rates for women who are in their first two years of school, have a disability, are bisexual, belong to a sorority, have numerous sexual partners, and drink more alcohol.[8] Such tendencies illustrate how external contexts related to individual characteristics and perhaps social expectations of the college experience could elevate assault risks. However, large-scale studies seem to indicate that non-students of the same age are somewhat more likely to be sexually assaulted.

Same-sex IPV creates similar pressures to those described earlier, though some unique concerns can influence the experience. For example, some IPA victims hesitate calling the police or telling others about the abuse out of the concern that either they or their partner will be discriminated against and treated unfairly. Similarly, an abusive partner can threaten to reveal the other partner's concealed sexual orientation or gender identity to employers, family members, or others whose knowledge could put the partner at greater risk for harm.

Improve Your Learning

Without peeking, take a moment to review in your mind (or say out loud) the key concepts from this chapter (this is a proven learning technique). Then review the "Chapter Preview" section at the top and compare. Skim Part A of the chapter with extra attention to the **bolded words**. Skip to the end of the chapter to find more learning resources.

Part B. Child Maltreatment Stressors

What Is Stressful About Child Maltreatment?

Again, we see what looks like a strange question. However, we will take a broad approach to understanding certain types of abuse as sources of stress for various family members. Abuse of children has some distinct elements compared to IPA for at least two reasons. First, children are **inherently vulnerable** because of their underdeveloped physical, cognitive, and emotional abilities and lack of experience, and therefore **depend** on others for their care. Second, these vulnerabilities, including underdeveloped verbal skills and uncertainty about the consequences of disclosing the abuse, also contribute to how children respond to and **cope** with abuse. Children are prone to **externalize** their frustrations, fears, and pain with impulsive and sometimes destructive behavior that can easily be interpreted as willful disobedience, immaturity, or bullying. Conversely, some children strive to avoid drawing attention to themselves or **internalizing** their concerns, which can be interpreted as shyness or a disposition to be well-behaved and cooperative. Sometimes well-intentioned teachers and other adults praise and reinforce these seemingly prosocial behaviors, making it even less likely they will learn about the child's victimization. Suspected child maltreatment is something that should be reported to the proper authorities.

What Constitutes Child Maltreatment?

A broader term for child abuse is **child maltreatment**, which also incorporates the concept of **neglect**. Parental neglect of children's needs seems to be the most common form of child maltreatment. What types of neglected needs come to mind? You might have first thought about basic needs of food, clothing, and shelter. Perhaps you thought of denying children of affection and nurture. Did you think of medical or educational neglect? What about hygiene neglect? Younger children, of course, are more at risk for neglect, and children who experience it for longer periods of time tend to have more detrimental outcomes. Imagine what the world looks like from the eyes of a neglected child—what would be stressful about such a world?

Children aren't always **aware** of their neglect; it is all they know. Imagine how children might interpret having frequent hunger, a complete lack of attention, or living in filth when they have nothing else to compare their experiences with. What might they conclude about life? How might they find motivation to excel? Conversely, awareness of their neglect might cause stress related to wondering whether they deserve such treatment, how their parents feel about them, and if they should feel resentment. Children who show up at school in dirty clothes, have poor hygiene, and lack basic social skills are likely to be **rejected or bullied**. Similar hardships could occur in one's neighborhood. Consider how it would feel to be deprived at home and isolated or picked on outside of home.

Maltreatment also includes abuse in various forms. Some children are hit and kicked, have their hair pulled and arms yanked, are purposely burned by cigarettes, are sexually fondled or penetrated (or are forced to do so to someone else), and/or are verbally demeaned or intimidated.

Being **threatened** with violence is also abusive—particularly when violence has occurred in the past. Several forms of maltreatment can happen at the same time. Abusers can verbally manipulate children to feel at fault for their treatment, or to feel worthy of nothing better.

Anything that **terrorizes** a child, especially on a regular basis, becomes **traumatizing**. As touched on in Chapter 1, living in a constant state of fear and high alert can overwhelm our natural stress management system and cause problems with anxiety, depression, and substance use. The early childhood years are especially sensitive to the effects of chronic stress and trauma.[9] In short, high and constant levels of adrenaline and cortisol hormones that get triggered to help us manage a threatening situation can affect the activation of certain genes during **brain development**. These hormones appear to influence parts of the brain that affect emotional reaction (amygdala), learning and memory (hippocampus), and regulation of impulsive or emotional behavior (prefrontal cortex). Research also suggests that traumatic-related brain development can also contribute to higher eventual obesity and the tendency to ruminate (i.e., the cognitive style of constantly focusing on the negative—see Chapter 2). Thus, abused children are at high risk (but not inevitably) for experiencing difficulty with emotions and behavior because of early trauma, and may have to work hard to compensate for the nature of specific brain architecture affected in early childhood.

How Does Child Maltreatment Influence Family Stress?

Consequences of child maltreatment can lead to stresses of **social rejection and isolation**, **fear of others**, and **harsher treatment** from family members, peers, and teachers. Many of us lack the tolerance to endure the apparent antics of frequent emotional outbursts, out-of-control or aggressive behavior, extreme passivity, or manipulative attempts to keep our attention and support, especially when we don't understand what is really driving such behavior. It should come as no surprise that maltreated children are at greater risk for depression, anxiety, suicide, academic problems, developmental delays, delinquent behavior (including legal problems), sleep problems, and various other psychological challenges. These outcomes are stressful for the children and they also become stressors for others around them. Maltreated children can be more difficult to raise or to encourage to thrive. They are prone to maladaptive coping strategies such as substance use or bullying that bring potentially unwanted attention to the family. Such stressors might trigger more maltreatment by parents and others.

In some (perhaps most) cases, abusive parents are **ashamed** themselves and experience frustrations about their apparent lack of control (though some abusers seem to feel justified in their behavior). Other family members might be embarrassed by the abuse and feel pressure to keep it **secret**. They might also worry that they could be the next victims if they were to openly talk about the abuse or do anything else to anger the abusive parent. Nonabusive parents who witness or know of their partner's maltreatment of their child can also feel tremendous stress about what to do about it. Questions similar to those in the table in Part A apply to such a situation. Some of the nonabusive parents are past or current victims of abuse, which can make it especially challenging for them to feel powerful and worthy enough to intervene. Some struggle with **denial** because the alternatives might seem worse than the current circumstances (e.g., homelessness, being alone, family rejection). Public opinion can be very harsh toward a parent who "stands by" a child abuser, which can add pressure to the decision about whether to disclose the abuse. Feeling torn between two seemingly difficult options can threaten one's mental health.

Just as with IPA, child maltreatment can be a reaction to stressors. Interviews of mothers who had experienced child maltreatment show that child maltreatment (especially neglect) can stem from the following:[10]

- Untreated depression levels or feeling suicidal
- Substance problems
- Frustration with medical professionals (e.g., neglecting to have a child take a prescription that the parent thinks is unnecessary or harmful)
- Having worries about a child's welfare at school (e.g., bullying) and thus allowing children to frequently stay home instead
- Struggling with poverty and a lack of resources
- Having experienced child maltreatment or IPA that has diminished capacity to patiently raise children without using violent threats or behavior

Also, children with **disabilities** or who have parents struggling with **mental illness** have higher rates of abuse and neglect, probably at least in part because of extra strain on family resources (e.g., time, energy, patience, money, specific knowledge).[11] Such risk factors likely contribute in other ways to a challenging **home environment and family relationships**, adding to the overall stress experienced by the children. Can you think of any examples?

What Is Unique About Child Sexual Abuse?

The information above about stress and trauma related to maltreatment also generally applies to children who are sexually abused by a family member, though sometimes with some subtle differences. Family sexual abuse especially is kept **secret**.[12] The legal and social consequences that can result if others find out about it can feel overwhelming and must be avoided. In the minds of some adults, perhaps as a way to protect themselves from the pain of acknowledging such a disturbing reality, it is the child who brings shame on the family through their allegedly "false allegations." Think about the stress sexually abused children feel if their traumatic experience is disbelieved and they get rebuffed by the person they reach out to for help.

Furthermore, sexual abusers often **manipulate** children to take the blame for the abuse or for hurting the family, causing feelings of guilt and shame. *You are just too beautiful to resist. You are breaking up the family by making a big deal about this.* Some children think they didn't resist hard enough, or because of their sexual arousal, they must have been cooperating. The child's other parent might know of the abuse and feel torn or incapacitated about doing anything to stop it. While some parents are quick to take action once child sexual abuse (or other maltreatment) is discovered, think about how the family stress theory concepts of resources, perceptions, and coping help make sense of why some parents are slower to stop the abuse. Whether you find such a decision excusable is a different matter and something to ponder.

As you would expect, stressful consequences of child sexual abuse are similar to the consequences of other child maltreatment. Additionally, some of the victimized children learn

poor boundaries around sexual behavior and **sexually victimize** other children, creating new pressures for the families to confront. Forming intimate, sexual relationships later in life can be more stressful if they trigger negative associations or memories or prior sexual trauma. Couples may need extra patience in this regard, being sure to strengthen trust in their relationship, not to take offense over hesitancy, and perhaps seek professional assistance to work through some of the barriers.

What Is Stressful About Abuse Involving Siblings?

If you grew up with a sibling close to your age, it is highly probable that you had incidents of yelling, teasing, arguing, name-calling, shoving matches, and possibly some bruising or bleeding. **Sibling violence** is known as the most common form of family violence, though sibling *abuse* requires a more one-sided pattern of domination (similar to the differences between SCV and IT mentioned in Part A). Parents might struggle to know whether the sibling maltreatment is normal or hurtful. Some parents downplay it, while others worry about whether siblings will grow up as enemies; it can be painful to watch someone you love hurt someone else you love. Older siblings in particular can use their size, strength, and experience to abuse a younger (or less able) sibling, which creates similar stressors and outcomes associated with any kind of family abuse. How might being abused by a sibling be interpreted differently than being abused by a parent?

Like witnessing IPA, witnessing a parent or another sibling abusing a child's sibling can also be traumatizing. Why would that be? Think about what the witnessing sibling might be thinking and feeling, and what might trigger a state of high alert. National data has indicated that 83% of children who witnessed a sibling being abused by a parent felt fear, especially when the parent was a father.[13] Children who witnessed the abuse were also at higher risk for mental distress. Any kind of abuse can threaten a family's ability to create a comfortable, safe atmosphere conducive to optimal child development that models how to respond to stress in healthy ways.

What Are Common Stressors Related to Foster Care?

Reports of child maltreatment that are substantiated by Child Protective Services (or the equivalent) can result in children being removed from their homes and placed into foster care. The vast majority of cases have to do with some form of neglect, often by parents who struggle with substance use problems. Data from the U.S. Department of Health and Human Services provide some context about the 632,000 children served by foster care in 2020 (the lowest amount since 2013) and the 224,000 children who exited foster care that year (Figure 7.1):[14]

Foster children leave much of their belongings behind and are most often placed with people they don't know (around a third are placed with other family members, though they might also have never met). Learning to trust a stranger or a less familiar relative can be stressful. Young children particularly lack an understanding of the reasons for their removal, but even children who knowingly suffered at home can miss the **familiarity** of former routines and spaces. Foster children might also be separated from siblings, creating anxiety over their whereabouts and welfare.

A key risk factor for foster children is **caregiving instability (or placement disruption)**—moving from one foster placement to another.[15] Children are sometimes moved because foster parents were

Children in Foster Care (on Sept. 30th)

Age	0-4	5-8	9-12	13-16	17-20		
Ethnicity	White	Black	Hisp.	Other			
Gender	Male	Female					
Placed After	Reunited W/ Parent(s)	Adopted	Guardian · Relative · Emancipated · Other				

0%   10%   20%   30%   40%   50%   60%   70%   80%   90%   100%

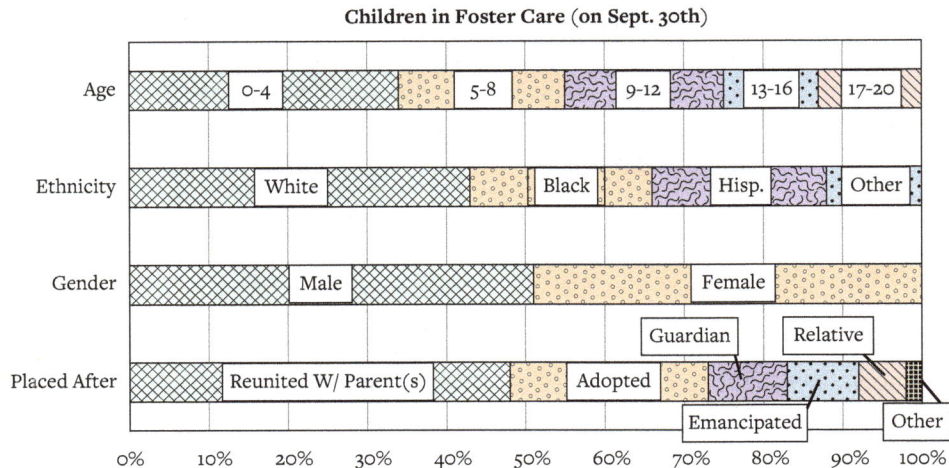

FIGURE 7.1 Children in Foster Care

unprepared or unwilling to continue in the current circumstances, perhaps having underestimated the level of trauma the children have endured and the resulting behavior challenges. As many as 80% of foster children experience mental health challenges—most frequent are PTSD and depression—and are prone to receiving inconsistent medical treatment and to arguably be overprescribed psychotropic medications.[16] Every change in environment requires the child to make new adjustments and new attempts and build **trust**.

When placements are a good match, children can get **attached** to foster families and face the stress of possibly losing those connections in the future if they go back home, losing the connections of their family of origin if they get adopted, and possibly having to choose (or feeling like they might have to choose) between two families. Foster children are subjected to regular visits from a variety of service providers who are intended as sources of support but place a high demand on schedules, possibly taking away from time completing school work, leisure activities, and just being a child.

How Resilient Are Maltreated Children?

Resilience is a reality and should not be overlooked. Nevertheless, it is important to understand the seriousness of the consequences of maltreatment, and how important it is to prevent if possible. Evaluations of child outcomes are not terribly encouraging.[17] In short, according to various evaluation data, proportions of maltreated children who do well in *one* type of outcome (e.g., physical, emotional, cognitive, academic, or social) can be quite high (66%, 56%, 49% of maltreated children), but when considering *multiple* types of outcomes at the same time, the numbers look more like 18%, 14%, or 11%. When looking at *consistent* resilience over *time* in *multiple* outcomes, some numbers are as low as 1.5% and 2%. However, many nonmaltreated children also fail to excel in multiple outcomes (e.g., 18% of maltreated children vs. 35% of nonmaltreated children in a comparative evaluation).

Some natural protective factors of child resilience might be suppressed by one's harsh environment. For example, children with certain genetic and intelligence factors tend to be highly resilient when confronting typical stressors, those advantaged diminished or disappeared when confronting maltreatment and serious family and neighborhood stressors. Hence, children can struggle with elements of well-being and competence for a variety of reasons, though those who experience maltreatment are especially likely to struggle in one or more ways for an extended time in their lives. Ultimately, survivors of childhood maltreatment can and do live satisfying and meaningful lives and are often able to stop the spillover of violence into the next generation.

How Do External Contexts Impact Child Maltreatment Stressors?

As noted earlier, children with disabilities are at elevated risk for maltreatment. Generally speaking, children with characteristics that are deemed as **less desirable** by certain parents are at higher risk of maltreatment, be it their physical attractiveness, not being the desired gender, their tendencies outside of heterosexual or gender-normative identities, or having a difficult temperament. Girls also tend to be at higher risk for sexual abuse than boys. Of course, these are only risk factors if parents are prone to be abusive.

Neighborhood and community contexts are potential risk factors for child maltreatment depending in part on levels of **social disorganization**.[18] Neighborhoods characterized as having low economic status, being more ethnically diverse, and having people frequently moving in and out lack the kind of stability that supports positive parenting and self-control. Studies indicate that indeed, parents who felt more socially isolated had more limited peer groups, perceived less neighborhood cohesion and trust, and tended to have a greater likelihood of aggressive punishment or abuse.

Some interesting nuance emerged when accounting for individual or family-level factors and neighborhood-level factors at the same time. Among mothers who were highly involved with community activities, if they perceived their communities positively, they were less likely to treat their children with psychological aggression, but if they perceived their communities negatively, they were more likely to do so. Also, more neighborhood turnover (moving in and out) increased the risk of child maltreatment in low-income families but not in higher income families from the same type of neighborhood. Conversely, believing it was likely that neighbors would get involved if they witnessed children acting out was linked to less child maltreatment for higher income families but not lower-income families. Some neighborhood risk and protective factors seem to apply more to families with certain resources or perceptions.

What Does All This Mean for You?

Your insights can be valuable to your personal life, your family relationships, and your professional roles. Take a few moments to ponder the following:

- How have you been feeling while engaging with this information? Why?
- How much of this topic can you personally relate to?

- What stereotypes about abusive families were challenged by what you learned in this chapter?
- What solutions come to mind when you think about preventing abuse and maltreatment in families?
- What other examples have come to mind that illustrate similar or diverse ways that families cope with stressors from abuse and maltreatment?

Reminders for Helpers

As a person of influence, you can help guide people through the coping processes and ideally help foster a **flourishing** life. However, take care to avoid letting your personal **interpretations** push you toward assuming too much about somebody else's circumstances, perceptions, and motivations. Always be ready to address issues that might be hard for you to face because of your own history.

Draw upon the elements of the **FIM framework** and other family stress concepts. Remember, **coping** refers to an action or response based on available or new resources and perceptions related to stressors. Families have either successfully **managed** a stressor's pressure through **adjustment coping** or reached crisis in which **adaptive coping** is needed to reestablish some level of **general family functioning**. **Resources** and **perceptions** are key concepts to focus on when confronting family stress. **Review the master table** in Chapter 4 as a guide for exploring the following ideas on how to help families with stressors.

What Are Some Ways to Encourage Effective Family Coping?

Drawing from the scholars mentioned earlier, with some additional insights based on other scholars noted next, we will explore **suggested resources and noteworthy perceptions** that can contribute to successful coping and more optimal family functioning.

How Can You Help Address Abuse and Maltreatment in Families?

While any form of maltreatment causes pressure and distress, and each form has some unique consequences, the frequency, severity, and level of one-sidedness influence the stressful impact and other consequences of the treatment. Such variability is important to keep in mind when addressing family maltreatment (including forms that were not covered in this chapter, such as adolescent children abusing their parents). For example, SCV, occasional use of spanking a child, and common sibling aggression bother some families and professionals more than others. Efforts to deter or prevent such interactions can emphasize learning alternative forms of coping with family disagreements and conflict. Learning to individually cope with stress can help those who are prone to lash out aggressively avoid reaching their **boiling point**.

Addressing situations that are more clearly abusive in nature—which usually means domination, intimidation, and control—might also involve promoting better conflict resolution and stress management skills but likely require additional intervention. **Denial** can be a major hurdle toward stopping abuse and promoting family healing. Abusers and victims need to truly understand their situations. Abusers must take responsibility for their actions and stop blaming others. Interventions can also involve helping abusers develop **empathy** for those whom they abuse. Victims might also need help to hold abusers accountable and let go of any **skewed perceptions** about somehow deserving the abuse or that no better options in life are possible.

Women who are more resilient to IPA have reported high levels of **informal and formal support** (see Chapter 2), relying on spiritual or religious faith, taking pride in their ability to rise above the violence, and recognizing personal growth and strength that helped them cope with their situations.[19] Deciding whether to leave an abusive situation is perhaps the most stressful part of the experience for some victims, and people will have all sorts of opinions about what should happen. Attempting to leave can be the most dangerous time for an abused woman, especially if she is doing it without support. She might need help to feel empowered enough to reach a decision on what to do and to find alternative places to live and resources to survive—especially if she has children. She might need help finding reasons to be optimistic about her future. Some families turn things around and discontinue the abuse, but it can be hard to predict whether it will happen.

Maltreated children, especially young children, need help **making sense** of the maltreatment they observed or experienced. Ideally, this is done in a way that eliminates self-blame but is also sensitive to children's potential desire to see their parents in a positive light.[20] Children who witnessed violence between parents can perceive their parents' relationship and the father-child relationship as less cohesive, which adds to anxiety and other post-trauma symptoms. Children might need extra assistance in processing difficult emotions. Victims of IPA and their children who witness it can benefit from **"emotions coaching"** (recognizing, allowing, showing empathy for, and helping children label negative emotions). This helps adults improve at regulating their own emotions, becoming more confident in their parenting, and engaging in less scolding/lecturing. Children can improve at regulating their emotions, become less negative while interacting with their mothers, and have fewer depression symptoms.

Various programs focus on preventing or stopping child maltreatment by promoting better parenting.[21] Some approaches focus on how parents define what it **means** (perceptions) to be a "good parent," which can help motivate more nurturing childrearing. Some emphasize learning to recognize and take responsibility for the maltreatment, to respectfully coparent with a partner, and to put the child's needs first. More holistic programs incorporate providing **resources** to address substance use problems, economic hardship, and childcare arrangements for employed single mothers. Other programs encourage parents to be more accepting of their child's emerging identity by better appreciating the trauma caused when a child feels rejected. They help parents maintain a strong connection with their children regardless of differing beliefs.

Improve Your Learning

Without peeking, take a moment to review in your mind (or say out loud) the key concepts from this chapter (this is a proven learning technique). Then review the "Chapter Preview" section at the top and compare. Skim Part B of the chapter with extra attention to the **bolded words**.

Do You Want to Learn More?

We have only touched on a portion of information related to some elements of this topic. **What really sparked your interest? What do you wish was covered more thoroughly?** Consider taking some time to further deepen your understanding of personal and professional issues related to helping families cope with stressors. Below are a variety of resources that you might find helpful, and some references directly or indirectly referred to in this chapter. You don't want to be accused of neglecting your learning, do you?

Videos

(Use links or do searches with the key words provided)
- *"What I See"—A Domestic Violence Short Film* (5 mins). Sutherland Shire Family Services. https://www.youtube.com/watch?v=B2h_PO9subA
- *Mark'd—Award-Winning Emotional Abuse Short Film* (7 mins). Danny Gibbons. https://www.youtube.com/watch?v=EavMqZ_6UvQ
- Why Domestic Violence Victims Don't Leave (16 mins). Leslie Morgan Steiner, TED. https://www.youtube.com/watch?v=V1yW5IsnSjo&t=614s
- Domestic Violence From a Son's Perspective (10 mins). Adam Herbst, TEDxYouth@Park Cityhttps://www.youtube.com/watch?v=bD52ne0rRw0
- Willis Clan Describes Healing After Their Father's Sexual Abuse (15 mins). *TODAY*. https://www.youtube.com/watch?v=S0oJGWHeGZM
- *Removed* (13 mins). A dramatization of a child removed from her traumatic home and placed in foster care. https://www.youtube.com/watch?app=desktop&v=lOeQUwdAjE0

Websites

- American Psychiatric Association. (n.d.). What is posttraumatic stress disorder? https://www.psychiatry.org/patients-families/ptsd/what-is-ptsd
- Centers for Disease Control and Prevention (n.d.). Violence prevention. https://www.cdc.gov/violenceprevention/datasources/nisvs/summaryreports.html#anchor_1535031475856
- Child Welfare Information Gateway. https://www.childwelfare.gov/topics/systemwide/statistics/foster-care/
- Children's Defense Fund. https://www.childrensdefense.org/state-of-americas-children/soac-2021-child-welfare/
- Dewar, G. (2021). Emotion coaching: Helping kids cope with negative feelings. *Parenting Science*. https://parentingscience.com/emotion-coaching/

Readings (Articles, Books, Book Chapters)

- Galano, M. M., & Graham-Bermann, S. A. (2019). Traumatic stress within the family. In B. H. Fiese, M. Celano, K. Deater-Deckard, E. N. Jouriles, & M. A. Whisman

(Eds.), *APA handbook of contemporary family psychology: Applications and broad impact of family psychology* (pp. 539–554). American Psychological Association. https://doi.org/10.1037/0000100-033

- Johnson, M. P. (2008). *A typology of domestic violence.* Northeastern University Press.
- Katz, L. F., Gurtovenko, K., Maliken, A., Stettler, N., Kawamura, J., & Fladeboe, K. (2020). An emotion coaching parenting intervention for families exposed to intimate partner violence. *Developmental Psychology, 56*(3), 638–651. http://dx.doi.org/10.1037/dev0000800
- Baker, L., Lalonde, D., & Tabibi, J. (2017, November). *Issue 21: Sibling violence.* Learning network. Centre for Research & Education on Violence Against Women & Children. https://www.vawlearningnetwork.ca/our-work/issuebased_newsletters/issue-21/index.html

Notes

1 https://www.acf.hhs.gov/cb/research-data-technology/statistics-research/afcars

2 Gelles, R. J. (1999). Family violence. In R. L. Hampton (Ed.). *Family violence: Prevention and treatment* (pp. 1–32). SAGE Publications.

3 Johnson, M. P. (2008). *A typology of domestic violence.* Northeastern University Press.

4 Askin, C. (2015, November 3). Abusive partners can change: We aren't doomed to repeat our mistakes. *Psychology Today.* https://www.psychologytoday.com/us/blog/hurt-people-hurt-people/201511/abusive-partners-can-change

5 Galano, M. M., & Graham-Bermann, S. A. (2019). Traumatic stress within the family. In B. H. Fiese, M. Celano, K. Deater-Deckard, E. N. Jouriles, & M. A. Whisman (Eds.), *APA handbook of contemporary family psychology: Applications and broad impact of family psychology* (pp. 539–554). American Psychological Association. https://doi.org/10.1037/0000100-033; Jaffee, S. R., Caspi, A., Moffitt, T. E., Polo-Tomás, M., & Taylor, A. (2007). Individual, family, and neighborhood factors distinguish resilient from non-resilient maltreated children: a cumulative stressors model. *Child abuse & neglect, 31*(3), 231–253. https://doi.org/10.1016/j.chiabu.2006.03.011; Jaffee, S. R., & Gallop, R. (2007). Social, emotional, and academic competence among children who have had contact with child protective services: Prevalence and stability estimates. *Journal of the American Academy of Child and Adolescent Psychiatry, 46*(6), 757–765. https://doi.org/10.1097/chi.0b013e318040b247

6 Erel, O., & Burman, B. (1995). Interrelatedness of marital relations and parent—child relations: A meta-analytic review. *Psychological Bulletin, 118,* 108–132. http://doi.org/10.1037/0033-2909.118.1.108; Tucker, C. J., Finkelhor, D., & Turner, H. (2021). Exposure to parent assault on a sibling as a childhood adversity. *Child Abuse & Neglect.* https://doi.org/10.1016/j.chiabu.2021.105310; National Council on Family Relations. (n.d.). Family focus. https://www.ncfr.org/ncfr-report/focus; Tucker, C. J., Sharp, E. H., Van Gundy, K. T., & Rebellon, C. (2019). Perpetration of sibling aggression and sibling relationship quality in emerging adulthood. *Personal Relationships, 26*(3), 529–539. https://doi.org/10.1111/pere.12288

7 Centers for Disease Control and Prevention (n.d.). Violence prevention. https://www.cdc.gov/violenceprevention/datasources/nisvs/summaryreports.html

8 Muehlenhard, C. L., Peterson, Z. D., Humphreys, T. P., & Jozkowski, K. N. (2017). Evaluating the one-in-five statistic: Women's risk of sexual assault while in college. *The Journal of Sex Research, 54,* 4–5, 549–576. http://doi.org/10.1080/00224499.2017.1295014; National Institute of Justice. (2008, September 30). Factors that increase sexual assault risk. https://nij.ojp.gov/topics/articles/factors-increase-sexual-assault-risk#alcoholuse

9 National Scientific Council on the Developing Child. (2009/2014). *Excessive stress disrupts the architecture of the developing brain.* Working paper 3, updated edition. Harvard University. Available at https://developingchild.harvard.edu/resources/wp3/; Osadchiy, V., Mayer, E. A., Bhatt, R., Labus, J. S., Gao, L., Kilpatrick, L. A., Liu, C., Tillisch, K., Naliboff, B., Chang, L., & Gupta, A. (2019). History of early life adversity is associated with increased food addiction and sex-specific alterations in reward network connectivity in obesity. *Obesity Science & Practice, 5*(5), 416–436. https://doi.org/10.1002/osp4.362; Peters, A. T., Burkhouse, K. L., Kinney, K. L, & Phan, K. L. (2019). The roles of early-life adversity and rumination in neural response to emotional faces amongst anxious and depressed adults. *Psychological Medicine, 49*(13), 2267–2278. https://doi.org/10.1017/S0033291718003203

10 Bundy-Fazioli, K., & Hamilton, T. A. D. (2013). A qualitative study exploring mothers' perceptions of child neglect. *Child & Youth Services, 34*(3), 250–266. https://doi-org/10.1080/0145935X.2013.826034

11 Brockington, I., Chandra, P., Dubowitz, H., Jones, D., Moussa, S., Nakku, J., & Ferre, I. Q. (2011). WPA guidance on the protection and promotion of mental health in children of persons with severe mental disorders. *World Psychiatry, 10*(2), 93–102. https://doi.org/10.1002/j.2051-5545.2011.tb00023.x; Legano, L. A., Desch, L. W., Messner, S. A., Idzerda, S., Flaherty, E. G., ABUSE, C. O. C., ... & Yin, L. (2021). Maltreatment of children with disabilities. *Pediatrics, 147*(5). https://doi.org/10.1542/peds.2021-050920

12 Gilgun, J. F., (2008, December). *Child sexual abuse: One of the most neglected social problems of our time.* Family Focus. National Council on Family Relations. https://www.ncfr.org/ncfr-report/focus

13 Tucker, C. J., Finkelhor, D., & Turner, H. (2021). Exposure to parent assault on a sibling as a childhood adversity. *Child Abuse & Neglect.* https://doi.org/10.1016/j.chiabu.2021.105310

14 Children's Bureau. (2021, October 4). Adoption & foster care statistics. Administration for Children and Families, U.S. Department of Health and Human Services. https://www.acf.hhs.gov/cb/research-data-technology/statistics-research/afcars

15 Proctor, L. J., Skriner, L. C., Roesch, S., & Litrownik, A. J. (2010). Trajectories of behavioral adjustment following early placement in foster care: Predicting stability and change over 8 years. *Journal of the American Academy of Child and Adolescent Psychiatry, 49*(5), 464–473. https://doi.org/10.1097/00004583-201005000-00007

16 National Conference of State Legislatures. (2019, November 1). Mental health and foster care. https://www.ncsl.org/research/human-services/mental-health-and-foster-care.aspx

17 Cicchetti, D., & Rogosch, F. A. (2012). Gene × Environment interaction and resilience: Effects of child maltreatment and serotonin, corticotropin releasing hormone, dopamine, and oxytocin genes. *Development and Psychopathology, 24*(2), 411–427. https://doi.org/10.1017/S0954579412000077; Jaffee, S. R., Caspi, A., Moffitt, T. E., Polo-Tomás, M., & Taylor, A. (2007). Individual, family, and neighborhood factors distinguish resilient from non-resilient maltreated children: A cumulative stressors model. *Child Abuse & Neglect, 31*(3), 231–253. https://doi.org/10.1016/j.chiabu.2006.03.011; Jaffee, S. R., & Gallop, R. (2007). Social, emotional, and academic competence among children who have had contact with child protective services: Prevalence and stability estimates. *Journal of the American Academy of Child and Adolescent Psychiatry, 46*(6), 757–765. https://doi.org/10.1097/chi.0b013e318040b247; Sattler, K., & Font, S. A. (2018). Resilience in young children involved with child protective services. *Child Abuse & Neglect, 75*, 104–114. https://doi.org/10.1016/j.chiabu.2017.05.004

18 Kim, B., & Maguire-Jack, K. (2015). Community interaction and child maltreatment. *Child Abuse & Neglect, 41*, 146–157. https://doi.org/10.1016/j.chiabu.2013.07.020; Maguire-Jack, K., & Negash, T. (2016). Parenting stress and child maltreatment: The buffering effect of neighborhood social service availability and accessibility. *Children and Youth Services Review, 60*, 27–33. https://doi.org/10.1016/j.childyouth.2015.11.016

19 Howell, K. H., Thurston, I. B., Schwartz, L. E., Jamison, L. E., & Hasselle, A. J. (2018). Protective factors associated with resilience in women exposed to intimate partner violence. *Psychology of Violence, 8*(4), 438–447. https://doi.org/10.1037/vio0000147

20 Paul, O. (2019). Perceptions of family relationships and post-traumatic stress symptoms of children exposed to domestic violence. *Journal of Family Violence, 34*, 331–343. https://doi.org/10.1007/s10896-018-00033-z; Katz, L. F., Gurtovenko, K., Maliken, A., Stettler, N., Kawamura, J., & Fladeboe, K. (2020). An emotion coaching parenting intervention for families exposed to intimate partner violence. *Developmental Psychology, 56*(3), 638–651. http://dx.doi.org/10.1037/dev0000800

21 Cohen, J. A. (2021, June 25). The trauma-focused CBT and family acceptance project: An integrated framework for children and youth. Psychiatric Times. https://www.psychiatrictimes.com/view/the-trauma-focused-cbt-and-family-acceptance-project; Daro, D., & Donnelly, A. C. (2002). Child abuse prevention: Accomplishments and challenges. *The APSAC Handbook on Child Maltreatment, 2*, 431–448. https://www.ojp.gov/ncjrs/virtual-library/abstracts/child-abuse-prevention-accomplishments-and-challenges-apsac; Ellenbogen, S., Klein, B., & Wekerle, C. (2014). Early childhood education as a resilience intervention for maltreated children. *Early Child Development and Care, 184*(9–10), 1364–1377. https://doi.org/10.1080/03004430.2014.916076; McConnell, N., Barnard, M., & Taylor, J. (2017). Caring dads safer children: Families' perspectives on an intervention for maltreating fathers. *Psychology of Violence, 7*(3), 406–416. http://dx.doi.org/10.1037/vio0000105

Image Credits

Fig. 7.1: Source: Adapted from https://www.acf.hhs.gov/cb/research-data-technology/statistics-research/afcars.

CHAPTER 8

Family Structural Complexity and Family Stress

About 85% of adults said they would feel "very obligated" to provide support to a biological parent in need; only 56% said the same about a stepparent.[1]

Chapter Preview

- Family structure indicates who is in a family and what transitions the family has undergone.
- Family structural complexity captures elements of diverse family structure resulting from multipartner fertility.
- Boundary ambiguity is a key concept that helps explain family structure stressors.
- Shifting attitudes about marriage and parenthood have contributed to the presence and acceptance of single parenthood.
- Family stress theory attends to differences in resources, perceptions, and family disruptions that help account for risk and protective factors of various family structures.
- Single-parent families have some unique stressors related to stigma, poverty, parental roles, and boundaries that increase risks for such families.
- Multiple transitions in family structure make it more challenging for parents and children to adjust to new family circumstances.
- Parental relationship dissolution contributes to emotional losses and boundary ambiguity that create family stress.
- The addition of family members (e.g., stepparent, step- or half-siblings) adds complexity to families that acts as a stressor.
- Various conceptual explanations contribute to our understanding of why relationship dissolution and family structural complexity put families at risk for negative outcomes.

What Is This Topic About?

Who is part of your family system? Do you have step-, half-, or adopted siblings? A stepparent? A hamster? Typically, the members who share a household are central figures for that family system, though other family members outside the household can play pivotal roles in our lives. When we talk of **family structure**, we tend to focus on family members with whom we live—the family in which we are raised or in which we have a committed partner. Family structure contributes to our family patterns (e.g., rules, roles, boundaries) and the nature of the personal relationships in the home. Family structure also reflects the history of family transitions.

Family transitions—or changes to the family structure—**disrupt** the typical family balance (**homeostasis**), thus creating pressure to adjust to added or subtracted family members and all the resulting shifts in family patterns. Family stress theory helps us understand that families in transition draw upon available resources and are guided by their perceptions of their circumstances as they establish a new sense of hemostasis or family functioning. Family transitions can also trigger a significant change in economic and social resources. Different types of family transitions can produce unique pressures—think about how a child might experience the removal of a parent from the home due to divorce compared to moving in with a single parent's new romantic partner. Generally speaking, children who experience more transitions tend to face more challenges that put them at risk for emotional, psychological, and behavioral problems.

Family transitions are common in places or cultures that have high rates of divorce, remarriage, and cohabitation (including cohabiting stepfamily arrangements). These transitions often lead to **sibling complexity**—siblings who share only one or no biological parents. The rise in **multipartner fertility**—having biological children with more than one person—increases sibling complexity. Family structure can be more complicated and diverse than we typically realize. In this chapter, we focus on what we call **family structural complexity** as a source for various family stressors. We primarily explore stressors associated with single parenthood, relationship dissolution (e.g., divorce), and subsequent relationship formation (e.g., stepfamilies).

Boundary ambiguity is also a helpful concept for understanding processes and consequences of family structural complexity.[2] As noted briefly in Chapter 1, boundary ambiguity refers to a lack of clarity regarding **who** is considered part of a family and what it means to be considered part of the family. It addressed who is **physically** and **psychologically** "there for you." For example, you might have a stepfather who is also a stepparent to another child—let's call her "Mariah"—who is 15 years older than you. Mariah might be the same as a stranger to you, but if she lived nearby and you both like watching international dart competitions, you might start hanging out. Are you more friends or family? You might view Mariah as family, but Mariah might view you as a friend (or Mariah's parents might disagree about whether the two of you should be considered siblings). Lack of clarity in family rules, roles, and (interpersonal) boundaries because of family transitions is also a part of boundary ambiguity and can prolong a **state of crisis** if families are unable to cope with it.

Sometimes **mismatches** exist between the physical and psychological presence of family members. For example, someone with Alzheimer's or who is in a coma is physically present in the lives of family members but isn't "there for you" psychologically—or, they aren't consistently psychologically present enough to count on. Conversely, someone who is missing for an extended period of time (kidnapped child, unaccounted for soldier at war) can still seem like part of the family (psychologically) regardless of their physical absence. Families find it more difficult to establish or maintain useful rules, roles, boundaries, and routines when somebody is only "kind of" an active participant in the family or home. Such ambiguity also makes it easier for family members to have contradictory **interpretations or meanings** of their circumstances (including who is considered family), opening the door to more family conflict. Families experiencing high levels of boundary ambiguity are at greater risk for experiencing stressors that threaten healthy individual and relationship development in the home.[3]

What Are the Assumptions?

Traditionally, a focus on family structure emphasized that the family unit made of certain components contributes to family well-being and subsequent societal stability. A bonded mother and father have been held up far and wide as a critical ingredient for meeting children's economic (and, somewhat more recently, emotional) needs. Marriage has commonly been institutionalized to help solidify the couple bond and protect children. As you well know, a **conservative** perspective is likely to value family and marital institutions and traditions as a proven means toward family and social stability. Religious conservatives especially view mothers and fathers as essential elements to child well-being and have thus been more critical of "alternative family forms."

Liberal perspectives have focused somewhat less on family structure and seem more supportive than conservatives of the idea that parents are interchangeable—in other words, parents' gender has much less to do with child welfare than how parents parent and a family's economic resources. Conservatives tend to see stronger **links** among family structure, the quality of parenting, and economic advantages for children—that family structure leads to certain parenting and economic outcomes. Liberals might acknowledge such links (especially between structure and poverty) but are more confident in the ability of government resources to compensate for the disparity of resources across family forms. Liberals also tend to be more concerned about reinforcing stigmas against diverse family forms, arguing that stigma makes conditions more difficult for marginalized families. Critics sometimes point out that some conservative regions of the United States have high levels of single parenthood or divorce, or that middle-class liberals tend to marry and wait until after marriage to have children. Do the critics have a point?

To some degree, ideological assumptions about family structure boil down to whether a parent is "**who** you are" or "**what** you do." Compared to their opposite ideology, conservatives tend to err on the side of "who" (or at least that the "who" and "what" are highly connected—a mom and a dad each bring something different to the table) while liberals tend to err more on the side of "what" (or at least that the "what" can be facilitated in a way to overcome any issues with the "who"—a single parent with proper support can provide all the parenting a child needs). These different perspectives can influence how family and professionals perceive or suggest solutions to certain family stressors—does the structure need to be adjusted and personal responsibility encouraged, or do certain families just need more assistance to counter disadvantages that are arguably out of their control? Can both be true—or neither?

As you **engage with** the rest of the chapter, remember the key elements of family stress theories (e.g., stressors, resources, perceptions, coping, and crisis) and consider the following:

- How might perceptions of family stressors be affected by family structure?
- Why might some families with similar structural complexity flourish while others are strained?
- How do the various pieces of information throughout the chapter fit together to help explain why certain family structures might be riskier for certain family outcomes?
- What experiences have you had or observed that help you relate to specific concepts?
- How might the ideological perspectives influence how people (including you) think about the relevance of family structure in explaining family stressors?

Part A. Family Structure and Single-Parent Family Stressors

How Does Family Structure Relate to Family Stress?

All family structures experience stressors that have the potential to become hardships. In the United States, the **nuclear** family—typically defined as a married male-female couple and their offspring—has somewhat decreased in prevalence in recent decades. For example, analyses of U.S. Census data show that in 2020 about 70% of children were living with two parents and 25% with a single parent compared to 88% and 9% in 1960, respectively.[4] When just looking at biological parents, about 63% of high school seniors in 2020 had been raised entirely by both their birth parents and another 5.3% by one biological parent and a stepparent.

Decades of research tend to show, on average, overall advantages and more positive outcomes for children and adults living in a two-parent household compared to a single-parent household, especially with married (usually biological) parents. Various factors account for why certain family structures tend to have greater disadvantages. While certain family patterns and processes could have a more direct influence on family outcomes, family structure also **signals** whether significant higher risk transitions or circumstances have occurred in that family (e.g., a stepfamily structure often indicates a history of divorce). How families cope with stressors associated with family structure also influences the effects of structure on family members.

What Contributes to Diverse Family Structures?

To avoid a long history or anthropology lesson, let's just focus briefly on major modern shifts in family structure in the United States. As society became more industrialized, families generally shifted from multigenerational households (extended families) to a more nuclear model. The default sequence of events was to marry and then have children (even if children were conceived first, hence the "shotgun wedding"). Over time, marriage became highly **romanticized**, and adult **gratification** and **personal expression** became more emphasized in mainstream culture. Divorce became a more viable and socially acceptable solution for individuals who felt less fulfilled (including because of abuse) in their marriage. With marriage still largely popular, divorced people commonly remarried and created stepfamilies.

In more recent decades, attitudes toward marriage have continued to shift, and marriage rates have somewhat declined. (Whether circumstances lead to attitude changes or the other way around is difficult to say.) Furthermore, nonmarital **cohabitation** has risen dramatically. Cohabitation is often perceived as a way to better prepare for marriage and avoid divorce, though for a growing number it has become an alternative to marriage—for some as a temporary condition while working toward establishing a more stable economic lifestyle and for others as a sign of indifference or opposition toward marriage. Changes in the economy have arguably made it more challenging for non-college-educated men especially to find consistent, good-paying jobs (which are generally expected in a marriageable man), while single mothers have become more able to live without marriage by either earning good wages or being supplemented by government programs.[5] Over time, the practices of marriage and parenthood have become somewhat detached.

According to national data, attitudes toward the importance of couples who have children marrying have been quickly declining. The chart in Figure 8.1 shows attitudes for those who find it "very important" (with chunks of people finding it "somewhat important" not reported here) by political ideology, race, marital status, religiosity (weekly church attendance vs. seldom/none), and age.[6] Of course, other factors contribute to family structure changes, such as the death of family members, but most of the shifts away from the nuclear family model have come as the result of avoiding or ending a marriage.

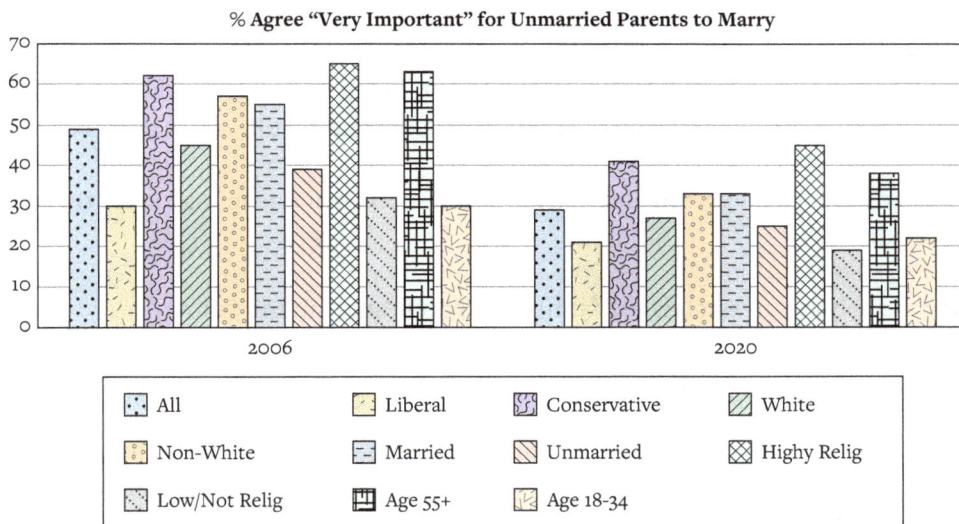

FIGURE 8.1 % Agree "Very Important" for Unmarried Parents to Marry

What Is It About Family Structure That Can Lead to Hardship?

You might have studied a foreign language in school or perhaps played around with a language-learning app for a few weeks. Imagine trying to live in a foreign country that uses that language after having just a little bit of preparation. Then, after you start to get the hang of it, get moved to another country with a different language and start the process again. Maybe you go through this several times. Each transition to another place requires different abilities, requiring time and effort while you struggle with your confidence and making connections with other people.

Changes to one's family structure can be a bit like learning a new language in a foreign land. We encounter new people who don't know our mannerisms, inside jokes, and communication styles. Perhaps we lose contact with someone who really did "speak our language," and we get a little rusty and lose some fluency. Each family system has a bit of its own culture, and adding and subtracting family members changes that culture. While families face normative changes anyway—children mature, life has its complications—there's something about a major and relatively sudden shift in family membership that can challenge our sense of belonging, our need for intimacy, and our social identity. The processes we go through to build trust with and really understand someone make us vulnerable to hurt feelings, self-doubt, and mistrust when things go wrong. We become more at risk of feeling alone, isolated, and fearful of connecting with others who might also leave us. Our whole **attachment** system can become more anxious or avoidant. Of course, sometimes changes in family structure are essential for optimal family functioning, but that doesn't mean the process will necessarily be free of hardships.

As mentioned in the introduction, **boundary ambiguity** is more likely to occur in certain family structures, especially when **multipartner fertility** is involved. Parents who only have biological children with only the same partner and who stay together to raise the children typically

- know the children from birth and can build off of early bonding to solidify a strong parent-child relationship,
- establish their parental identity (and co-parental identities) at a gradual pace and ease into some aspects of parenting as children develop and require more constant attention, and
- are clearly identified within and outside the home as being responsible for the welfare of the children.

In contrast, joining an established family as a parental or sibling figure

- is a quicker transition with fewer clear expectations of how to identify with and participate in the family system;
- increases the likelihood of having children shift between living with different parents, which can lead to inconsistent and sometimes competitive expectations from each household about one's parental role; and
- could expose children to adults and children from other parental relationships (like Mariah discussed earlier), which could create confusion and jealousy.

Ambiguity over family member identity and expected contributions makes it difficult for all involved to know how to participate in a family system and develop reliable and trusting relationships.

From a **family stress perspective**, family structure can be conducive to different types or amounts of **resources** to manage family stressors. For example, having more adults share the parenting load can lighten physical and emotional demands. Multiple adults can also provide social support and encouragement to one another, though they can also disagree on how to manage a home. Financial resources can vary depending on how many adults are earning income. Having multiple parents can help children experience greater and more diverse forms of support and guidance.

Perceptions might also differ based somewhat on family structure. As noted, boundary ambiguity is largely about perception, and family structures that result from the relatively quick addition or subtraction of family members are especially prone to boundary ambiguity. Major **disruptions to family patterns** (e.g., divorce) increase the likelihood that existing resources and default interpretations will be insufficient for avoiding **crisis**. After all, those resources and perceptions were based on supporting a certain family structure, which apparently wasn't going very well. We will focus on how family processes and internal and external contexts can vary within key types of family structures that potentially affect the type of stressors certain families could face and how families might cope with such circumstances.

Why Are Single-Parent Families Stressful?

Single parenthood can vary dramatically in whether children experience disruptive family transitions. Some children are born to a single parent who never pursues intimate partner relationships and therefore avoids bonding with new adult members who might only build temporary relationships with the child. Other single parents have been in committed relationships or marriages that ended, sometimes several of them, some of which resulted in multiple children through multi-partner fertility (usually producing half-sibling relationships). Some might live with a partner (cohabitation) but still think of themselves as single and resist any attempts by the partner to be an active parental figure. Single parents also vary in the number of family members or friends who are availing and willing to step in and assist with parenting. Recognizing such **differences in single-parent family structures** helps us understand the stressors such families might face.

Reviews of research and interviews with parents and children help identify why children of single-parent families have elevated risks for various internalizing, externalizing, and academic problems.[7] Here we focus more on stressors related to the **persistent absence of a second parent** in a household (especially a father), whereas in Part B we focus more on stressors related to the subtraction and addition of a second parent and on ongoing co-parental relationships, some of which also apply to single-parent families.

- Single-parent families can feel **stigmatized** by others, adding to anxiety and a lack of support. Some young children have reported the stress of trying to explain their family situation to other children who can't relate. Children sometimes reject sympathy and pity from others who attribute any child or family difficulties to single parenthood, feeling like their family was being put down in some way.
- Lesser economic stability and greater work-family conflict are more common for single parents, meaning that they and their children could struggle with various **poverty**

stressors (see Chapter 4). Poorer parents tend to have lower levels of **self-efficacy**—a perceived sense of mastery or control they have over their circumstances. Lower self-efficacy can correspond to greater stress and child behavioral problems.

- Declines in **parental mental health** because of difficult stressors are more common and contribute to children's higher risk for distress and developing mental health problems. Single-parent families might lack an available companion to help compensate for a depressed parent not fully attending to children's emotional needs.

- Single parents might not be able to **share parenting duties**. This can create extra burdens on the parent and less attention for the children. **Low parental monitoring** (parental knowledge of whereabouts and activity, supervision, communication) is a key predictor of children's misbehaviors, especially regarding adolescent risky sexual and substance use activities and delinquency. Children with less monitoring also spend more time with peers who engage in risk-taking behavior. Single parents have less opportunity to closely monitor their children when no other trustworthy adults are around to help, especially if they are working extra hours to make ends meet. Some have also reported being overly **lenient or permissive** with their children because they didn't have a partner who could back them up to enforce rules.

- With only a single parent to take on daily parenting responsibilities, children can be expected (or feel obliged) to compensate. Older children especially have mentioned their awareness of the pressure their single parent (especially a mother) feels and can become more protective of the parent. Some tried to reduce their own demands on the parent to lighten the pressure, even to the point of not disclosing their needs. Some worried about a single mother's future well-being once the children grow up and leave the home. **Boundaries** that perhaps more naturally form between parents and children in a two-parent household can become less hierarchical and more peer- or spouse-like in a single-parent household. For example, some single mothers have described adult-like communication with children out of "pure desperation" for adult conversation. Consequently, parental authority can be weakened and children who take on parental responsibilities—including as an emotional companion to a parent—are exposed to adult pressures and are at risk of becoming overburdened (i.e., **parentified**). Parentified children can feel so much pressure that they struggle to recognize and advocate for their own needs, miss out on parental guidance and mentorship, can come across to others as aggressive or arrogant, and struggle with the inconsistency of being treated as an adult at home but a child at school.[8]

How Do External Contexts Impact Families With Single-Parenthood Stressors?

Parent and child **gender** can contribute to some distinct single-parent family processes or risk factors.[9] Given that most single-parent households are led by mothers, one might suspect that sons and daughters have somewhat different experiences in such homes. Indeed, **daughters** of absent and low-invested fathers are especially at greater risk for earlier age of sexual intercourse, teen pregnancy, and a higher number of sexual partners. They tend to have more negative attitudes about men, see men as less reliable, and are less interested in forming committed relationships with men. Single mothers, on average, indicate spending more time with and feeling more warmth toward their daughters than their sons, who can be at greater risk for parentification associated with emotional support and communication.

Sons raised in single-mother households can be thought of as "the man of the house" and be at risk for parentification involving instrumental tasks and support. They are more likely to be diagnosed with attention deficit hyperactivity disorder, act out in school, be suspended, have lower grade point averages, and not go to college (when compared to children in two-parent homes and girls from single-parent homes). Differences in educational outcomes between boys and girls with single mothers might be at least partially due to girls in general being better readers and having fewer behavioral problems and thus more able to navigate classroom expectations even with less parental involvement. Because single-parent households tend to cluster in the same (more affordable) neighborhoods, boys are less likely to have mentoring and role modeling from men who otherwise can help them be more resilient.

The distribution of single-parent families varies dramatically by **ethnic group** in the United States: 64% of Black children, 52% of Native American children, 42% of Hispanic children, 24% of White children, and 15% of Asian and Pacific Islander children live with a single parent.[10] Risk factors of single-parent families are generally similar across ethnic groups, though some argue that the risks to minority children (especially Black children) raised by single parents are smaller than they are for White children raised by single parents, perhaps because Black children are more used to childhood stressors.[11] For example, college graduation rates are similar for Black children regardless of family structure (though high school graduation rates are lower for Black children than White children from single-parent households). Black and Hispanic families tend to lean on extended family or other family-like figures for support, which could counter some of the challenges of single-parent households.

Only about 20% of single-parent households with children under age 18 are led by a **father**.[12] Such households tend to be wealthier than single-mother households (e.g., about half as likely to be in poverty). Child outcomes are generally similar for single-father and single-mother households, though some evidence shows that children in single-father households are at greater risk for externalizing behaviors and substance use. Most of the research on single fathers is dated, however, and contemporary changes to gendered expectations for parents could contribute to unforeseen differences or similarities in the future.

Improve Your Learning

Without peeking, take a moment to review in your mind (or say out loud) the key concepts from this chapter (this is a proven learning technique). Then review the "Chapter Preview" section at the top and compare. Skim Part A of the chapter with extra attention to the **bolded words**. Skip to the end of the chapter to find more learning resources.

Part B. Family Structure Transitions and Complexity Stressors

How Do Family Transitions Influence Family Stress?

Recall in Part A we considered that changes to family structure pressure a family to adjust its patterns, and that such adjustments can be disorienting and take time to establish. Frequent **transitions** can make it difficult for a family to ever fully adjust to changes in family patterns and routines—kind of like having to quickly learn new languages with little time to master any of them. Transitions can contribute to greater financial problems, harsher parental discipline, child aggression, and other externalization problems, school difficulties, and more family moves (moving can interfere with having friends and keeping up in school).[13] Besides the pressures that come with forming and losing relationships, children are potentially exposed to multiple adults who apparently struggle to maintain long-term couple relationships, and such parental figures might not model ideal relationship skills.

We noted that transitions that involve the subtraction of parental figures, or at least a major decrease in involvement or presence, can contribute to difficult attachment and trust-building processes, especially for children. Interrelationships among all family members can change dramatically when relationships between parents or parental figures change or dissolve. Whether it be between unmarried or formerly cohabiting parents—one or both of whom head a single-parent household—or divorced parents, the subtraction of a parent from a household is typically a major stressor. Similarly, heavily cutting back on contact with a now nonresidential parent can threaten the parent-child relationship.

Continuing to co-parent after the couple separates has some unique challenges that can also test a family's resilience. Of course, some of the difficulties that come with a transition are created by problematic family relationships and circumstances that led to the transition (e.g., a conflicted marriage leading to divorce). Sometimes the circumstances after the transition are much healthier than those before the transition, though the transition itself has its own challenges. In this next section, we focus more on transitions that involve the **subtraction of a residential parent** such as through a divorce or other breakup—referred to as **relationship dissolution** (RD).

What Is Stressful About Parental RD?
Virtually everyone knows that divorce has been common in the last several decades. Nonmarital cohabiting relationships have become more normative but tend to last even shorter than marriages. Some single parents dissolve relationships with individuals who play a parental role of some sort for a time. If you have ever broken up with somebody or lost a connection to a close family member, you can probably relate to the idea that **RD** can be emotionally painful. Even when it is clearly the best decision for an individual or family, the emotional, psychological, and instrumental interdependency we create in relationships can make us **vulnerable** to feeling lonely, insecure, and fragile, at least for a time.

Children, depending on their ability to understand and make sense of the missing or relocated parent, can struggle with interpreting and expressing their feelings. Other RD pressures for children could come from the following:

- Blaming themselves for the relationship change and carrying the burden of guilt for years to come
- Feeling abandoned and wondering who will desert them next, causing them to be extra clingy or to act out in ways to test their parents' commitment to them
- Being used as a go-between for their co-parenting communication and frustration
- Receiving less optimal parenting and additional parentification when separating parents experience mental health problems (something they are at greater risk for)
- Losing quality interaction with a parent (and potentially grandparents and other extended family members), thus being denied any benefits that come from such relationships

Overall, children who have experienced parental divorce (or similar RD) are generally at **increased risk** for various internalizing and externalizing behavior problems, academic challenges, risk-taking behaviors (e.g., early sex and substance problems), and relationship problems.

Children with **siblings** prior to RD can experience some unique risk and protective factors with the transition.[14] Siblings potentially understand better than anyone else what the other is going through and have someone to connect with when parents are preoccupied. Sibling relationships can thus become closer through such a bond, but they can also increase in conflict when children exhibit bothersome externalizing behavior as they cope with the RD. Some siblings unite over a common cause, such as vilifying the parent they perceive as being at fault for the RD or a potential stepparent viewed as breaking up the family or playing favorites toward their own children. Older siblings sometimes filter information for younger siblings—help spare them from more traumatic details, help distract younger children from focusing on their loss, and provide instrumental support. However, as noted, such children are at risk for parentification stress.

Applying the **FSS integrated model (FIM) of family stress and crisis framework** to families experiencing RD can give us a sense of why children might be more apt to struggle in such situations. RD would be a sign that a family has reached **crisis** (all members' needs are not met through typical coping processes), and unresolved stressors continue to **pile up** while in crisis. For example, financial stressors or witnessing interpersonal violence can continue to impact family members after a divorce. What other examples come to your mind? Additionally, stressors owing to the divorce transition itself add to the pileup, like potentially moving, having fewer people to share household tasks, having less access to a parent, and restructuring family patterns in light of an absent family member (at least from the household). **Adjustment coping** requires additional effort, patience, and probably compromise. Some of what was mentioned as stressors for single-parent families also apply to RD.

What Are Some Stressful Decisions Regarding RD?

From a parent's perspective, deciding whether to separate can be very challenging. It is common to have mixed feelings, and being unable to restore a previously satisfying relationship can be painful. As discussed in Chapter 7, even in cases of interpersonal abuse, the decision to leave a relationship can be complicated, especially when the relationship had positive qualities and the alternatives to staying seem worse. **Second-guessing** the decisions also adds pressure to the experience. Struggling with regret can lead to self-blame, especially if children appear to suffer from the experience—*Did I make the wrong decision because of my own stubbornness?* Family and friends aren't always supportive of whatever decision is made, which can diminish much-needed social support and confidence. What else might make such a decision difficult?

Deciding if, when, and how to **tell children about RD** is often stressful and the manner in which it happens can impact children in various ways.[15] Imagine if an affair was the reason for a divorce—at what age is a child old enough to hear such information, if ever? What about hidden abuse, mental illness, or addiction problems? Children exposed to developmentally inappropriate information could suffer undue psychological stress and might unfairly vilify one or both parents. How many parents really know the best way to disclose this information to avoid as much misunderstanding and pain as possible?

Young children especially can be caught off guard by RD. Many children don't find out about a divorce until the day the parents separate, and some are told alternative stories about a parent's absence that makes little sense to the children. Older siblings are more often told the truth and take on part of the responsibility of obscuring the facts for younger siblings. Adults who experienced parental divorce in their childhood have suggested that

- parents jointly tell their children about the divorce with maturity and calmness,
- both adults take responsibility for contributing to relationship problems,
- children have an opportunity to express themselves and ask questions, and
- children need help to feel secure, know that the divorce is not their fault, and understand what to expect in the divorce process.

Consider the pressures that occur when such advice is not followed. Overall, children have reported a variety of emotional responses to the news, sometimes with mixed feelings, particularly when they get relief from high conflict but will also miss frequent interaction with each parent.

How Can Boundary Ambiguity Contribute to RD Stress?

RD can also trigger high levels of **boundary ambiguity**, especially given the **mismatch** between the psychological and physical presences in the home, which creates confusion and uncertainty. For example, consider the following:

- A father moving out after a divorce still has a psychological presence in the family and home—he is still a child's parent and the adult's co-parent and is likely in the hearts and minds of those still in the home even though his physical presence has changed.
- A mother who remains in the home might still feel emotionally connected to the father, especially if she had not wanted to divorce.
- As they work to co-parent the children, the separating couple might still feel like spouses in some ways but not in other ways, creating uncertainty about who they really are to

one another. The mother will also need to adjust her roles around the house while the father adjusts his parent identity to suit his nonresidential location; if the couple can't stand to be around one another, they might have to figure out how to parent the children while avoiding the other parent.

- Children have to adjust their expectations of what it means to be a father if he doesn't live there anymore and what it means to have their parents have some kind of ongoing relationship that is different from before. Though some children feel relief after a highly hostile marriage ends, most if not all children arguably prefer that their parents happily stay together and have a well-defined, harmonious family household.

The challenges associated with this boundary mismatch can make the reorganization of the family structure and parenting more difficult.[16] While divorce has become common, there is no clear set of accepted **norms** to follow to manage the transition and establish a new structure. Defining what it means to be a divorced spouse/parent takes time. Strong emotions, incompatible expectations, limits to communication, and jealousy can complicate working through the ambiguity. **Disagreement** over child support and custody issues, including friction over how the parents use their time with the children, can slow the process of minimizing boundary ambiguity and expose children to toxic interactions between parents. Money is also a touchy subject, and some separated parents might be reluctant to help pay for an additional living space or for the other parent's expenses. Some noncustodial parents don't want to financially support a home that includes children that they rarely get to see.

In-depth interviews with divorced adults highlight some likely stressors that occur for parents while they navigate boundary ambiguity during the transition from marriage to single parenthood.[17] Findings suggested the following:

- Divorce can seem like a personal failure and can lead to feeling discouraged, isolated, and brokenhearted.
- Divorced parents can feel uninvited to socialize with married people, struggle with a clear sense of identity, lose support from a partner and partner's social system, and lose friendships (some friends were seemingly stressed about having to choose sides, so they avoided the former spouses altogether).
- The loss of social support particularly pressured mothers to lean more on their children for comfort and motivation.
- Postdivorce adjustment can include a "hazy period" that is highly unstructured, chaotic, and overwhelming. Parents are uncertain about how they would get by as single parents, and the details of this period can be difficult to remember or seem hazy.
- After initial adjustments, custodial parents establish new routines to at least temporarily counter the early chaos and ambiguity. Some parents embrace an independent approach to parenting, while others surround their family with supportive individuals to share some of the parenting roles.
- Eventually, adjustments can become more sustainable by aligning work and family roles and creating major routines to guide family patterns.

Well-adjusted families create a new **homeostasis** and **acceptance** of their realities and find reasons for contentment and hope. Though parents have stated the necessity of changing some of their values and belief systems to make the new lifestyle work for them, doing so commonly felt preferable to remaining in their prior marriage.

What Is Stressful About Transitions Involving Adding Family Members?

The addition of family members through new relationship formation also requires changes to the family system and household routines. From never-partnered single parenthood to cohabitation or marriage, or from post-RD single parenthood to remarriage/re-partnering, parents and children face the pressures of getting to know someone new in their lives, sometimes begrudgingly. Such transitions often produce diverse types of sibling relationships or **sibling complexity**. **Stepsibling** identities form when children from prior relationships are brought into the same family through a new couple relationship. Typically, a divorce and then remarriage to someone who already has children would be the key path to this arrangement, though high rates of cohabitation and never-married single parents add to diverse ways of forming such relationships. **Half-siblings**, on the other hand, share one biological parent and commonly result from parental RD followed by one or both parents having a biological child with a different partner.

About 12% of children in the United States live with a step- or half-sibling, and about 30% of remarried stepfamilies include both spouses having children from prior relationships.[18] Children in stepfamilies and children born to cohabiting parents (compared to married parents) are more likely to experience sibling complexity. Similar to single-parent and divorced-parent households, children who experience sibling complexity—many or most of whom will have transitioned from a single-parent or divorced household—are generally at higher risk for behavior problems (e.g., internalizing, externalizing, delinquency, aggression), poorer educational achievement, and substance use problems.[19] Both the stressors of former family transitions and the stressors of living in a family that has sibling complexity likely contribute to the elevated risk for negative outcomes.

What Is Risky About Sibling Complexity?

So, someone has a half- or stepsibling—big deal, right? Of course, it may not be a big deal at all, and such siblings can be important sources of support. However, if we think about the fact that the presence of step- or half-siblings indicates that families have undergone stressful relationship transitions and that families that include sibling complexity have some additional ... complexity, we might suspect that the children in such families face challenges that test their resilience. For example, additional pressures come from having a new residential parent figure, especially when that person is in some way replacing some functions of someone who has since left the household.

A new residential stepparent also faces **boundary ambiguity** that is amplified by having an unclear psychological presence in the home that might compete with the psychological presence of the nonresidential biological parent. Furthermore, it takes time and effort to determine whether the new parent figure should act more like a parent, friend, or mere acquaintance to each child in the household—potentially having a different role for each child. The new parent figure might also have children from a prior relationship, and each of the biological parents might produce more children, adding further complexity toward establishing clear boundaries and expectations for these various interconnected lives.

Table 8.1 includes a compilation of explanations that help account for the somewhat unique risk factors associated with sibling complexity.[20] Several common conceptual explanations provide general frameworks for interpreting family processes likely to result from sibling complexity. Some of the processes could be compatible with more than one explanation. The last column provides examples of how the family processes could contribute to negative family or child outcomes. Take some time to come up with some of your own ideas or observations that could be added to the table, particularly the last column.

TABLE 8.1 Conceptualizations of Sibling Complexity Risk Factors

Conceptual Explanation	Concepts	Family Processes	Family/Child Outcomes
Disruption	Disrupt equilibrium	Must create new patterns for family unit.	Lose sense of predictability.
	Diminished parenting	Parental depression is more common in complex family structures.	Children get less attention.
	Father involvement	Drops off when either partner re-partners, can feel pressure from current partner to focus on residential children over nonresidential children.	Children have fewer tangible and intangible resources.
	Co-parenting	Disagreements over parenting styles and involvement among three or more parent figures.	Exposure to conflict.
	New parent	Imposes rules or values on stepchildren, personality differences, excludes stepchildren in family events (preferential treatment or ignoring children's preferences).	Children resent new parent and stepsiblings.
Biology/ Evolution	Parental investment/ favoritism	Natural tendency to invest more in own biological child (maintain own biological family line).	Creates inequality among children and households.
	Sibling competition	Naturally have more conflict when they don't share (or share less) biology.	Sibling conflict adds to a hostile family environment.
Stress	Pileup	Transitions and adjustments cumulate (e.g., divorce, remarriage).	At risk of becoming overwhelmed with strains.
	Resources	Stepfamilies tend to be larger and experience more economic strain.	Resources/attention spread thinner for each child.
	Relationships	More subsystems (e.g. stepparent and child; stepchild, parent, and stepparent) for negotiating over space, privacy, and communication issues.	Strain from relational challenges.

(Continued)

Conceptual Explanation	Concepts	Family Processes	Family/Child Outcomes
Boundary Ambiguity	Few norms	Stepfamilies have fewer established norms to follow.	Uncertainty about roles and relationship expectations.
	Competing presences	Psychological presences of nonresidential parent and stepparent.	Feeling compared to nonresidential biological parent.
	Multipartner fertility	Addressing needs of children in multiple households.	Disparity of attention and resources across children.
	Unfamiliarity	New parent entering home that has established routines and relationships.	Difficulty for new parent to fit in.
	Quick transition	Stepsiblings lack a shared history, must quickly adapt to one another.	Relationship may feel forced.
	Support diminishes	Mother's family support drops off when she has a child with a new partner.	Feelings of isolation.
	Jealousy	Between biological parents, stepparents and biological parents, stepparents and extended family, and stepparents and stepchildren.	Makes communication in the family more difficult.
	Awkwardness	Watching biological parent connecting with stepchildren.	Questioning loyalty.
Residency	Paternal investment	Nonresidential fathers invest less in complex families.	Less access to father figure.
	Changing locations	Child living in two different households with different rules, roles, boundaries, and relationships.	Inconsistency of parenting.
	Visitation issues	Older children may prefer staying home with friends instead of visiting nonresidential parent on weekend.	Feeling resentment from child and/or nonresidential parent.
	Caught in the middle	Child exposed to hostility between nonresidential parent and residential parent (including the stepparent).	Feeling responsible for smoothing out relationships.

Adapted from: Brown, S. L., Manning, W. D., & Stykes, J. B. (2015). Family structure and child well-being: Integrating family complexity. *Journal of Marriage and Family, 77*(1), 177–190. https://doi-org.proxy.bsu.edu/10.1111/jomf.12145; Degreeff, B. L., & Platt, C. A. (2016). Green-eyed (step) monsters: Parental figures' perceptions of jealousy in the stepfamily. *Journal of Divorce and Remarriage, 57*, 112–132. https://doi.org/10.1080/10502556.2015.1127876; Kinniburgh-White, R., Cartwright, C., & Seymour, F. (2010). Young adults' narratives of relational development with stepfathers. *Journal of Social and Personal Relationships, 27*(7), 890–907. https://doi.org/10.1177/0265407510376252; National Council on Family Relations. (n.d.). Family focus. https://www.ncfr.org/ncfr-report/focus; Sanner, C., & Jensen, T. M. (2021). Toward more accurate measures of family structure: Accounting for sibling complexity. *Journal of Family Theory & Review, 13*(1), 110–127. https://doi-org.proxy.bsu.edu/10.1111/jftr.12406; Schrodt, P. (2016). Coparental communication with nonresidential parents as a predictor of children's feelings of being caught in stepfamilies. *Communication Reports, 29*(2), 63–74. https://doi.org/10.1080/08934215.2015.1020562

As a reminder, many families and children are **resilient** and avoid major negative outcomes. And, having additional adults around—when able to support one another and avoid creating drama—can be an asset to families. Sometimes children respond better to a stepparent who has more of a friend-like relationship when addressing emotionally charged topics like dating and career choices than they would to biological parents.

How Do External Contexts Impact Families With Transition and Complexity Stressors?

A child's **age** appears to contribute to the stressful effects of RD.[21] Generally speaking, children who are younger at the time of the transition appear to be more vulnerable to negative outcomes. This could be due to spending more of their lives in a complex family structure, developmental limits to processing and making sense of their circumstances, or a lesser ability to clearly and directly communicate their needs. Speaking of age, married adults over the age of 55 have been divorcing at record-high rates.[22] With an increasing life expectancy and cultural values that promote personal gratification, older people appear less willing to remain in unsatisfying marriages. Consequently, more families are likely exposed to additional transitions and complexity in the form of multiple in-law and stepgrandparent relationships.

Gender also appears relevant to the impact of transitions and complexity.[23] Girls appear to have more negative outcomes from divorce, on average, including intimate relationship problems. For adults whose parents had divorced, women seem especially prone to struggle with confidence in their own marriages. For adults who themselves have experience RD, men seem especially prone to isolate themselves and to use substances as a coping mechanism (which could have implications for nonresidential father involvement). Stepmothers tend to have more depression and anxiety compared to biological mothers and more stress compared to stepfathers. Any thoughts as to why?

Sibling complexity and stepfamily transitions also appear to vary by **ethnicity**.[24] Black residents, followed by Hispanic residents of the United States, are more likely than White residents to have a step- or half-sibling (available data from Pew shows the percentages to be 45%, 38%, and 26%, respectively, in 2010). Black and Hispanic families are somewhat more likely to end in divorce than White families (a disparity typically attributed by scholars to **minority stress/poverty**). Scholars suggest, however, that racial minority families, especially Black families, are more accustomed to having nonrelated parenting figures involved with raising children, making transitions and sibling complexity less of a new adjustment for such families. A sizable proportion of Black stepfamilies are actually formed by the mother's first marriage, but not to the biological father of her children. Thus, stressors associated with a longer history of single parenthood tend to be especially relevant to Black stepfamilies. Black stepfathers also appear to back off and yield more to biological mothers in times of parental discipline, which might contribute to some unique elements of boundary ambiguity.

Same-sex couples with children typically include sibling complexity and are thus arguably similar to male-female stepfamilies, with both family types having experienced similar kinds of transitions. Specifically, in the case that children were at least partially raised by a mother and father, the family structure change to same-sex parents could require some unique adjustments and expectations. Same-sex couples also experience RD and re-partnering, and even fewer social norms exist for same-sex stepfamilies than male-female stepfamilies. They are also at greater risk for confronting challenges related to **minority stress** (e.g., stigma), and negative attitudes toward same-sex unions held by the nonresidential parent could also put same-sex stepfamilies at risk for relational conflict.

What Does All This Mean for You?

Your insights can be valuable to your personal life, your family relationships, and your professional roles. Take a few moments to ponder the following:

- How have you been feeling while engaging with this information? Why?
- How much of this topic can you personally relate to?
- Did you grow up around others who experienced family complexity stressors? What did you observe about them?
- What opinions do you have about single parenthood or divorce that might differ from other peoples' opinions?
- What other examples have come to mind that illustrate similar or diverse ways that families cope with family structural complexity stressors?

Reminders for Helpers

As a person of influence, you can help guide people through the coping processes and ideally help foster a **flourishing** life. However, take care to avoid letting your personal **interpretations** push you toward assuming too much about somebody else's circumstances, perceptions, and motivations. Always be ready to address issues that might be hard for you to face because of your own history.

Draw upon the elements of the **FIM framework** and other family stress concepts. Remember, **coping** refers to an action or response based on available or new resources and perceptions related to stressors. Families have either successfully **managed** a stressor's pressure through **adjustment coping** or reached crisis in which **adaptive coping** is needed to reestablish some level of **general family functioning**. **Resources** and **perceptions** are key concepts to focus on when confronting family stress. **Review the master table** in Chapter 4 as a guide for exploring the following ideas on how to help families with stressors.

What Are Some Ways to Encourage Effective Family Coping?

Drawing primarily from citations and insights noted in the chapter thus far, we will explore **suggested resources and noteworthy perceptions** that can contribute to successful coping and more optimal family functioning.

How Can You Help With Family Structure Complexity Stressors?

Single-parent families can benefit from plenty of social and emotional support, particularly in helping parents gain confidence and increase self-efficacy. By helping cultivate perceptions of having more control over their lives, single parents likely cope more actively with their circumstances and strengthen family functioning. Additionally, helping single parents identify and minimize potential parentification of their children can ease children's burdens.

As families transition to the **subtraction** of a household partner/parent through RD, some key things families could use help with could include the following[25]:

- Establishing a workable structure, including rules, roles, boundaries, and routines that might involve multiple households.
- Separating their former marital roles from current co-parental roles; this could mean letting go of the past and constructing new ways of thinking about a former partner to achieve harmonious co-parenting.
- Attending to diverse meanings and interpretations of the transition across different family members, finding ways to honor divergent perceptions while addressing misunderstandings.
- Learning to regulate hostile emotions toward a former partner and curtailing aggressive or passive-aggressive behavior toward the partner, especially in front of children; learning to anticipate what will trigger negative emotions or behavior and preparing to respond in a more helpful way.
- Improving parenting skills, particularly in light of trying to parent through and after the transition.
- Fostering a new, satisfying identity as a single or nonresidential parent.
- Focusing on the future after establishing initial stability and not getting stuck in a state of constant adjustment without long-term goals.

Some of what has already been mentioned also applies to the complexity that increases when **adding** members to the family and household. Some additional key things families could use help with could include the following[26]:

- Accepting that having challenging transitions and circumstances is normal for stepfamilies
- Finding ways to hand off children for visitation, such as neutral places that don't evoke strong reactions from either parent
- Learning to negotiate patterns and routines across two households, likely requiring compromise and altered expectations
- Nourishing new subsystem relationships, such as a remarriage and stepparent/stepchild relationships
- Adjusting perceptions to think of new people as true family members; doing so tends to promote more positive attitudes and behavior toward one another

- Developing greater empathy for what others in the family are going through; doing so can foster more patience and understanding
- Becoming more flexible with parenting approaches to facilitate adjusting to changes and complexity as needed; this might include more of a team approach of three or more parental figures

Improve Your Learning

Without peeking, take a moment to review in your mind (or say out loud) the key concepts from this chapter (this is a proven learning technique). Then review the "Chapter Preview" section at the top and compare. Skim Part B of the chapter with extra attention to the **bolded words**.

Do You Want to Learn More?

We have only touched on a portion of information related to some elements of this topic. **What really sparked your interest? What do you wish was covered more thoroughly?** Consider taking some time to further deepen your understanding of personal and professional issues related to helping families cope with stressors. The following are a variety of resources that you might find helpful and some references directly or indirectly referred to in this chapter. Go for it—add more structure to your study habits.

Videos

(Use links or do searches with the key words provided)
- I Am Tired of Being a Single Mom … (21 mins). Mary Gissell Barahona. https://www.youtube.com/watch?v=feuOKrKOZU4
- How Do Children Cope With Divorce? A Journey Through the Kid's Eyes (55 mins). Real Families. https://www.youtube.com/watch?v=CvHML5NmloM
- The Impact of Divorce on Children: Tamara D. Afifi (20 mins). TEDxUCSB. https://www.youtube.com/watch?v=cKcNyfXbQzQ
- Step-Kids, Family Boundaries and Stress-Eating (first 20 mins). *The Dr. John Delony Show.* https://www.youtube.com/watch?v=lvA2q9C9cPM
- Parents Tell Stepparents What They Really Think (6 mins). Participant. https://www.youtube.com/watch?v=v8Ffgctm3zQ
- The Dos and Don'ts of Stepparenting (4 mins). *The Real Daytime.* https://www.youtube.com/watch?v=uxOyc_EV-QY

Websites

- Hymowitz, K. (2020, August 4). Disentangling the effects of family structure on boys and girls. Institute for Family Studies. https://ifstudies.org/blog/disentangling-the-effects-of-family-structure-on-boys-and-girls
- The Annie E. Casey Foundation. (n.d.). Kids count data center: Children in single-parent families by race in the United States (2019). https://datacenter.kidscount.org/data/tables/107-children-in-single-parent-families-by-race#detailed/1/any/false/1729,37,871,870,573,869,36,868,867,133/10,11,9,12,1,185,13/432,431
- U.S. Census Bureau. (2022, March 21). National Single Parent Day: March 21, 2022. https://www.census.gov/newsroom/stories/single-parent-day.html

Readings (Articles, Books, Book Chapters)

- Brown, S. L., Manning, W. D., & Stykes, J. B. (2015). Family structure and child well-being: Integrating family complexity. *Journal of Marriage and Family, 77*(1), 177–190. https://doi-org.proxy.bsu.edu/10.1111/jomf.12145
- Carroll, J. S., Olson, C. D., & Buckmiller, N. (2007). Family boundary ambiguity: A 30-year review of theory, research, and measurement. *Family Relations, 56*(2), 210–230. https://doi-org.proxy.bsu.edu/10.1111/j.1741-3729.2007.00453.x
- Fomby, P., & Osborne, C. (2017). Family instability, multipartner fertility, and behavior in middle childhood. *Journal of Marriage and Family, 79*(1), 75–93.
- Sanner, C., & Jensen, T. M. (2021). Toward more accurate measures of family structure: Accounting for sibling complexity. *Journal of Family Theory & Review, 13*(1), 110–127. https://doi-org.proxy.bsu.edu/10.1111/jftr.12406
- Van Gasse, D., & Mortelmans, D. (2020). Reorganizing the single-parent family system: Exploring the process perspective on divorce. *Family Relations, 69*, 1100–1112. https://doi.org/10.1111/fare.12432

Notes

1 Pew Research Center. (2011, January 3). A portrait of stepfamilies. https://www.pewresearch.org/social-trends/2011/01/13/a-portrait-of-stepfamilies/

2 Boss, P. (2002). *Family stress management: A contextual approach.* SAGE Publications; Carroll, J. S., Olson, C. D., & Buckmiller, N. (2007). Family boundary ambiguity: A 30-year review of theory, research, and measurement. *Family Relations, 56*(2), 210–230. https://doi-org.proxy.bsu.edu/10.1111/j.1741-3729.2007.00453.x

3 Beckmeyer, J. J., Krejnick, S. J., McCray, J. A., Troilo, J., & Markham, M. S. (2021). A multidimensional perspective on former spouses' ongoing relationships: Associations with children's postdivorce well-being. *Family Relations, 70*(2), 467–482. https://doi-org.proxy.bsu.edu/10.1111/fare.12504; National Council on Family Relations. (n.d.). Family focus. https://www.ncfr.org/ncfr-report/focus

4 Zill, N. (2021, June 18). Growing up with mom and dad: New data confirm the tide is turning. Institute for Family Studies. https://ifstudies.org/blog/growing-up-with-mom-and-dad-new-data-confirm-the-tide-is-turning

5   Baer, D. (2020, January 23). American men are getting less marriageable—here's why. *Business Insider*. https://www.businessinsider.com/why-american-men-are-getting-less-marriageable-2018-1

6   Jones, J. M. (2020, December 28). Is marriage becoming irrelevant? Gallup. https://news.gallup.com/poll/316223/fewer-say-important-parents-married.aspx?_hsmi=2&_hsenc=p2ANqtz--5GObG0WBgHQEsNH6VJubyaDVs-TyDwCVHbwkFumRT4yJpRbto7-N4J-TzP8l-01T78RkaL-9dHQcK0n5nsqbSezvmstCTAa8k2pyee9RbXJ6CT6qU

7   DelPriore, D. J., Shakiba, N., Schlomer, G. L., Hill, S. E., & Ellis, B. J. (2019). The effects of fathers on daughters' expectations for men. *Developmental Psychology, 55*(7), 1523–1536. https://doi.org/10.1037/dev0000741.supp; Jackson, A. P., Choi, J., & Franke, T. M. (2009). Poor single mothers with young children: Mastery, relations with nonresident fathers, and child outcomes. *Social Work Research, 33*(2), 95–106. https://doi.org/10.1093/swr/33.2.95; Sieh, D. S., Visser-Meily, J. M. A., & Meijer, A. M. (2013). The relationship between parental depressive symptoms, family type, and adolescent functioning. *PLoS ONE, 8*(11). https://doi.org/10.1371/journal.pone.0080699; Nixon, E., Greene, S., & Hogan, D. M. (2012). Negotiating relationships in single-mother households: Perspectives of children and mothers. *Family Relations, 61*(1), 142–156. https://doi.org/10.1111/j.1741-3729.2011.00678.x; Nixon, E., Greene, S., & Hogan, D. (2015). "It's what's normal for me": Children's experiences of growing up in a continuously single-parent household. *Journal of Family Issues, 36*(8), 1043–1061. https://doi.org/10.1177/0192513X13494826

8   Burton, L. M. (2007). Childhood adultification in economically disadvantaged families: A conceptual model. *Family Relations*, 56, 329–345. https://doi.org/10.1111/j.1741-3729.2007.00463.x

9   Cole, R. L. (2015). Single-father families: A review of the literature. *Journal of Family Theory & Review, 7*(2), 144–166. https://doi.org/10.1111/jftr.12069; DelPriore, D. J., Shakiba, N., Schlomer, G. L., Hill, S. E., & Ellis, B. J. (2019). The effects of fathers on daughters' expectations for men. *Developmental Psychology, 55*(7), 1523–1536. https://doi-org.proxy.bsu.edu/10.1037/dev0000741.supp; Hymowitz, K. (2020, August 4). Disentangling the effects of family structure on boys and girls. Institute for Family Studies. https://ifstudies.org/blog/disentangling-the-effects-of-family-structure-on-boys-and-girls

10   The Annie E. Casey Foundation (n.d.). Kids count data center: Children in single-parent families by race in the United States (2019). https://datacenter.kidscount.org/data/tables/107-children-in-single-parent-families-by-race#detailed/1/any/false/1729,37,871,870,573,869,36,868,867,133/10,11,9,12,1,185,13/432,431

11   Cross, K. (2020). Racial/ethnic differences in the association between family structure and children's education. *Journal of Marriage and Family, 82*, 691–712. https://doi.org/10.1111/jomf.12625

12   Cole, R. L. (2015). Single-father families: A review of the literature. *Journal of Family Theory & Review, 7*(2), 144–166. https://doi.org/10.1111/jftr.12069; U.S. Census Bureau (2022, March 21). National Single Parent Day: March 21, 2022. https://www.census.gov/newsroom/stories/single-parent-day.html

13   Brown, S. L., Manning, W. D., & Stykes, J. B. (2015). Family structure and child well-being: Integrating family complexity. *Journal of Marriage and Family, 77*(1), 177–190. https://doi-org.proxy.bsu.edu/10.1111/jomf.12145; Fomby, P., & Osborne, C. (2017). Family instability, multipartner fertility, and behavior in middle childhood. *Journal of Marriage and Family, 79*(1), 75–93. https://doi-org.proxy.bsu.edu/10.1111/jomf.12349; Sanner, C., & Jensen, T. M. (2021). Toward more accurate measures of family structure: Accounting for sibling complexity. *Journal of Family Theory & Review, 13*(1), 110–127. https://doi-org.proxy.bsu.edu/10.1111/jftr.12406

14   Chapman, F. S. (2022, March 13). Siblings may grow closer when parents divorce: Siblings are the only constant in divorce and often grow closer in the upheaval. https://www.psychologytoday.com/gb/blog/brothers-sisters-strangers/202203/siblings-may-grow-closer-when-parents-divorce; Jacobs, K., & Sillars, A. (2012). Sibling support during post-divorce adjustment: An idiographic analysis of support forms, functions, and relationship types. *Journal of Family Communication, 12*(2), 167–187. https://doi-org.proxy.bsu.edu/10.1080/15267431.2011.584056

15   Cohen, O., Leichtentritt, R. D., & Volpin, N. (2014). Divorced mothers' self-perception of their divorce-related communication with their children. *Child & Family Social Work, 19*(1), 34–43. https://doi.org/10.1111/j.1365-2206.2012.00878.x; Westberg, H., Nelson, T. S., & Piercy, K. W. (2002). Disclosure of divorce plans to children: What the children have to say. *Contemporary Family Therapy: An International Journal, 24*(4), 525–542. https://doi.org/10.1023/A:1021271411917

16   Beckmeyer, J. J., Krejnick, S. J., McCray, J. A., Troilo, J., & Markham, M. S. (2021). A multidimensional perspective on former spouses' ongoing relationships: Associations with children's postdivorce well-being. *Family Relations, 70*(2), 467–482. https://doi-org.proxy.bsu.edu/10.1111/fare.12504; Carroll, J. S., Olson, C. D., & Buckmiller, N.

(2007). Family boundary ambiguity: A 30-year review of theory, research, and measurement. *Family Relations*, 56(2), 210–230. https://doi-org.proxy.bsu.edu/10.1111/j.1741-3729.2007.00453.x; Moore, E. (2016). Delaying divorce: Pitfalls of restrictive divorce requirements. *Journal of Family Issues*, 37(16), 2265–2293. https://doi-org.proxy.bsu.edu/10.1177/0192513X14566620

17 Van Gasse, D., & Mortelmans, D. (2020). Reorganizing the single-parent family system: Exploring the process perspective on divorce. *Family Relations*, 69, 1100–1112. https://doi.org/10.1111/fare.12432; Thomas, C., & Ryan, M. (2008). Women's perception of the divorce experience: A qualitative study. *Journal of Divorce & Remarriage*, 49(3–4), 210–224. https://doi.org/10.1080/10502550802222394

18 Brown, S. L., Manning, W. D., & Stykes, J. B. (2015). Family structure and child well-being: Integrating family complexity. *Journal of Marriage and Family*, 77(1), 177–190. https://doi-org.proxy.bsu.edu/10.1111/jomf.12145; Stykes, B., & Guzzo, K. B. (2015). FP-15-10 *Remarriage & stepfamilies*. National Center for Family and Marriage Research Family Profiles. 75. https://scholarworks.bgsu.edu/ncfmr_family_profiles/75

19 Fomby, P., & Osborne, C. (2017). Family instability, multipartner fertility, and behavior in middle childhood. *Journal of Marriage and Family*, 79(1), 75–93. https://doi-org.proxy.bsu.edu/10.1111/jomf.12349; Sanner, C., & Jensen, T. M. (2021). Toward more accurate measures of family structure: Accounting for sibling complexity. *Journal of Family Theory & Review*, 13(1), 110–127. https://doi-org.proxy.bsu.edu/10.1111/jftr.12406

20 Brown, S. L., Manning, W. D., & Stykes, J. B. (2015). Family structure and child well-being: Integrating family complexity. *Journal of Marriage and Family*, 77(1), 177–190. https://doi-org.proxy.bsu.edu/10.1111/jomf.12145; Degreeff, B. L., & Platt, C. A. (2016). Green-eyed (step) monsters: Parental figures' perceptions of jealousy in the stepfamily. *Journal of Divorce and Remarriage*, 57, 112–132. https://doi.org/10.1080/10502556.2015.1127876; Kinniburgh-White, R., Cartwright, C., & Seymour, F. (2010). Young adults' narratives of relational development with stepfathers. *Journal of Social and Personal Relationships*, 27(7), 890–907. https://doi.org/10.1177/0265407510376252; National Council on Family Relations. (n.d.). Family focus. https://www.ncfr.org/ncfr-report/focus; Sanner, C., & Jensen, T. M. (2021). Toward more accurate measures of family structure: Accounting for sibling complexity. *Journal of Family Theory & Review*, 13(1), 110–127. https://doi-org.proxy.bsu.edu/10.1111/jftr.12406; Schrodt, P. (2016). Coparental communication with nonresidential parents as a predictor of children's feelings of being caught in stepfamilies. *Communication Reports, 29*(2), 63–74. https://doi.org/10.1080/08934215.2015.1020562;

21 Beckmeyer, J. J., Krejnick, S. J., McCray, J. A., Troilo, J., & Markham, M. S. (2021). A multidimensional perspective on former spouses' ongoing relationships: Associations with children's postdivorce well-being. *Family Relations*, 70(2), 467–482. https://doi-org.proxy.bsu.edu/10.1111/fare.12504; Windle, M., & Windle, R. C. (2018). Parental divorce and family history of alcohol disorder: Associations with young adults' alcohol problems, marijuana use, and interpersonal relations. *Alcoholism: Clinical and Experimental Research*, 42(6), 1084–1095. https://doi.org/10.1111/acer.13638

22 National Council on Family Relations. (n.d.). Family focus. https://www.ncfr.org/ncfr-report/focus

23 Besharat, R., Azemat, E. S., & Mohammadian, A. (2018). A comparative study of rumination, healthy locus of control, and emotional regulation in children of divorce and normal children. *Journal of Practice in Clinical Psychology, 6*(4), 207–214. http://dx.doi.org/10.32598/jpcp.6.4.207; Yárnoz-Yaben, S., & Garmendia, A. (2016). Parental divorce and emerging adults' subjective well-being: The role of "carrying messages." *Journal of Child and Family Studies, 25*(2), 638–646. https://doi.org/10.1007/s10826-015-0229-0; Gustavsen, G. W., Nayga, R. M., Jr., & Wu, X. (2016). Effects of parental divorce on teenage children's risk behaviors: Incidence and persistence. *Journal of Family and Economic Issues, 37*(3), 474–487. https://doi-org.proxy.bsu.edu/10.1007/s10834-015-9460-5; https://www.sciencedirect.com/science/article/pii/S2667321522000014?via%3Dihub; Gates, A. L. (2018). Stepmothers' coparenting experiences with the mother in joint custody stepfamilies. *Journal of Divorce & Remarriage*, 60(4), 253–269. https://doi.org/10.1080/10502556.2018.1488124

24 Adler-Baeder, F., Russell, C., Kerpelman, J., Pittman, J., Ketring, S., Smith, T., Lucier-Greer, M., Bradford, A., & Stringer, K. (2010). Thriving in stepfamilies: Exploring competence and well-being among African American youth. *Journal of Adolescent Health*, 46(4), 396–398. https://doi.org/10.1016/j.jadohealth.2009.10.014; Jensen, T. M., & Pace, G. T. (2016). Stepfather involvement and stepfather-child relationship quality: Race and parental marital status as moderators. *Journal of Marital and Family Therapy*, 42(4), 659–672. https://doi:10.1111/jmft.12165; Pew Research Center (2011, January 3). A portrait of stepfamilies. https://www.pewresearch.org/social-trends/2011/01/13/a-portrait-of-stepfamilies/

25 National Council on Family Relations. (n.d.). Family focus. https://www.ncfr.org/ncfr-report/focus; Willén, H. (2015). Challenges for divorced parents: Regulating negative emotions in post-divorce relationships. *Australian and New Zealand Journal of Family Therapy*, 36(3), 356–370. https://doi-org.proxy.bsu.edu/10.1002/anzf.1115; Van Gasse, D., & Mortelmans, D. (2020). Reorganizing the single-parent family system: Exploring the process perspective on divorce. *Family Relations*, 69, 1100–1112. https://doi.org/10.1111/fare.12432

26 Cubitt, R. (2019). Finding the right support: One size doesn't fit all. *Family Court Review*, 57(3), 327–331. https://doi.org/10.1111/fcre.12425; Higginbotham, B., Davis, P., Smith, L., Dansie, L., Skogrand, L., & Reck, K. (2012). Stepfathers and stepfamily education. *Journal of Divorce & Remarriage*, 53(1), 76–90. https://doi.org/10.1080/10502556.2012.635972; National Council on Family Relations. (n.d.). Family focus. https://www.ncfr.org/ncfr-report/focus

Image Credits

Fig. 8.1: Source: Adapted from https://news.gallup.com/poll/316223/fewer-say-important-parents-married.aspx?_hsmi=2&_hsenc=p2ANqtz--5GObG0WBgHQEsNH6VJubyaDVsTyDwCVHbwkFumRT4yJpRbto7-N4J-Tz-P8l-01T78RkaL-9dHQcK0n5nsqbSezvmstCTAa8k2pyee9RbXJ6CT6qU.

CHAPTER 9

Disability and Family Stress

Among caregivers of a chronically ill/disabled family member, 45% reported having their own chronic health problems (e.g., heart disease, cancer, diabetes, arthritis), 58% said their eating habits worsened since caregiving, and 78% said they neglected going to the doctor as much as they should have for their own health.[1]

Chapter Preview

- Diverse assumptions about disability lead to disagreement about terminology and interpretations of disability.
- Family stress theory helps explain why some families with disabled children experience greater strain.
- Having a disabled child can have a powerful impact on parental identities and expectations with potentially stressful and painful consequences.
- Parents of disabled children experience a variety of challenging thoughts and feelings and can face some difficult decisions.
- Parents' lifestyles can become restricted and overwhelming due to close monitoring of disabled children and dealing with school systems and other people's involvement.
- Cultural views on disability and parenthood can shape stigma that parents experience.
- Caring for a disabled child can put pressure on parent-child, sibling, couple, and extended family relationships to adjust to specific child needs and circumstances.
- Disabled parents face pressures inside and outside the home that can impact parenting and family relationships.
- Having a disabled spouse can challenge a couple to uniquely define their relationship.
- Adult children caring for a disabled parent face particularly difficult pressures when the parent suffers from dementia.
- Caregiver perceptions can vary dramatically and are an important target for intervention.

What Is This Topic About?

Have you ever wondered what it would be like to live without being able to see, hear, talk, or walk? Maybe you don't have to wonder or have lived with someone who was **impaired** in some way. Families that include one or more members with a form of **disability** face some unique stressors. Some such stressors are similar across a variety of disability circumstances while others are more particular to a certain type or severity of disability.

The Americans With Disability Act defines disability as "a physical or mental impairment that substantially limits one or major life activities."[2] A disability is more than just a person's condition but the **interaction between the person and the environment**. A person without legs 300 years ago was much more disabled than a similar person today. We have technological advancements and structural accommodations that can enable a person in a wheelchair to access buildings, attend events, and play sports. If someday we all move around by hover-chair, a lack of legs might no longer be considered a disability, at least in certain contexts. At the same time, not all disabilities are equally accommodatable, particularly intellectual disabilities, and not all people believe that all disabilities should be "cured" were it possible.

The focus of this chapter is on stressors that are created or intensified due to having a family member with a disability. Of course, many disabilities are along some kind of **spectrum**—a limp versus having no legs, a mild reading disability versus the inability to communicate or understand others. Generally speaking, the more disabling the impairment, the more **pressure** it places on family members to compensate and care for the disabled person. Some disabilities are developmental, meaning they begin during childhood (or at birth) and will have a lifelong impact. Others can happen as part of the deterioration of the body or mind that tends to come with old age, though some are not age-specific—like paralysis from a car accident.

Our approach is to include physical, emotional, intellectual, and behavioral illnesses, disorders, or characteristics that create a state of significant disability in a family. Examples will lean toward the **more serious** end of the spectrum that seems more conducive to triggering **crisis** since those families are most likely to need assistance. However, the intent is not to make things seem worse than they really are. Some higher functioning individuals and their families are understandably sensitive to stereotypes that seem to diminish their abilities and resilience—something to keep in mind. And, as you will see (and should not be surprised by given what we know about family stress), families can find great joy and satisfaction in these high-pressure circumstances. Keep a special eye out for **similarities** throughout the chapter despite the different types of disabilities and family relationships highlighted.

What Are the Assumptions?

You might believe you are a pretty normal person. The concept of "**normal**" is highly debated, and it can reflect many different assumptions about life. If you think about it, being abnormal can sometimes seem attractive—after all, many people like to stand out or rebel. But deep down, perhaps we all get a bit nervous about whether something is "wrong" with us. As you may have noticed, we live in an age in which great efforts are made to make everyone feel important, accepted, and essentially normal—as if to say there is no such thing as "normal." Yet, we recognize that some tasks are inherently more difficult for some people, even if we make helpful accommodations.

What we assume to be normal shapes how we interpret our reality, what we expect from ourselves and others, and how we address deviations from the norm. We don't always agree on the boundaries of normal. For example, disagreement exists regarding autism and the extent to which autistic thinking is a form of **neurodiversity**—in other words, whether we should consider or even celebrate autistic brain functioning as falling within a "normal" range of intellectual processing. It seems likely that some of the disagreement depends on the level of the cognitive differences a given person might have, with family caregivers of people who have more severe challenges seeing the uniqueness as disabling.

Assumptions can also differ about whether a disability is more an **illness** or an **identity**. For example, is there a person trapped inside or underneath a mental disability—such as schizophrenia—or is the mental disability a central characteristic of the person? Furthermore, deafness, which has become a culture in itself (people share a common language, seek each other out for socialization, and have a relatively similar perspective on life), can be seen as essential to one's identity. Some worry that if deafness were completely avoidable or healable that a group of people—a rich social identity—would disappear. We should be cautious when assuming that the exitance of a disability is something inherently undesirable or tragic. Yet, critics of the identity perspective encourage a cautious approach toward normalizing debilitating conditions, pointing to potential harm caused by groups that promote eating disorders (anorexia and bulimia) as legitimate identities that should be affirmed.[3]

In a similar vein, there is also disagreement about **terminology**. "Special needs" is viewed by some as having a negative connotation, and they argue that "disability" should be used and understood more neutrally as a way to destigmatize disabled people. **Person-first language**—saying "a person with autism" instead of "an autistic person"—is intended to focus on the universally human element of one's identity, but some argue that this approach ends up stigmatizing the condition by making it sound like a disease. Thus, there seems to be a growing preference for saying "autistic child" or "blind adult." Choices in terminology often reflect our assumptions, but many assumptions continue to be debated. Given the lack of consensus, this chapter will use "disabled" and similar terms as adjectives that precede the noun that indicates a person (e.g., autistic child) merely for the sake of efficiency.

Whether **political ideology** influences assumptions about disability is unclear. People with disabilities appear very similar to everyone else in their political views.[4] However, given the especially high emphasis of liberals on the **care foundation**, including an overall tendency to advocate for the inclusion of various minority populations, it is possible that liberals err more on the side of recognizing disability and perhaps supporting the identity argument (e.g., the neurodiversity movement). The conservatives' emphasis on **authority** and **loyalty** could play into ideals about family caregiving that more negatively views the placement of disabled family members in care centers.

As you **engage with** the rest of the chapter, remember the key elements of family stress theories (e.g., stressors, resources, perceptions, coping, and crisis) and consider the following:

- How can assumptions and perceptions about disability and disabled family members shape the impact of disability stressors on families?
- Why might some families with disabled family members flourish while others are strained?
- How do the various pieces of information throughout the chapter fit together to help explain why each family might be affected differently by disability stressors?
- What experiences have you had or observed that help you relate to specific concepts?
- How might the ideological perspectives influence how people (including you) think about potential ways to understand and help families facing disability stressors?

Part A. Child Disability Stressors

What Is Stressful About Raising a Disabled Child?

Some people, long before becoming a parent, imagine what their children will look like and accomplish. Once pregnancy is confirmed, the imagination kicks into full gear. The anticipation of meeting this new person grows daily and the future is full of possibilities. Once the child is born, we solidify some of our suspicions and hopes based on the child's characteristics—*It's a girl! Ten fingers and ten toes*. While the real future remains unknown, hopes are high—*She could be president someday!* But wait, something seems off. Her leg seems odd, and she isn't responding well to external cues—*What if she can't walk? What if she can't learn to communicate? Why is this happening to us?*

It seems only natural for parents to feel distressed over the prospect of their child not living what the parents perceive to be a normal, if not high-achieving, life. Having a disabled child need not be considered a tragedy, nor does it mean the child has any less value as a human being or won't contribute to a fulfilling family life. Consistent with the **FSS integrated model (FIM) of family stress and crisis framework**, disability becomes a family stressor in that it places **pressure** on the family to respond to extra or unusual and often unanticipated needs of a child. The family might view this pressure as a **hardship** when the disability is severe and threatens their hopes and expectations for the child and themselves. Disability can also be perceived as an **opportunity** for strengthening families or having special experiences, particularly by parents who have optimistic dispositions or perhaps certain belief systems. Are you aware of any types of beliefs that might have this effect?

A family with a disabled child can avoid **crisis** or (prolonged crisis) through effective coping, but many families are insufficiently prepared for such circumstances and find that additional resources and more helpful interpretations are needed to maintain healthy family functioning. Established family rules, roles, and boundaries might no longer work for the new circumstances. Adjusting and creating new patterns takes time and some experimentation—parents who were raised in families with no disabled members have little modeling to draw from, and what their new families need might feel awkward at first.

This section is heavily informed by the work of Andrew Solomon who interviewed over 300 families and numerous experts to understand families with children who are distinctly different from their parents, in most cases because of some form of disability.[5] What seems clear from the interviews (and other research) is that parents differ dramatically in the meanings they draw from their experiences. Any examples that come across as highly negative or positive need not imply that everyone in similar circumstances perceives things the same way.

What Pressures Do Parents of Disabled Children Experience?

Each family is different, and each disability has its own characteristics, but generally speaking, several types of pressures appear common for parents of disabled children. These next subsections can alert you to possible pressures and outcomes to look out for when interacting with families dealing with disability stress.

How Are Parental Identities and Expectations Affected?

We typically assume that if we have children they will share some meaningful similarities—like language, skin tone, and at least some common preferences or values. Having a disabled child typically creates some dissimilarity in the parent-child relationship, and parents can struggle to relate to **the child's perspective**. If the disability is associated with a subculture, like being deaf, parents can feel like an outsider to a child who embraces an identity as part of a subculture that hearing parents can't fully relate to. Parents might feel a bit reluctant about giving up some of their control and trusting others to socialize their child. The child might feel pulled between two cultures, adding concern and stress to the whole family.

Parents also inherit the **identity** as *parents of a disabled child*, and, as illustrated earlier, likely have some **expectations** for their child and family that will need to be adjusted if not completely abandoned. Some parents go through a **mourning** period when they feel they lost the child that they never had (see Chapter 11). Perhaps even more challenging, disabilities that begin sometime after birth can feel like a loss of the child the parents once knew. For example, signs of autism might not appear until a child is a toddler; schizophrenia—a mental disorder that creates disconnection from reality and typically includes voices in one's head and even hallucinations—usually first manifests itself in late adolescence or early adulthood. Imagine believing that your child is typically abled and on a trajectory to live the kind of life you had anticipated and then discovering you had drawn premature conclusions. How easy would it be for you to adjust your thinking and behavior?

However, the **severity** of a disability is not always clear early on. Sometimes medical professionals are unable to come up with a clear diagnosis, at least for a while. As you likely recall, **ambiguity** is particularly stressful because we don't know precisely how to adjust our expectations and how to respond. A diagnosis can be a huge relief for parents in that it helps eliminate such ambiguity, but it also makes the disability more real, which can trigger other strong emotions. But even with a diagnosis, we might not know precisely how a disabled child fits in with the family system. As noted previously (see Chapter 8), **boundary ambiguity** occurs when there is a mismatch between one's physical and psychological presence. A child with a severe intellectual disability might have a clear physical presence at home but the extent to which family members' efforts to connect with the child have the desired effect could be unclear, making it hard for the family to know how to incorporate the disabled child into their interconnected social lives.

Ambiguity also exists when, for example, in some cases of autism, children appear very competent in certain skills but lacking in others, which can give parents and others an unclear sense of what the child is actually **capable of achieving**. A major parenting challenge is to know how hard to push a child because of limitations. When limitations aren't clear or consistent, parents risk putting undue pressure on children to perform or failing to help children reach their potential by not pushing them enough. Children can complicate things by using their disability as an excuse to avoid undesirable tasks—*My muscles are hurting today*—and parents can struggle with identifying when that is the case.

Similarly, boundary ambiguity can emerge as parents face uncertainty about their own **roles** as parents, specialized caregivers, and advocates. Parents often wonder where to draw the line in taking charge of a disabled child's health and treatment versus leaving things up to specialized medical professionals. They might find that if they don't actively advocate for medical and other resources, their child will be short-changed. *What exactly is my job in making sure his medical needs are met? I'm just a parent!* Some parents are criticized by service professionals as being both too aggressive and not aggressive enough, so it can feel like a no-win situation.[6]

How Are Parental Thoughts and Feelings Affected?

Parents can be quick to wonder whether they are to **blame** for the disability. *Should I have taken more vitamins? Did I push myself too much during pregnancy?* Imagine how you might feel if you believe that you were the cause of perceived child suffering. Some parents are indeed responsible for the condition, such as those who cause fetal alcohol syndrome. But even when our decisions had no impact on the disability, it is stressful to wonder if we could have avoided it. Furthermore, people around us might wonder and verbalize the same thing, suspecting substance misuse during pregnancy or that we neglected prenatal screening or unwisely chose not to abort, creating an uncomfortable **stigma** surrounding childhood disability.[7]

Parents also typically have various reasons to **worry** about their disabled child's physical and mental well-being.[8] *Is my child in pain? Will her life span be shortened? Is she happy?* For some conditions, like cystic fibrosis, parents are constantly concerned about exposing their children to germs. Some children are in and out of hospitals, which can induce fear in some children and expose them to the stresses of seeing other people in pain or who pass away. Of course, a major worry is how other people, especially children, will treat their disabled children. Besides mockery and teasing, disabled children can also be taken advantage of, including sexually. Parents also worry about how their children will be cared for as parents become frail with age or pass away.

The thought and feeling processes involved with **decision-making** can also be taxing. Some key decisions can include the following:

- Parents might have to decide whether to **give birth or choose abortion**, and whether to keep a child or give them up for **adoption**.

- Some parents can feel subtle or immense pressure from doctors, family members, and their social communities regarding such decisions.[9]
- Parents might struggle with deciding on the balance between **accepting** a child and trying to **improve** the child. Some children with greater awareness of their disability can feel like a parental attempt to cure them of their condition is a personal rejection. Expressing any regret about the child's condition feels hurtful to some children. At the same time, parents typically want to ease their children's suffering and help them reach their full potential, and some children appreciate that. Can you do one without the other? Where is the line between wanting the best for your child and stigmatizing your child? When parents pursue various treatments to more "normalize" their child, deciding when to stop can be complicated, giving opportunity for later **regrets**—*If I had only tried one more experimental treatment.*
  - Such decisions are made harder when family members, friends, and advocacy groups have different perspectives. For example, helping deaf children improve their hearing through cochlear implants is frowned upon by some within the deaf community. Such a procedure is more effective when it happens early in life, but its success is hard to predict, and the child's eventual preferences are unknown—*Will he want to be immersed within the deaf community?* A child who is assisted with hearing can be **stigmatized** by both the hearing and deaf communities, not fully fitting in anywhere. Limb extensions for dwarf children, which are often done for medical reasons, can also create tensions within a community of little people.
- The decision of whether to **institutionalize** a child can also be pressure-packed. In some cases, a child's needs are so major that parents are unable to continue being effective primary caregivers. Some might question their motives—*What kind of parent would give up their child to live in a group home or care facility?* As you might suspect, parents can struggle with guilt and feeling like failures in such circumstances and are likely to hear opinions from others that reinforce such feelings.
  - Even when parents are confident about their decision to place the child outside the home, the paperwork and **bureaucracy** involved in the care system can feel overwhelming, and sometimes people are on wait lists for years. While having a child in a facility tends to ease parents' physical burdens, emotions can feel very mixed. Interviewed parents of a Down syndrome child felt like they competed with facility staff members for the child's attention and love, which was hard to accept. Conversely, other parents worried that professional caregivers don't love their severely disabled child like they do and about missing high points in the child's life that they only hear about when they visit.

How Are Parental Lifestyles Affected?

As you might expect, disabled children can add major **expenses** to a family's budget.[10] Not only are medical care and specialized equipment expensive (e.g., electric wheelchair), some parents cut back on employment hours or quit their jobs to accommodate heavy caregiving tasks. Insurance companies can be challenging to work with, and children with more chronic, complex conditions often need care outside of the insurance company's provider network, which makes the treatment more expensive for families. Hospitals are also notorious for their lack of transparency on prices, even though it appears that a large majority of parents want hospital employees to discuss costs.[11] Paying professional home caregivers is also costly and less affordable for poorer families. Parents' concerns about expenses can lead to children feeling guilty or distressed about their contribution to the family's financial challenges.

Solomon concluded, "The birth of a healthy child usually expands the parents' social network; the birth of a child who is disabled often constricts that network."[12] Specifically, parents of disabled children are at higher risk for social isolation for various reasons, including the following:

- They have difficulty finding parents who can relate to their circumstances.
- People are often uncertain about how to act around disabled children and keep their distance.
- Some parents are put off by the pity and negativity they receive from others who see the situation as tragic, while other parents are frustrated with the lack of empathy they receive from others.
- They can get bombarded with all sorts of advice that people read about somewhere, which can be a tiring and frustrating experience.
- Parents avoid public places in which they receive stares or potential consternation for noisy or otherwise disruptive behavior from a disabled child. (Children with behavioral disorders, such as oppositional defiance disorder or attention deficit hyperactivity disorder (ADHD), or severe intellectual disorders, can be especially difficult to deal with in public and can be difficult for other people to connect with and tolerate.[13])
- For similar reasons, finding people to watch the children at home so the parents can take a break can be difficult, especially potential caregivers who have the competencies to address the child's specific needs.

Dealing with **schools** can also significantly tax parents' resources.[14] About 14% of public school children have a disability, about two thirds of which are **males**. Learning disabilities are the most common. Even though schools work to be accommodating, it can take time to receive a doctor's official diagnosis and to help school administrators and teachers to understand a child's needs. Children with severe conditions can act out in school and create difficulties for teacher and peer relationships. Chronic illness can contribute to regular school absences, falling behind at school, and attracting bullying. Sometimes families make sacrifices to move to where they can find specialized schools for their children, like schools for the deaf. The chart in Figure 9.1 indicates percentages of specifically disabled students served in schools in accordance with the Individuals with Disabilities Education Act (IDEA).[15]

Parents often sacrifice leisure time when disabled children need **constant monitoring and care**. For example, some children have physical needs related to getting dressed, eating, and bodily waste. Some can be a danger to themselves, like those with severe intellectual disabilities who go days without sleeping; can hurl themselves into furniture; or could injure themselves with sharp

Percentages of Students (Ages 3-21) Served Under the IDEA

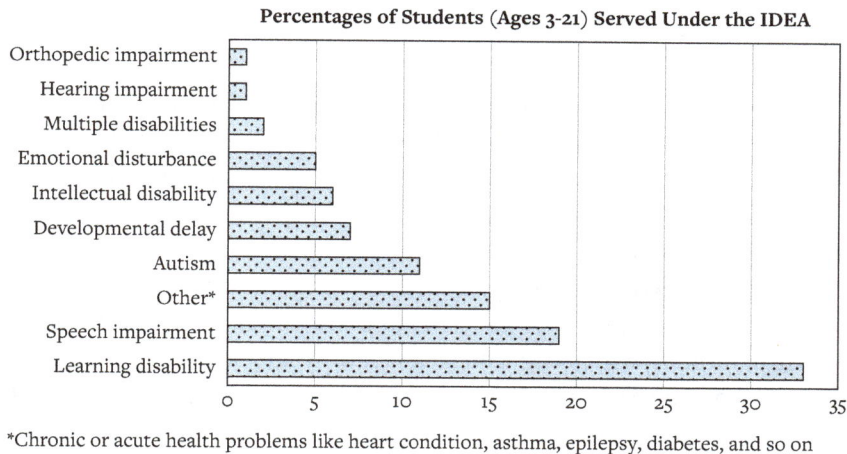

*Chronic or acute health problems like heart condition, asthma, epilepsy, diabetes, and so on

FIGURE 9.1 Percentages of Students (Ages 3–21) Served Under the IDEA

objects. They can also be a danger to others—schizophrenic individuals have elevated rates of making threats and perpetrating violence against family members.[16] Parents can be on constant **high alert** because of frequent door slamming, yelling, mess making, and emotional meltdowns; trying to create structure can feel futile. Monitoring **medication** can also be challenging. Medicine for serious mental illness can dull senses and feel undesirable to a child, and sometimes children (and adults) quit taking medication after starting to feel better. Symptoms then return, and it might require hospitalization to get back on the medication.

Some parents get very little back from their children (e.g., few loving gestures) to help keep them motivated, and some children appear to lack appreciation for the parents' efforts. One parent of an autistic child desperately proclaimed that she "waited eleven years to hear him say, 'I love you, Mom.'"[17] Feelings of despair can easily seep in under such conditions, especially when parents see nothing on the horizon for their children—college, marriage, parenthood, home ownership, and so on. Some children pick up on those feelings, which makes parents feel even more guilty about their despair.

Unsurprisingly, parents of disabled children as a whole are at heightened risk for poorer physical and mental health, especially in cases of severe disability, fewer resources, and more years of intense supervision. Sleep deprivation can be a key contributor to poor health. Such parents are at risk for **burnout**—emotional, mental, and physical exhaustion, making it harder to relax, find satisfaction in caregiving, and avoid feeling helpless.[18] Disabled children are consequently at greater risk for abuse and even being killed by a family member.[19] Some "filicidal" parents have claimed they intended to spare their child a lifetime of suffering and meaninglessness. How sympathetic would you be if you were on a jury for such a case?

While this section has skewed toward negative family outcomes related to disability, Part B includes some reminders about how perceptions and resources can contribute to more typical if not desirable elements of family stressors.

How Do External Contexts Impact Parents With Child Disability Stressors?

Much of the variation in experiences for parents with disabled children have been discussed regarding different types of disabilities and different levels of their severity. As noted, issues of **stigma** exist when people hold negative views toward disability or toward parents' perceptions and decisions regarding disability. **Social and cultural norms** related to beliefs and attitudes are important contexts in which families manage their circumstances.

Ethnic (or cultural) heritage specifically seems to inform views and experiences related to disability.[20] For example, in some places—such as in parts of Pakistan, child disability is thought to result from a sinful mother, which can lead to less family and social support. Similarly, in some Asian cultures, people perceive a particularly strong stigma toward parents of children with cognitive or emotional disabilities, often rooted in assumptions about parents causing the disability. However, some Asian American parents appeared to have a more positive outlook on raising an autistic child than other Americans. Black parents of autistic children have seemed especially impacted by their levels of family solidarity (e.g., talking with one another, working together, recognizing family strengths) compared to White and Hispanic families; among families with low solidarity, Black families experienced the most stress, but among families with high solidarity, Black families experienced the least stress. Some racial minority parents have also reported being accused of causing a child's disability due to prenatal drug use and believed that White parents were less likely to face such accusations.

Some challenges associated with **poverty** have already been noted, particularly in that poorer or **lower class** families can face more extreme financial stress given the expenses associated with raising a disabled child. In some ways such families might be more accepting of the child's conditions and less tempted to "fix" the child given the lack of resources—and thus lack of control—that wealthier families have. **Religious** families sometimes find deep meaning in suffering or believe a divine will guides their circumstances, consequently increasing motivation or positivity when it comes to caring for disabled children.[21]

Improve Your Learning

Without peeking, take a moment to review in your mind (or say out loud) the key concepts from this chapter (this is a proven learning technique). Then review the "Chapter Preview" section at the top and compare. Skim Part A of the chapter with extra attention to the **bolded words**. Skip to the end of the chapter to find more learning resources.

Part B. Family Caregiving Relationship Stressors

How Are Family Relationships Affected by Caregiving Stress?

Thinking of the family as a system, the behavior and well-being of a disabled family member impact every other member of the family in some way. In this section, we focus on how family caregiving of a disabled child, spouse, and an aging parent can put pressure on other family members and relationships that influence family functioning.

How Can Caring for a Disabled Child Put Pressure on Family Relationships?

The quality of the **parent-child relationship** can depend on numerous factors, including the attitude and health of the parent and the nature of the child's disability. Some disabilities directly impact the potential emotional nature of the relationship. Severe autism, schizophrenia, and oppositional defiance disorder can make children seem disconnected, cold, ungrateful, grumpy, rude, purposefully defiant, and as one parent put it, like an "unpleasant stranger."[22] When parents feel they receive very little love in return, they can struggle to feel like they have an intimate connection with the child. Merely the presence of the child can be a constant reminder of the hardships of caregiving and trigger negative feelings. Conversely, some parents develop a profound love for their child that is enhanced through the limitless sacrifices and investments made for the child. Many parents find great joy in their relationship with a disabled child and can feel very moved by the seemingly unconditional love and acceptance they receive.

Siblings of disabled children can similarly develop deep, loving relationships and are prone to develop greater empathy and openness toward others who have disabilities. They can also struggle to make an intimate connection for similar reasons mentioned earlier. Common contributing factors to sibling stress and relationship dynamics include the following: [23]

- Abled siblings might have extra duties at school protecting a disabled sibling and helping teachers and students understand their sibling's needs.
- While any set of siblings can be a source of embarrassment for one another, some disabled siblings create even more opportunities to funnel unwanted attention to an abled sibling.
- Siblings have been found to have increased school absences when they have a hospitalized sibling.
- Both older and younger siblings of children with developmental disabilities have been shown to be at higher risk for distress, depression, and other mental health challenges, especially sisters. Older siblings with a greater age difference and younger siblings with a smaller age difference were also especially at risk, possibly because of higher levels of caregiving responsibilities.
- Siblings can become parentified when they take on excessive parental-type responsibilities (see Chapter 8). This could also lead to less participation in leisure and extracurricular activities.

- People might pay more attention to an abled sibling who is perceived as more responsive and easier to connect with, which can contribute to discomfort and sorrow for children and parents.
- Some siblings have expressed a lack of desire of coming home from school to a house full of chaos and potential violence.
- Abled siblings are at risk of having their needs neglected when parents are consumed with caring for a severely disabled child.
- Removing a disabled child from home can be distressful for siblings who have a meaningful relationship.

Married parents (or who are otherwise coupled) can find their relationship significantly impacted when raising a disabled child.[24] While it may seem logical that caregiving stress and burnout can take a toll on a marriage, studies have mixed findings in that regard. Indeed, some find lower marital satisfaction or higher divorce rates among parents who have disabled children, while others are inconclusive or show that the difference is not nearly as large as one might expect. One study found that the range of marital satisfaction scores was broader (higher highs and lower lows) for parents of disabled children than for other parents (i.e., higher highs and lower lows), even though the averages were the same. Taken together, it appears that some parents are better able than others to maintain or even enhance a marriage in the face of stressors, and some circumstances are probably more difficult than others on parents' relationships.

Regardless of the ultimate impact, couples can face certain pressures that are somewhat unique to raising disabled children that have the potential to disrupt their relationship. For example,

- worrying about a partner's caregiving stress and consequences,
- frustration over a lack of a partner's caregiving involvement,
- disagreement on proper care and treatment of a disabled child (including whether to pursue certain treatments or to place the child in an institution),
- jealousy toward a parent who "escapes" the home through employment,
- feeling unable to leave an unsatisfying marriage because neither spouse can handle the disabled child alone,
- missing out on other things to focus on in their relationship besides caregiving, and
- if a spouse has the same disability as the child (e.g., blindness), the abled spouse's preference (if indeed the case) to have an abled child or negative feelings about raising a disabled child can feel rejecting and hurtful to the disabled spouse.

Extended family members—like grandparents or aunts and uncles—could struggle with connecting with a disabled child because of less time with the child to learn how to communicate. They can cause friction by disagreeing with how the parents handle the situation, though they can also provide much-needed support. Concerns over passing along genetics that contribute to disability (e.g., schizophrenia) can scare off **potential mates** for family members who are biologically related to a disabled child.

How Can Being a Disabled Parent Put Pressure on Family Relationships?

Do you know any parents in a wheelchair, or who are blind, or who struggle with serious mental illness? Consider how having a disability might influence parenting duties and parent-child relationships. Of course, the nature of the disability is highly relevant to the parenting circumstances, as is the presence of a co-parent and other supportive individuals who can do the tasks a disabled parent might be unable to complete. When investigating the impact of parental disability on children, one encounters strong feelings about disabled people's rights to be a parent and assumptions about parental inadequacy.[25] Of greatest concern is the welfare of children who have parents with psychiatric or intellectual disabilities. Generally speaking, children with such parents tend to be at greater risk for health and behavioral problems, though some argue that issues of poverty, inadequate support, and social isolation that can accompany such disabilities account for at least some portion of that elevated risk.[26]

Parental disability can contribute to various pressures **within the home**.[27] For example, a mother in a wheelchair found that she had to compensate for the bond that comes from rough-and-tumble play with her toddler with more creative verbal communication. While some parents are limited in their physical activity, others might struggle with helping with homework or communicating with their children. Families with a disabled parent lack role models and often need to be more flexible and innovative with family rules, roles, and boundaries, which many certainly do so with great success. Some families find that children develop enhanced coping and problem-solving skills, find meaning and purpose in their contributions, develop stronger family bonds, better learn to appreciate life, and adopt more positive attitudes and empathy toward others with challenges. Conversely, parents need to guard against the possibility of depending too much on abled children to take on inappropriate roles that could lead to **parentification**.

Interviews with children raised by a parent with a serious mental disability (e.g., bipolar or major depression, schizophrenia) further enlighten us as to the pressures that such families face within the home.[28] Table 9.1 (next page) summarizes what the children described happens on "bad days" in the first two columns, and I offer some examples of potential pressures families consequently experience. See if you can add a few more of your **own ideas** for the third column and then consider how the pressures could influence family relationships.

Disabled parents also confront barriers **outside the home**—in a "society not built for them"—that adds pressure to the family.[29] For example,

- feeling like others doubt their capacity to be a parent;
- having to deal with their children being ostracized or bullied by their peers because of having a disabled parent;
- feeling judged by others as being lazy because of asking for accommodations (like having children brought to the car when picked up at a childcare center so the parent can avoid climbing the stairs to get them);
- having difficulty accessing some of the venues that children perform or compete at (and not knowing ahead of time how accessible the places—and bathrooms—will be for a wheelchair, creating anxiety);

TABLE 9.1 Experiencing a "Bad Day" When Having a Parent With a Serious Mental Disability

On a "Bad Day"		Potential Pressures
Parental Behavior	Low affection	Other parent worries that child feels rejected.
	Grumpy, yelling	
	Avoids reading books, playing games, helping with homework	
	Low communication or showing interest	
	All day in bed or sitting alone	
Child Responses	Ignore or avoid parent	Child feels the need to be perfect.
	Be sure not to cause problems (have a clean room)	
	Take responsibility for younger siblings and be sure they don't cause problems	
Child Perceptions	Interpret parental withdrawal as less attention to the child (instead of a symptom of an illness)	Parent worries that the child will think badly of the parent.
	Blame self for symptoms (should have monitored medicine better or should have been better behaved)	
	Confusion about parent's condition (often not told about the illness; some figure it out gradually; comparing their own family to others; for some, it is a family secret)	
Child Concerns	Feel sad, worry about parent's and child's welfare	Child is unsure whether the parent will continue to be present.
	Confusion over why the parent is hospitalized; associates hospital with death	
	Removed from home and placed with extended family or in foster care	
	Worry about inheriting the illness/turning out like the parent	

Data from: Riebschleger, J. (2004). Good days and bad days: The experiences of children of a parent with a psychiatric disability. *Psychiatric Rehabilitation Journal, 28*(1), 25–31. https://doi.org/10.2975/28.2004.25.31

- facing restrictive policies at amusement parks that don't allow a child to sit on the lap of a parent who is operating a motorized wheelchair or to pull a wagon behind a mobility scooter;
- being considered the "problem parent" at the child's school for insisting on accommodations that help the parent engage the child during homework (like having documents

digitized for a computer-aided reading or communication system or replicated with extra-large print);
- feeling ignored by other parents at school events because it seems they aren't comfortable around the disabled parent;
- seeming to be on display when in public and people complimenting them for their parenting ability or needlessly trying to assist them; or
- worrying that someone will call Child Protective Services (which happens) and potentially have their children removed because of assumptions about their parenting capacity.

Caring for **a disabled spouse** or partner also exerts pressure on the couple's relationship.[30] The potential for caregiver burnout likewise applies to couples, especially if the caregiving spouse has to remain on constant high alert. Household tasks might be difficult to divide equally, so spouses could contend with feelings of guilt and resentment. The disabled spouse might have minimal employment, creating the potential for extra economic pressure. Psychologically, couples can go through a grieving period for the loss of the type of relationship they would hope to have, which can produce anger and discouragement. Some spouses feel like they lost their best friend and future, depending on the nature and timing of the disability. Couples can struggle with creating realistic expectations for their relationship that also push them to continue to grow. They also have to work through what can feel like incompatible roles as a spouse and caregiver or care recipient; some caregivers feel more like a parent than a spouse, and some disabled spouses feel more like a to-do list than an intimate companion.

Couples can **isolate** themselves because of the time constraints or hassles of dealing with going out in public (e.g., getting a spouse into a wheelchair and into a vehicle). Constant contact with one another can build tension, especially if the caregiving spouse feels overly restricted from pursuing personal interests and self-care. Feelings of shame and resentment by either party can erode their intimacy. Caregiving spouses can also struggle with understanding that their companion's moods and withdrawal are symptoms of the disability and not meant to be taken personally. Yet, as you have certainly suspected, many **resilient** couples are able to adapt to their circumstances and find ways to flourish despite them, or because of them (e.g., develop greater intimacy and empathy through their joint trials).

How Can Caring for a Disabled Parent Put Pressure on Family Relationships?

Much of what you have learned regarding caregiver stress also applies to adult children caring for a disabled parent:

- Caregiver burdens that can strain family members' resources (e.g., physical, emotional, social, financial) and lead to burnout.
- Women are prone to doing more of the hands-on caregiving (in this case adult daughters and daughters-in-law; men tend to do more of the financial and home maintenance tasks).
- Adjusting to seemingly incompatible roles as child and caregiver (i.e., a somewhat role reversal in caregiving).

- Experiencing boundary ambiguity (e.g., a parent with a mental disability may not be psychologically present).
- Grief for the loss of certain types of joint activities or relational connection (e.g., grandchildren limited in their relationship with grandparents).
- Deciding whether to place the parent in institutionalized care—facing guilt and possible stigma if doing so.
- An elevated risk of abuse (e.g., vulnerable parents can be taken advantage of financially and be verbally, emotionally, and physically victimized by caregivers).
- Potentially experiencing satisfaction and relationship closeness through family caregiving.

Caring for aging family members who have cognitive disabilities, such as **dementia**, is especially challenging for caregivers because disabled individuals struggle with memory and can even become violent in their confusion.[31] How would you feel if you cared for a parent who can't remember you, doesn't show appreciation for your sacrifices, and even strikes out at you verbally or physically? What would keep you motivated to continue?

Consider the unique pressures that come with caring for a disabled parent. Does the caregiving child truly become the parent? How might stigma be different when an elderly adult has mental challenges from when a child has similar challenges? How might it feel to manage the hygiene of a parent, particularly of a different sex? What other responsibilities might the adult child be balancing along with the caregiving role? What might siblings and other parents disagree about that creates conflict in the family? How might family structural complexity impact caregiving? How might a declining birth rate impact caregiving? What unique personal and family benefits might come from caring for a needy parent?

How Do External Contexts Impact Families With Caregiving Stressors?

Given that mothers are likely to take on more of the family caregiving work, especially regarding direct emotional and physical care of a child, **women** tend to report greater levels of caregiving stress than **men**.[32] Some male-female couples can struggle to establish or maintain what both partners perceive as an equitable division of labor, perhaps dealing with feelings of resentment or jealousy. Having two full-time careers is likely incompatible with a desire to provide parent-based care to a highly needy child, so at least one partner might give up a dream job—more typically a mother. The couple might have to come to terms with a lower standard of living than they had anticipated, placing more pressure on the full-time employed parent as an earner—more typically a father.

Parent-child relationships might also be subtly influenced because of **gender** issues related to disability. Boys are more likely to be diagnosed with certain developmental disabilities, including learning disabilities, autism, and ADHD. They also have more behavioral disorders, whereas girls have more mood disorders. Consider how different gender combinations of parents and disabled children could shape how each combination interacts and emotionally connects. For example, a mother-son relationship might have some distinct qualities given her propensity to be the primary caregiver and his tendency to struggle with learning and controlling his behavior.

Culture can also play an important role in family caregiving relationships.[33] For example, Asian cultural values—especially in China—have long endorsed the concept of **filial piety**, which emphasizes parent-child relationship harmony and dutiful caregiving. Social norms and policies reinforce these cultural values. In more Western societies, the couple bond tends to supersede the parent-child relationship, and individualism is highly pursued and rewarded. Asian American adult children who have internalized these Asian values or live in Asian American communities might feel more pressure to care for disabled parents and experience greater guilt and shame over placing frail parents in an institution. Consequently, they might experience more friction in their relationship with their parents when they don't fully embrace the caregiving role.

Some cultural influences might impact the level of caregiver burden family members experience, which could influence their family relationships.[34] For example, a sample of Black adults caring for parents with dementia reported less perceived burden than similar White adults, at least partially explained by their greater involvement with their church community. Many Native American adults in North America embraced the caregiving role with joy, an attitude that may have been aided by living in close-knit kin systems. However, this population tended to have less knowledge about dementia, which created confusion and ambiguity in their caregiving roles, which could lead to less helpful interpretations of the care recipient's behavior (e.g., taking harsh comments personally and damaging the relationship).

What Does All This Mean for You?

Your insights can be valuable to your personal life, your family relationships, and your professional roles. Take a few moments to ponder the following:

- How have you been feeling while engaging with this information? Why?
- How much of this topic can you personally relate to?
- Did you grow up in a home with a disabled family member? What was it like?
- What opinions do you have about family caregiving that might differ from other peoples' opinions?
- What other examples have come to mind that illustrate similar or diverse ways that families cope with disability stressors?

Reminders for Helpers

As a person of influence, you can help guide people through the coping processes and ideally help foster a **flourishing** life. However, take care to avoid letting your personal **interpretations** push you toward assuming too much about somebody else's circumstances, perceptions, and motivations. Always be ready to address issues that might be hard for you to face because of your own history.

Draw upon the elements of the **FIM framework** and other family stress concepts. Remember, **coping** refers to an action or response based on available or new resources and perceptions related to stressors. Families have either successfully **managed** a stressor's pressure through **adjustment coping** or reached crisis in which **adaptive coping** is needed to reestablish some level of **general family functioning**. **Resources** and **perceptions** are key concepts to focus on when confronting family stress. **Review the master table** in Chapter 4 as a guide for exploring the following ideas on how to help families with stressors.

What Are Some Ways to Encourage Effective Family Coping?

Drawing primarily from citations and insights noted in the chapter thus far, we will explore **suggested resources and noteworthy perceptions** that can contribute to successful coping and more optimal family functioning.

How Can You Help With Disability and Caregiving Stressors?

As noted at the beginning of the chapter, disability can tax a family's various resources. Advocating for workplace flexibility and private or public funding of medical and caregiving resources could help more families successfully cope with disability stressors. Resources of time, energy, and patience can be enhanced or rejuvenated when family caregivers get a break—or **respite**—from their tasks. They need to practice **self-care** (see Chapter 2) to avoid burnout, and a break from caregiving tasks might be essential for their well-being. However, what if people aren't available who can be trusted to provide particularly specialized care—or, in the case of professionals, what if a family can't afford to pay for respite services? Having access to reliable family members and trained volunteers can be an invaluable resource for exhausted caregivers, especially when affordable professional services (or subsidies that fund them) are scarce.

Solomon argued, "Everyone would be better off if we could destigmatize parental ambivalence. ... There is no contradiction between loving someone and feeling burdened by that person; indeed, love tends to magnify the burden."[35] Guilt and stigma have been repeatedly mentioned throughout this chapter. Perhaps you can help with **normalizing** the presence of disability and the mixed feelings that family caregivers might have toward their situations. If mothers feel less blamed for their children's infirmities and exhausted parents feel less judged for their desires to escape or to hand a loved one over to people better equipped to constantly monitor them, more families might be open about their needs, seek help, and be less self-critical. Whatever they ultimately decide to do would hopefully be more intentional and based on well-thought-out reasoning that produces the greatest benefits.

As hinted at throughout the chapter, **perceptions** can vary dramatically among family caregivers in ways that seem to have a meaningful impact on the caregiving experience. While some people find dread and resentment, others find deeper meaning, purpose, growth, and joy through their burdens. A mother of a deaf child declared that her life now had a cause to fight for, and she enjoyed empowering people. A parent of a Down syndrome child noted the blessing of living life a little slower. A couple looked on the bright side that though they worried about the future of their seriously disabled child, at least they didn't worry about their child getting into trouble at school or with drugs or pregnancy. Conversely, a father with a schizophrenic son who had tried to kill him mourned that he was never able to bring joy to his son. A mother was unable to enjoy her long-awaited respite care because she felt humiliated that someone else was "better at loving" her disabled child than she was. Some parents felt like their love was squandered or rejected by their unresponsive child as if they were just a piece of furniture in the child's mind. Having mixed perceptions is perhaps most common—leaning more toward hope or despair depending on the day.

Families may need help analyzing their perceptions and **cognitive coping strategies**. Choosing more helpful interpretations and attitudes should facilitate better coping and finding reasons for hope, though circumstances matter. A higher proportion of couples raising autistic children reported having caregiver burden and less satisfying marriages than did couples raising a Down syndrome child—the latter of which is more likely to want to please parents and show affection.[36] Nevertheless, addressing problematic thoughts can help families interpret their experiences in ways that help avoid burnout. For example, some research suggests that mindfulness training (i.e., learning to focus on the present without judgment; see Chapter 2) has helped parents of children with ADHD improve in self-control, self-compassion, mental health, well-being, and their own ADHD symptoms.[37]

Positive attitudes, hopeful perceptions, and social support also help adults who care for a disabled spouse or parent. Furthermore, experts have recommended that couples with a disabled spouse consider the following:[38]

- Learn to view the disability as something this is shared and that should be addressed as a couple (i.e., thinking of it as a third party outside of the disabled spouse).
- Find and preference activities the couple can do together while also allowing the abled spouse to have some separate leisure.
- Creatively divide up tasks in the household as much as possible so both feel like they are contributing (especially so the disabled spouse isn't only playing the passive role of care recipient).
- Openly and respectfully communicate feelings and grief instead of holding them in to protect the others' feelings—expressing them more about the disability than about the disabled person.

Couples might need help working through some of these negotiations and processes, especially if they already have relationship problems. Ultimately, a strong marriage is a helpful resource and protective factor against burnout and distress related to any form of family caregiving.[39]

Improve Your Learning

Without peeking, take a moment to review in your mind (or say out loud) the key concepts from this chapter (this is a proven learning technique). Then review the "Chapter Preview" section at the top and compare. Skim Part B of the chapter with extra attention to the **bolded words**.

Do You Want to Learn More?

We have only touched on a portion of information related to some elements of this topic. **What really sparked your interest? What do you wish was covered more thoroughly?** Consider taking some time to further deepen your understanding of personal and professional issues related to helping families cope with stressors. The following are a variety of resources that you might find helpful, and some references directly or indirectly referred to in this chapter. I have full confidence in your ability to make the most of this learning opportunity.

Videos

(Use links or do searches with the key words provided)
- Parenting Twins With Disabilities (My Perfect Family: Twins) (29 mins). Attitude. https://www.youtube.com/watch?v=kYULF0AdFXo
- Two Kids. Two Undiagnosed Disabilities (30 mins). *The Atlantic*. https://www.youtube.com/watch?v=CFlzCPAdKC8
- Why Can't She Talk?—Nonverbal Autism (14 mins). FatheringAutism. https://www.youtube.com/watch?v=8O3FC86WjWU
- Parents of Children With Special Needs Have Needs, *Too* (13 mins). Debra Vines, TEDx. https://www.youtube.com/watch?v=AC9Q3IJeH1w
- Glass Children (11 mins). Jamie Guterman (siblings of disabled children). TEDxYouth. https://www.youtube.com/watch?v=J3-uT2OCd30
- How This Couple Is Planning Their Future With 2 Adult Children With Autism (6 mins). *Today*. https://www.youtube.com/watch?v=jeOf2n9ZO2M
- Dad Living With Parkinson's (28 mins). Attitude. https://www.youtube.com/watch?v=8bp9n60m3AY
- She Gets Paid to Be Her Paralyzed Boyfriend's Caregiver, but Marriage Could Change That (6 mins). *Washington Post*. https://www.youtube.com/watch?v=adccBN1y3E0
- *Experiencing the Virtual Dementia Tour®* (4 mins). Second Wind Dreams. https://www.youtube.com/watch?v=Nsne9-QZQH4

Websites

- National Center for Education Statistics. (2021, May). Students with disabilities. U.S. Department of Education, Institute of Education Sciences. https://nces.ed.gov/programs/coe/indicator/cgg
- Powell, R. (2019, June 4). What it's like to be a disabled parent in an inaccessible world. Rewire Newsgroup. https://rewirenewsgroup.com/article/2019/06/04/what-its-like-to-be-a-disabled-parent-in-an-inaccessible-world/
- PsychGuides.com (2022). Behavioral disorder symptoms, causes and effects. https://www.psychguides.com/behavioral-disorders/

- Russo, F. (2022, January 5). How a spouse's physical disability impacts a relationship. Next Avenue. https://www.nextavenue.org/how-a-spouses-disability-impacts-a-relationship/
- U.S. Department of Justice (2020, February). A guide to disability rights laws. https://www.ada.gov/cguide.htm
- Zeittlow, A., (2018, December 13). An aging society needs caregiving superheroes. Institute for Family Studies. https://ifstudies.org/blog/an-aging-society-needs-caregiving-superheroes

Readings (Articles, Books, Book Chapters)

- Legano, L. A., Desch, L. W., Messner, S. A., Idzerda, S., Flaherty, E. G., Council on Child Abuse and Neglect; Council on Children With Disabilities; Haney, S. B., Sirotnak, A. P., Gavril, A. R., Girardet, R. G., Hoffert Gilmartin, A. B., Laskey, A., Mohr, B. A., Nienow, S. M., Rosado, N., Kuo, D. Z., Apkon, S., Davidson, L. F., Ellerbeck, K. A., Foster, J. E. A., et al. (2021). Maltreatment of children with disabilities. *Pediatrics, 147*(5). https://doi.org/10.1542/peds.2021-050920
- Marquis, S., McGrail, K., & Hayes, M. V. (2020). Using administrative data to examine variables affecting the mental health of siblings of children who have a developmental disability. *Research in Developmental Disabilities, 96.* https://doi.org/10.1016/j.ridd.2019.103516
- Solomon, A. (2012). *Far from the tree: Parents, children, and the search for identity.* Scribner.
- Unson, C., Flynn, D., Glendon, M. A., Haymes, E., & Sancho, D. (2015). Dementia and caregiver stress: An application of the reconceptualized uncertainty in illness theory. *Issues in Mental Health Nursing, 36*(6), 439–446. https://doi.org/10.3109/01612840.2014.993052

Notes

1   Ingber, R. (n.d.). Caregiver stress syndrome. Today's Caregiver. https://caregiver.com/articles/caregiver-stress-syndrome/

2   U.S. Department of Justice. (2020, February). A guide to disability rights laws. https://www.ada.gov/cguide.htm

3   Solomon, A. (2012). *Far from the tree: Parents, children, and the search for identity.* Scribner.

4   Igielnik, R. (2016, September 22). A political profile of disabled Americans. Pew Research Center. https://www.pewresearch.org/fact-tank/2016/09/22/a-political-profile-of-disabled-americans/

5   Solomon, A. (2012). *Far from the tree: Parents, children, and the search for identity.* Scribner.

6   National Council on Family Relations. (n.d.). Family focus. https://www.ncfr.org/ncfr-report/focus

7   National Council on Family Relations. (n.d.). Family focus. https://www.ncfr.org/ncfr-report/focus

8   Hall, G. N., Coun, M., Sanders, D., Noel, C., & Fife, S. T. (2020). Treating systemic issues in families affected by cystic fibrosis: A solution-focused approach. *Families, Systems, & Health, 38*(4), 464–475. http://dx.doi.org/10.1037/fsh0000544

9   National Council on Family Relations. (n.d.). Family focus. https://www.ncfr.org/ncfr-report/focus

10 Hall, G. N., Coun, M., Sanders, D., Noel, C., & Fife, S. T. (2020). Treating systemic issues in families affected by cystic fibrosis: A solution-focused approach. *Families, Systems, & Health, 38*(4), 464–475. http://dx.doi.org/10.1037/fsh0000544; Carlton, E. F, Donnelly, J. P., Prescott, H. C., et al. (2021). School and work absences after critical care hospitalization for pediatric acute respiratory failure: A secondary analysis of a cluster randomized trial. *JAMA Network Open*, 4, e2140732. http://doi.org/10.1001/jamanetworkopen.2021.40732;

11 Bassett, H. K., Beck, J., Coller, R. J., et al. (2021). Parent preferences for transparency of their child's hospitalization costs. *JAMA Network Open*, 4, e2126083. https://doi.org/10.1001/jamanetworkopen.2021.26083

12 Solomon, A. (2012). *Far from the tree: Parents, children, and the search for identity.* Scribner. (p. 363).

13 National Council on Family Relations. (n.d.). Family focus. https://www.ncfr.org/ncfr-report/focus; PsychGuides.com (2022). Behavioral disorder symptoms, causes and effects. https://www.psychguides.com/behavioral-disorders/; Wingrove, C., & Rickwood, D. (2019). Parents and carers of young people with mental ill-health: What factors mediate the effect of burden on stress? *Counselling Psychology Quarterly, 32*(1), 121–134. https://doi.org/10.1080/09515070.2017.1384362

14 Carlton, E. F, Donnelly, J. P., Prescott, H. C., et al. (2021). School and work absences after critical care hospitalization for pediatric acute respiratory failure: A secondary analysis of a cluster randomized trial. *JAMA Network Open*, 4, e2140732. http://doi.org/10.1001/jamanetworkopen.2021.40732; Schaeffer, K. (2020, April 23). As schools shift to online learning amid pandemic, here's what we know about disabled students in the U.S. Pew Research Center. https://www.pewresearch.org/fact-tank/2020/04/23/as-schools-shift-to-onlin

15 National Center for Education Statistics. (2021, May). Students with disabilities. U.S. Department of Education, Institute of Education Sciences. https://nces.ed.gov/programs/coe/indicator/cgg.

16 Nordström, A., & Kullgren, G. (2003). Victim relations and victim gender in violent crimes committed by offenders with schizophrenia. *Social Psychiatry and Psychiatric Epidemiology: The International Journal for Research in Social and Genetic Epidemiology and Mental Health Services, 38*(6), 326–330. https://doi-org.proxy.bsu.edu/10.1007/s00127-003-0640-5; Short, T., Thomas, S., Mullen, P., & Ogloff, J. R. P. (2013). Comparing violence in schizophrenia patients with and without comorbid substance-use disorders to community controls. *Acta Psychiatrica Scandinavica, 128*(4), 306–313. https://doi.org/10.1111/acps.12066

17 Solomon, A. (2012). *Far from the tree: Parents, children, and the search for identity.* Scribner. (p. 294).

18 https://www.helpguide.org/articles/stress/caregiver-stress-and-burnout.htm

19 Legano, L. A., Desch, L. W., Messner, S. A., Idzerda, S., Flaherty, E. G., Council nn Child Abuse and Neglect; Council on Children with Disabilities; Haney, S. B., Sirotnak, A. P., Gavril, A. R., Girardet, R. G., Hoffert Gilmartin, A. B., Laskey, A., Mohr, B. A., Nienow, S. M., Rosado, N., Kuo, D. Z., Apkon, S., Davidson, L. F., Ellerbeck, K. A., Foster, J. E. A., et al. (2021). Maltreatment of children with disabilities. *Pediatrics, 147*(5). https://doi.org/10.1542/peds.2021-050920

20 Chang, C., Su, J., Chang, K., Lin, C., Koschorke, M., Rüsch, N., & Thornicroft, G. (2019). Development of the Family Stigma Stress Scale (FSSS) for detecting stigma stress in caregivers of people with mental illness. *Evaluation & the Health Professions, 42*(2), 148–168. https://doi.org/10.1177/0163278717745658; Kim, I., Dababnah, S. & Lee, J. (2020). The influence of race and ethnicity on the relationship between family resilience and parenting stress in caregivers of children with autism. *Journal of Autism and Developmental Disorders, 50*, 650–658. https://doi.org/10.1007/s10803-019-04269-6 ; Kim, I., Wang, Y., Dababnah, S., & Betz, G. (2020). East Asian American parents of children with autism: A scoping review. *Review Journal of Autism and Developmental Disorders.* https://doi.org/10.1007/s40489-020-00221-y; National Council on Family Relations. (n.d.). Family focus. https://www.ncfr.org/ncfr-report/focus

21 Baider, L. (2012). Cultural diversity: Family path through terminal illness. *Annals of Oncology, 23*(Suppl 3), iii62–iii65. https://doi.org/10.1093/annonc/mds090

22 Solomon, A. (2012). *Far from the tree: Parents, children, and the search for identity.* Scribner.

23 Carlton, E. F, Donnelly, J. P., Prescott, H. C., et al. (2021). School and work absences after critical care hospitalization for pediatric acute respiratory failure: A secondary analysis of a cluster randomized trial. *JAMA Network Open*, 4, e2140732. http://doi.org/10.1001/jamanetworkopen.2021.40732; Marquis, S., McGrail, K., & Hayes, M. V. (2020). Using administrative data to examine variables affecting the mental health of siblings of children who

have a developmental disability. *Research in Developmental Disabilities, 96.* https://doi.org/10.1016/j.ridd.2019.103516; Rum, Y., Genzer, S., Markovitch, N., Jenkins, J., Perry, A., & Knafo-Noam, A. (2022). Are there positive effects of having a sibling with special needs? Empathy and prosociality of twins of children with non-typical development. *Child Development.* http://doi.org/10.1111/cdev.13740.

24 Mitchell, D. B., Szczerepa, A., & Hauser-Cram, P. (2016). Spilling over: Partner parenting stress as a predictor of family cohesion in parents of adolescents with developmental disabilities. *Research in Developmental Disabilities,* 49–50, 258–267. https://doi.org/10.1016/j.ridd.2015.12.007; Parker, J. A., Mandleco, B., Roper, S. O., Freeborn, D., & Dyches, T. T. (2011). Religiosity, spirituality, and marital relationships of parents raising a typically developing child or a child with a disability. *Journal of Family Nursing,* 17(1), 82–104. https://doi.org/10.1177/1074840710394856; Risdal, D., & Singer, G. H. S. (2004). Marital adjustment in parents of children with disabilities: A historical review and meta-analysis. *Research and Practice for Persons With Severe Disabilities,* 29(2), 95–103. https://doi.org/10.2511/rpsd.29.2.95; Wieland, N., & Baker, B. L. (2010). The role of marital quality and spousal support in behaviour problems of children with and without intellectual disability. *Journal of Intellectual Disability Research,* 54(7), 620–633. https://doi.org/10.1111/j.1365-2788.2010.01293.x

25 National Council on Disability. (n.d.). Rocking the cradle: Ensuring the rights of parents with disabilities and their children. https://ncd.gov/publications/2012/Sep272012; Powell, R. (2019, June 4). What it's like to be a disabled parent in an inaccessible world. Rewire Newsgroup. https://rewirenewsgroup.com/article/2019/06/04/what-its-like-to-be-a-disabled-parent-in-an-inaccessible-world/

26 Peay, H. L., Rosenstein, D. L., & Biesecker, B. B. (2013). Adaptation to bipolar disorder and perceived risk to children: A survey of parents with bipolar disorder. *BMC Psychiatry,* 13. https://doi.org/10.1186/1471-244X-13-327

27 National Council on Disability (n.d.). Rocking the cradle: Ensuring the rights of parents with disabilities and their children. https://ncd.gov/publications/2012/Sep272012; Powell, R. (2019, June 4). What it's like to be a disabled parent in an inaccessible world. Rewire Newsgroup. https://rewirenewsgroup.com/article/2019/06/04/what-its-like-to-be-a-disabled-parent-in-an-inaccessible-world/

28 Riebschleger, J. (2004). Good days and bad days: The experiences of children of a parent with a psychiatric disability. *Psychiatric Rehabilitation Journal,* 28(1), 25–31. https://doi.org/10.2975/28.2004.25.31

29 Collings, S., & Llewellyn, G. (2012). Children of parents with intellectual disability: Facing poor outcomes or faring okay? *Journal of Intellectual and Developmental Disability,* 37(1), 65–82. https://doi.org/0.3109/13668250.2011.648610; National Council on Disability (n.d.). Rocking the cradle: Ensuring the rights of parents with disabilities and their children. https://ncd.gov/publications/2012/Sep272012; Powell, R. (2019, June 4). What it's like to be a disabled parent in an inaccessible world. Rewire Newsgroup. https://rewirenewsgroup.com/article/2019/06/04/what-its-like-to-be-a-disabled-parent-in-an-inaccessible-world/

30 Graham, J. (2019, November 7). When caring for a sick spouse shakes a marriage to the core. Kaiser Family Foundation. https://khn.org/news/when-caring-for-a-sick-spouse-shakes-a-marriage-to-the-core/; Ritter, D. B. (2013, October 10). 10 marriage challenges caregivers of people with disabilities face. The Mobility Resource. https://www.themobilityresource.com/blog/post/10-marriage-challenges-caregivers-of-people-with-disabilities-face/; Russo, F. (2022, January 5). How a spouse's physical disability impacts a relationship. Next Avenue. https://www.nextavenue.org/how-a-spouses-disability-impacts-a-relationship/

31 Hopwood, J., Walker, N., McDonagh, L., Rait, G., Walters, K., Iliffe, S., Ross, J., & Davies, N. (2018). Internet-based interventions aimed at supporting family caregivers of people with dementia: Systematic review. *Journal of Medical Internet Research,* 20(6), e216. https://doi.org/10.2196/jmir.9548; Unson, C., Flynn, D., Glendon, M. A., Haymes, E., & Sancho, D. (2015). Dementia and caregiver stress: an application of the reconceptualized uncertainty in illness theory. *Issues in Mental Health Nursing,* 36(6), 439–446. https://doi.org/10.3109/01612840.2014.993052

32 Jones, T. (2022, March 22). Study: Increasing "uplifts" leads to better marital outcomes for parents of children with autism, Down syndrome. Medical Express. https://medicalxpress.com/news/2022-03-uplifts-marital-outcomes-parents-children.html; National Council on Family Relations. (n.d.). Family focus. https://www.ncfr.org/ncfr-report/focus

33 Hanzawa, S., Bae, J., Bae, Y. J., Chae, M., Tanaka, H., Nakane, H., Ohta, Y., Zhao, X., Iizuka, H., & Nakane, Y. (2013). Psychological impact on caregivers traumatized by the violent behavior of a family member with schizophrenia. *Asian Journal of Psychiatry,* 6(1), 46. https://doi.org/10.1016/j.ajp.2012.08.009; Ren, P., Emiliussen, J., Christiansen,

R., Engelsen, S., & Klausen, S. H. (2022). Filial piety, generativity and older adults' wellbeing and loneliness in Denmark and China. *Applied Research in Quality of Life.* https://doi-org.proxy.bsu.edu/10.1007/s11482-022-10053-z

34 Jacklin, K., Pace, J. E., & Warry, W. (2015). Informal dementia caregiving among indigenous communities in Ontario, Canada. *Care Management Journals, 16*(2), 106–120. http://doi.org/10.1891/1521-0987.16.2.106; Kaufman, A. V., Kosberg, J. I., Leeper, J. D., & Tang, M. (2010). Social support, caregiver burden, and life satisfaction in a sample of rural African American and White caregivers of older persons with dementia. *Journal of Gerontological Social Work, 53*(3), 251–269. https://doi.org/10.1080/01634370903478989

35 Solomon, A. (2012). *Far from the tree: Parents, children, and the search for identity.* Scribner. (p. 21)

36 Jones, T. (2022, March 22). Study: Increasing "uplifts" leads to better marital outcomes for parents of children with autism, Down syndrome. Medical Express. https://medicalxpress.com/news/2022-03-uplifts-marital-outcomes-parents-children.html

37 Sohn, E. (2021, July 13). Mindfulness benefits kids with ADHD, and their families. WebMD. https://www.webmd.com/add-adhd/news/20210713/mindfulness-benefits-kids-with-adhd-and-their-families

38 Graham, J. (2019, November 7). When caring for a sick spouse shakes a marriage to the core. Kaiser Family Foundation. https://khn.org/news/when-caring-for-a-sick-spouse-shakes-a-marriage-to-the-core/; Ritter, D. B. (2013, October 10). 10 marriage challenges caregivers of people with disabilities face. The Mobility Resource. https://www.themobilityresource.com/blog/post/10-marriage-challenges-caregivers-of-people-with-disabilities-face/

39 Kersh, J., Hedvat, T. T., Hauser-Cram, P., & Warfield, M. E. (2006). The contribution of marital quality to the well-being of parents of children with developmental disabilities. *Journal of Intellectual Disability Research, 50*(12), 883–893. https://doi.org/bsu.edu/10.1111/j.1365-2788.2006.00906.x

Image Credits
Fig. 9.1: Source: Adapted from https://nces.ed.gov/programs/coe/indicator/cgg.

CHAPTER 10

Addiction, Compulsion, and Family Stress

Over the past 5 years, an average of more than 70,000 people died each year of a drug overdose.[1] In 1994, over 40% of eighth graders said it was highly risky to try LSD or "acid" just once or twice; in 2020, that number dropped to 20%.[2]

Chapter Preview

- Substance and behavioral compulsions can interfere with family life and create stressors.
- Various conflicting perspectives interpret issues about the meaning of a substance problem differently.
- Substance use can alter brain functioning, which contributes to addiction.
- Growing up in a home with substance problems puts children at risk for several long-term challenges.
- Children's use of substances places multiple pressures on parents.
- Childhood trauma often contributes to why adults develop substance compulsions.
- Treatment for substance problems is also stressful for families, especially early on.
- Behaviors related to gambling and sex can also be compulsive and problematic.
- Excessive screen time and social media use can increase risks for of negative individual and family outcomes.

What Is This Topic About?

Have you ever had a craving so strong you felt like you had no willpower to fight it? Maybe toward something simple like an ice cream cone, or more serious like shoplifting or injecting an illegal substance? Then after you give in to that craving, you find only temporary relief or pleasure and maybe even feel worse about yourself afterward. While the formal diagnosis of **addiction** requires that specific criteria be met, the primary concern of this chapter is family stress related to substance use problems and other problematic behavior that seems difficult to stop. Let's use the broader concept of "**compulsion**"—an irresistible urge or impulse that can counter a person's more conscious desires—which could be a component of addiction. A **problematic compulsion** interferes with everyday living and one's general well-being. When it comes to family stress, we will emphasize how compulsive substance use and other compulsive behaviors affect families—and how family problems might contribute to such compulsions. What's the first specific example that comes to mind when you think of someone having a problematic compulsion? Why was that the first example?

What Are the Assumptions?

What does each of these words imply about consuming alcohol or drugs?

- experiment
- recreation
- use
- misuse
- abuse
- disorder
- disease

The language used to describe problematic substance use has changed over time, and we have no universal agreement on terminology. "**Substance use disorder (SUD)**" has become increasingly popular; how is that different from "substance abuse?" Which one sounds more like the person is the problem or that the person is more in control of one's own actions? Terminology changes are at least partially intended to affect the way we think about addictions or compulsions—you know, our perceptions.

A key assumption about this topic has to do with the **amount of choice or power** one has in controlling compulsions. Or, how much is someone to **blame** for giving in to compulsions? On the one hand, with blame comes **shame** and **stigma**, two concepts that are commonly thought of as barriers to overcoming a compulsion. When people feel worse about themselves they sometimes turn toward the temporary comfort they find in feeding the compulsion. On the other hand, people usually choose whether to try a substance or to engage in a problematic behavior for the first time (and perhaps beyond). Furthermore, it seems impossible to **empower** people to change their lives if they are indeed completely powerless toward the compulsion.

We lean toward certain ways of thinking (or have biases) about compulsions and blame based perhaps on experiences and ideological perspectives. From a **conservative** viewpoint that generally emphasizes family and societal **stability** and personal accountability (and possibly religious beliefs related to righteous living or **sanctity**), compulsive substance use might be seen as immoral behavior that should be discouraged and even punished. The emphasis on the **fairness** dimension can push perceptions toward seeing victims as suffering the natural consequences of poor decisions. That is not to say this perspective has a complete lack of sympathy—in fact, people with substance problems might be viewed as victims of the societal breakdown of the family or permissive government policy. Conversely, from a **liberal** perspective, with emphases on the **care** dimension and on societal inequities, problematic substance use might be seen as a symptom of unfair social structures that marginalize certain groups. The correct government policies that address issues such as poverty—not necessarily the choices of those with the compulsions—would alleviate much of the causes of substance problems. Such ideological assumptions inform the types of professional prevention and intervention efforts that we will discuss later.

As you **engage with** the rest of the chapter, remember the key elements of family stress theories (e.g., stressors, resources, perceptions, coping, and crisis) and consider the following:

- What do different types of compulsions have in common? Why might they also have different consequences?
- How do the various pieces of information throughout the chapter fit together to help explain why each family might be affected differently by the stressors?
- What experiences have you had or observed that help you relate to specific concepts?
- How might the ideological perspectives influence how people (including you) think about potential causes of and solutions to families' problematic compulsions?

Part A. Substance Use Compulsion Stressors

What Is Stressful About Substance Use Compulsions?

Think of a fictional character from a book, TV show, or movie who has a drinking problem. Ready? What about the person or situation made you conclude there was a **problem**?

Data from the National Survey on Drug Use and Health reveal the percentages of adults of different ages who have had five alcoholic beverages in a row at least once during the prior two weeks, and who have taken an illegal substance within the prior 30 days (see chart in Figure 10.1).[3] While most adults who use substances don't report serious problems or dependency, it is estimated that over 14 million adult Americans have a drinking problem, and about 21 million have at least one substance addiction. Chances are you know a few.

Much of the research on problem drinking or alcoholism mirrors research on problems with other substances, whether it be the misuse of prescription medications or using illicit drugs like cocaine, LSD, or (in many places) marijuana. In some ways, a compulsion is a compulsion—it doesn't really matter what the specific substance or behavior is, just whether it interferes with having a good life. However, substances differ in their physiological effects and their legal and social implications. One's motivations, personal vulnerabilities, and social circumstances are also relevant to a compulsion's power and impact. Nevertheless, this chapter emphasizes **similarity** of conditions and consequences across various substances.

Scientific breakthroughs in the study of the brain have helped explain why substances can become so addictive.[4] Not everyone who uses a given substance develops a SUD and it is not completely clear why. Even so, when casual use of a substance turns into unhealthy use, or when medical use of a substance turns into chronic dependence, addiction becomes the next potential step. Some people seem to be at greater risk for developing addiction based on their biological makeup and their environmental experiences (e.g., traumatic stress). The brain is susceptible to developing patterns that make self-control especially difficult. Brain changes can endure well after substance use has stopped, and it is not clear how much of the change can be reversed.

The path to a SUD begins with the pleasurable sensations of intoxication. Many substances appear to trigger our natural **dopamine** (and comparable) system, which produces pleasure associated with things like eating and sexual activity. At some point, the pleasure wears off (withdrawal) and is followed by neutral or negative emotional sensations that can then lead to a preoccupation with seeking to use the substance again. The pleasurable sensations reinforce the desire to continue substance use, as can approval of others (e.g., treated as one of the group, backing off peer pressure). However, addictive substances seem to essentially overload our dopamine receptors, causing them to work at a diminished capacity. As substance use becomes a habit, things that had typically brought pleasure don't seem to trigger pleasure as much, if at all, including the substance. Thus, cravings for the substance become more powerful, and higher amounts of the substance are used in an attempt to recover the pleasure of intoxication.

Furthermore, it appears that withdrawal activates **stress neurotransmitters** that essentially cause an overreaction of the brain's stress system, leading to negative sensations. Thus, substance use can become motivated by merely the need to soothe these negative symptoms, to try to just feel normal. Cravings can be triggered by being around familiar people or places that serve as reminders of the substance, by nearby use of a substance, or by experiencing stress. The executive functions of the brain (prefrontal cortex) seem to be manipulated by the cravings in ways that stimulate powerful urges, disrupt decision-making processes, and interfere with regulating impulsive behavior. Even after people have been through addiction recovery, triggering can still occur and lead to persistent relapse. Adolescence appears to be an especially high-risk period for developing brain-altering substance use habits given the tendency for youth to experiment with substances and the vulnerability of their actively developing brains.

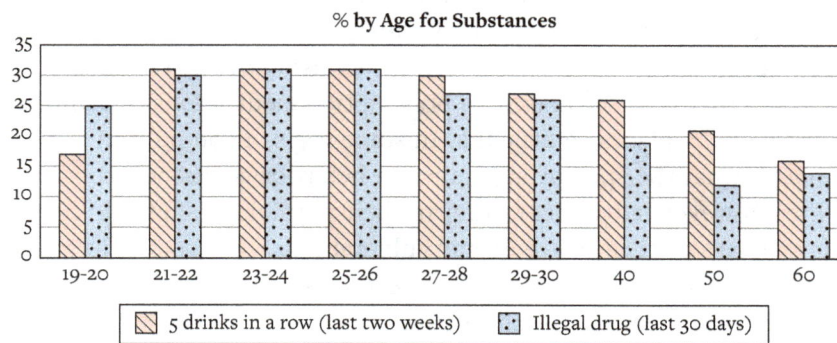

FIGURE 10.1 % by Age for Substances

What Does This Have to Do With Family Stress?

Remember that stressors put **pressure** on families to change or to act. A family with long-term substance compulsions has established patterns (e.g., rules, roles, boundaries) that likely have negative consequences for one or more family members. For example, a young child may feel distressed about having to step in for an inebriated parent to prepare meals for the rest of the family. It is difficult for families to **flourish** when a compulsion interferes with meeting the needs of family members, though some families can show signs of stability for a time. **Strained families** are less prepared for stressors in general, including compulsions. The presence of a substance compulsion can be a sign that a family has reached **crisis**. New substance compulsions can create unfamiliar or intense pressures that push families to adapt in ways that alter the quality of general family functioning.

What Specific Effects Can a Substance Compulsion Have on a Family?

Substance-related stressors put children and families at higher risk for a variety of negative outcomes.[5] Specifically, when a parent has the substance problem, children are more likely to suffer from **neglect**. For example, consider the following:

* Prenatal substance problems increase the likelihood of **fetal alcohol syndrome** and babies born with drugs in their system, putting children at risk for developmental delays and other difficulties.
* Mothers with substance problems sometimes neglect proper premedical care in fear of having their drug problem discovered, also increasing the likelihood of their babies being born with health problems.
* Young children in need of regular and loving attention struggle when highly intoxicated parents are physically or emotionally unavailable, or when parents are preoccupied with obtaining and using a substance.
* The physiological stimulation of a mothers' drug usage can overpower or neutralize the typical psychological and emotional pleasures of engaging with children, making the drug the more appealing option.
* Interaction with children tends to be harsher and less positive. Children might not feel loved, safe, and important because of barriers to forming healthy attachments with parents.
* Families with substance problems are at higher risk for intimate violence, thus creating fear and potential trust issues for the children.

Parents with substance problems can also struggle to support older children and monitor their behavior. Some of these children tend to struggle with having too much unsupervised freedom, increasing risks of causing trouble for others, hurting themselves, and neglecting school work. Others become **parentified**—having adult responsibilities too early, which can lead to high anxiety, self-neglect, and difficulty establishing healthy levels of responsibility as an adult. As described in previous chapters, these adult responsibilities are often physical (e.g., cleaning up a parent's mess, dressing siblings, putting a parent to bed) and emotional tasks (e.g., soothing a distraught parent or sibling, communicating on the parent's behalf to another family member or professional).

Children are apt to flourish when raised in a nurturing environment with significant consistency, predictability, and safety. The moods and actions of an intoxicated parent can be unreliable and even terrifying, which disrupts children's meal and sleep patterns and causes children to consistently be on high alert for negative treatment, neglect, or the need to step in and compensate for the unavailable parent. Think about how being raised in such a household affects the identity of children. Why might such children be more **vulnerable** to having similar challenges in their own potential, future families?

Families with substance problems might also face certain financial pressures. The costs of substances, loss of parental employment, and in some cases expensive treatment programs diminish resources used to meet other family needs. Parents and children might feel ashamed of a parent's substance problems, so **secrecy** becomes a major family theme. Children don't learn how to trust others and to talk about their feelings, if they are allowed to express them at all. Parental behavior that makes a public scene, damages property, or injures others can cause **embarrassment**, **shame**, and **hopelessness** for family members.

Remember the concept of **ambiguous** stressors? Explaining a parent's substance compulsion to a child is complicated, and children can have many misunderstandings about what is going on with the parent. Such ambiguity makes it especially difficult to cope with situations—how do you respond to something you don't understand? How do you know if you did something wrong? For any family member, uncertainty about how best to help someone with a substance compulsion brings its own set of stressors, which will be described later in the chapter.

In addition to—or because of—the challenges already mentioned, children of parents with substance problems are at higher risk for exposure to conflict and violence between parents, their parents splitting up, a parent being imprisoned, and the premature death of a parent. Children might also be removed from their home and placed in foster care, which can have its own set of challenges (see Chapter 7). Consequently, children of parents with substance problems are overall at higher risk for the following:

- Struggling with healthy development (physical, emotional, psychological, social)
- Academic underachievement
- Mental health problems
- Suicidal ideation
- Relationship problems
- Adolescent and adult substance problems
- Concerns about being an adequate parent themselves

Remember, however, that families and children can be **resilient**. While substance problems put families at risk for a variety of challenges, some families **cope** with the challenges better than others. Nevertheless, if our goal is to help families flourish, we need to understand what is at stake, what families might need, and how to prevent as many barriers as possible to flourishing.

What Is Going on With These Parents?

Did you notice any patterns in how stressors created by (or amplified by) parental substance problems typically impact children? What happens when those children become parents? **Childhood trauma** (see Chapter 1)—including that which is related to family substance problems—is thought of as a common cause of adulthood substance compulsions. Childhood trauma elevates the risk of later mental health problems such as depression and anxiety. Survivors of childhood trauma might turn to substances to help **dampen** emotional pain, feelings of self-doubt or loathing, and a sense of helplessness. Parents with substance problems commonly report having been mistreated as children, and the numbing effects of certain substances (e.g., opioids) may be attractive in times of distress.

It has been said that parenting is the hardest job there is. Now imagine experiencing the typical stressors of raising children while also battling all sorts of negative thoughts and feelings about yourself and powerful cravings for an intoxicating substance. Parents tend to feel inadequate much of the time anyway, so struggling with compulsions that inhibit their ability to be fully present and engaged as a parent can really inflate feelings of shame and guilt. Remember our earlier discussion about accountability and control? How much blame you assign to such parents depends somewhat on your own worldview—your own biases. Putting aside the issue of blame, it should seem unsurprising by now that substance problems can pass on from one generation to the next (from parent to child).

How Can Recovery Be Stressful for Families?

Recovery from substance compulsions (or addiction) can take many years with multiple setbacks. This can be extremely discouraging for a family, especially if this is not realized upfront. A **setback** might feel like a personal failure to family members; it can make it difficult to know if the person can be trusted. Families are often unsure of the best way to support their loved one who is trying to recover. Do they insist on complete abstinence from the substance? Do they enforce tough consequences for violating rules or agreements? Are they unintentionally enabling the substance use by showing some acceptance and helping to avoid catastrophes that put the family in jeopardy (e.g., job loss)? Even experts disagree on such issues—imagine how confused family members might be. Families benefit by finding **social support** and getting educated about the potential consequences of their responses to substance problems, and realizing it is normal to be so confusing and complicated.

The **early stages of a parent's recovery** are often highly stressful for children.[6] Why might that be? Think about family rules, roles, boundaries, and routines. Even when general family functioning is strained due to substance problems, children can find ways to cope with the family patterns and figure out how best to meet some basic needs (if possible). A parent in early recovery will need to make major behavioral changes that can dramatically disrupt the family patterns and alter expectations for family member responses. The family loses the comfort of a familiar atmosphere and the coping strategies they are accustomed to using may no longer apply. This can be confusing and unsettling for family members who now have to develop new family patterns, revise parts of their identities, and learn new coping strategies that ideally lead to better overall family functioning. Some children prefer the certainty of the former environment over the ambiguity of the changing environment, at least for a time.

How Is Adolescent Substance Abuse a Stressor for Families?

Children with substance problems can create many stressors for their parents, regardless of whether their parents have substance problems themselves. **Adolescence** is a key time in which children experiment with some substances. Why might that be? National data show the following:[7]

- Some 61.5% of adolescents have had more than just a few sips of alcohol by the time they finish high school (26% had done so by eighth grade).
- About 40% of 12th graders had used an illegal drug within the prior 12 months.
- Over the past two decades, adolescents have increasingly viewed some substances as less dangerous (LSD, crack), though some substances have gone the other direction (meth-amphetamines, heavy smoking). Misusing prescription drugs (including sedatives and opioids) is viewed by adolescents as less dangerous since the drugs can be legally used and thus have legitimate purposes.
- The number of adolescents who said most substances were easy to get has also been dropping in that time span, however.
- Vaping took off for the first three years it was introduced and then it dropped off a bit, illustrating a common pattern for new drugs—a quick rise with experimentation and then some of the appeal lessens over time.

For some parents, **any substance use** by their children would cause pressure, such as worry about health consequences and forming addictions, concerns about how others may view their children or themselves (stigma), and the violation of legal, moral, or religious standards. Others share only some of these concerns and see substance use as a normal part of adolescence. Some parents feel hypocritical if they prevent their children from doing what they themselves may have done in the past. Hence, parental **perceptions** of substance use and the surrounding circumstances contribute to whether and how parents respond. Given our focus on problematic compulsions, the most relevant point here is that families are especially prone to perceive adolescent substance use as a stressor when it is believed to contribute to academic, social, legal, or health-related problems.

Within the home, we might expect adolescent substance use pressures to create extra tension and conflict in parent-child and sibling **relationships**. If multiple parental figures live in the home, each might react differently to the circumstances and have distinct (or contrary) ideas about how to address them, causing conflict in their relationship with each other. Children suspended or expelled from school for **delinquent behavior**, or who get in trouble with the law, could demand major amounts of time from parents who may already be stretched thin with caring for other family members and fulfilling employment responsibilities. Additionally, parents can be consumed with self-blame for a child's misbehavior, experiencing the pressures of guilt and regret. Siblings can be embarrassed by the adolescent's behavior, resent the disruption created by the substance use problems, and contend with each other's differing perspectives regarding the substance use and its consequences.

Can you imagine a home in which a parent *and* an adolescent experience substance problems? The compulsions can feed into one another. In some cases, parents share their substances and even use them with their child, and in others, the adolescent secretly takes the substances from a parent's or sibling's supply, including prescription drugs that the adolescent uses for nonmedical purposes. Be it a parent, a child, or both struggling with a substance compulsion, general family functioning is at elevated risk of becoming strained, making the family more vulnerable to detrimental impacts of any other stressors that **pile up**.

How Can Substance Use Stressors Be Avoided in the First Place?

Ideally, substance use compulsions would be **prevented** from occurring. Childhood trauma, economic desperation, and a lack of healthy coping skills are common **risk factors** for developing substance problems. Successful prevention efforts would help decrease risk factors and increase **protective factors** such as education, responsive caregivers or intimate partners, and opportunities for growth and thriving. Within the home, parents can engage in the following to help prevent the risk of child and adolescent substance use:[8]

- Learn about healthy child development and how to identify warning signs of problems that could contribute to at-risk behavior.
- Build strong, trusting parent-child relationships.
- Respectfully monitor children's behavior and their whereabouts (where they are, who is with them, what they are doing).
- Have frequent and open communication (including about substances and parents' expectations).
- Have an authoritative parenting style (high standards mixed with parental warmth and nurture) rather than a permissive (low standards) or authoritarian one (high standards mixed with parental harshness and rigid punishment).
- Become educated about substances and the risk factors for their use.
- Teach and model healthy coping skills for dealing with frustration, disappointment, and negative peer pressure (including with social media).

None of these will guarantee desirable results, and influences outside the home also play a large role in the choices people make and the risk- and protective factors they face, but these are time-tested elements of generally successful prevention and early intervention efforts. Helping families identify their **strengths** and think through their successful coping examples from their past can also help boost the **resilience** of families facing the prospect of substance problems.

How Do External Contexts Impact Families With Substance Use Stressors?

Studies from across various countries and subgroups within the United States tend to show many similarities in the types and impacts of the stressors described earlier.[9] However, as has been the case with other topics, **social class** can contribute to increased stressors with fewer resources to combat them. Substances might become a form of **coping** with the discouragement that comes with poverty. Conversely, some substance issues (e.g., binge drinking) tend to be more common for adolescents from wealthier families. Similarly, college students (especially men) tend to report more past and recent alcohol use—including being drunk—than do non-college students of the same age. Nonmedical use of substances such as Adderall and Ritalin that are prescribed for treating attention deficit hyperactivity disorder (ADHD) can also tempt students who feel pressure to keep up with homework and other obligations. In some regions of the United States (e.g., Appalachia), low-income parents are especially likely to misuse and die from opioids. Think about the **intersection of wealth and social norms** as they contribute to substance problems.

Adolescent and adult **females** generally have lower rates of substance usage, but the gap has been decreasing some due to **males** using less and females using more (though adolescent females may have higher rates of misuse of prescription drugs like tranquilizers).[10] When there are **gender** differences, men are more likely to use drugs with male friends while women are more likely to use drugs with an intimate partner. Women also tend to be at greater risk for poorer physical and mental health because of family substance problems, at least in part because they also tend to provide more care to a loved one with a substance problem, and to children suffering the consequences of the substance problem.

White adolescents have historically had the highest rates of illegal drug usage in the United States, though **Black** adolescents' increasing use of marijuana has helped narrow the gap.[11] Black and **Hispanic** adolescents tend to report less misuse of prescription drugs. While Hispanic youth tend to be somewhere between White and Black adolescent substance use trends, they report the highest use of cocaine, crack, and crystal. Interestingly, for Hispanic youth, those who speak better English than their parents (who are thus probably immigrants) may be especially likely to drink alcohol. Belonging to cultures or communities that tend to view personal and family issues as highly private (e.g., Irish) can contribute to shame and stigma that prevents open discussion of family substance problems. What differences might groups have in access to various substances? What legal and social implications do certain drugs have compared to others?

As one would expect given what you have learned about **minority stress**, **LGBT** adults tend to struggle more with substance problems than the general population, estimates are around 7% compared to just over 5% of all adults. Sexual minority women appear to especially be at higher risk for substance problems. Lack of family support and using substances as a coping mechanism can be key contributors to these patterns. Some have also pointed to an element of "queer coming of age" that contributes to high alcohol usage in queer social settings.[12]

Older adolescents living in **rural** areas have generally reported a lower rate of ever having tried an illegal drug than those who live in larger cities. However, when marijuana is excluded from those numbers, those in larger cities have tended to have a lower rate of having ever tried an illegal drug.[13] Generally speaking, **religious** families tend to have lower rates of substance use. **Veterans** may be vulnerable to certain substance use problems; about 10% of young adult veterans misuse prescription pain relievers, nearly twice the rate of the general population of the same age. Veterans also tend to have higher rates overall of problematic use of illegal drugs and alcohol (see Chapter 11 for more insight).

Improve Your Learning

Without peeking, take a moment to review in your mind (or say out loud) the key concepts from this chapter (this is a proven learning technique). Then review the "Chapter Preview" section at the top and compare. Skim Part A of the chapter with extra attention to the **bolded words**. Skip to the end of the chapter to find more learning resources.

Part B. Behavioral Compulsion Stressors

What Other Compulsions Are Problematic for Families?

Have you heard about people who are controlled by their urges to overeat or shop? A variety of compulsive behaviors can lead people to feelings of **euphoria** (a high). The thrill, risk, or comfort of certain sensations could seem like a needed distraction from life's pressures or disappointments, and sometimes the sensations become too compelling to ignore. We will focus briefly on the compulsions of gambling, sex-related issues, and personalized technology usage to illustrate.

What Does This Have to Do With Family Stress?

Similar to powerful cravings for addictive substances, behavioral compulsions can become habits that interfere with individual and family well-being. Time and energy that could be used toward maintaining and improving family relationships are used up in activities that prevent optimal family functioning. Furthermore, the compulsions can put heavy pressure on family members that end up increasing the risk of reaching **crisis**.

How Can a Gambling Compulsion Influence Family Stress?

Winning can be such a thrill. The anticipation of an outcome could be even more exciting. Imagine a parent, however, who can't feel good unless some money is on the line—*I just need one big win to finally make things better.* Why might this be a stressor for families? Assuming the person is struggling with a powerful compulsion, it is likely that the family's financial stability is at risk. Consequently, family members may suffer because of[14]

- **neglect:** The person may have less time and attention to dedicate toward caring for children, supporting a spouse or partner, or assisting aging parents;
- **financial difficulties:** Basic needs of food, clothing, and shelter are at risk; parents may take on extra jobs to help make ends meet, resulting in less time to meet other family needs; and
- **relationship challenges:** Arguments over the gambling problem bring tension in the home; family members, including extended family, may struggle with decisions about giving or lending money to the family, worried that it will be spent to feed the gambling problem.

Unsurprisingly, children in such families likely struggle with emotional and mental health problems, physical health problems (e.g., headaches, digestion, exhaustion), and substance use. Just as with substance compulsions, and possibly more so, explaining a gambling compulsion to a child is difficult. Again, **ambiguity** about the problem leads to confusion and misunderstandings about the tension and financial struggles in the home.

How Can a Sexual Compulsion Influence Family Stress?

You can probably quickly imagine how a compulsion to have sex could lead to cheating and potentially ending couple relationships. Cybersex, or some kind of virtual sexual interaction with one or more individuals from a distance, might also seem like an obvious cause of tension in a relationship. Though some people see virtual sex as meaningfully different from real, physical sex, committed partners nevertheless commonly feel insecure, jealous, and betrayed in both cases. Does it make a difference if no "real" people are involved on the other side of the screen?

Pornography has become a major focus related to sexual compulsions, probably because of its abundance and ease of access due to the internet. People have various perceptions about if and how pornography is harmful to children and adults, but here we are discussing compulsions—be they based on actual sexual behavior or on viewing sexually explicit content. This is a good example of the importance of one's **perceptions of the stressor**. For some spouses, compulsive pornography viewing might not seem like a critical threat to their relationship quality. For others, it is somewhere down the path toward cheating. The extent to which people interpret their partner's viewing to mean the partner is dissatisfied with or rejecting them could make a difference in how they are affected. It appears that for many spouses, there are unpleasant outcomes.

Various experts have explained the potential hardships for families that include someone with a sexual compulsion.[15] Popular pornographic videos tend to depict messages that could be counter to relationship commitment and harmony. For example, sexual **infidelity** is shown more often than sex within a committed relationship. Sexual encounters focus more on women pleasuring men rather than mutual pleasure. Women tend to play a more submissive role with sex and are even depicted as recipients of sexual violence. More times than not, such acts and attitudes are met by neutral or positive responses by the depicted women. Such messaging can arguably influence attitudes and expectations that lead to relational conflict and perhaps betrayal.

Pornographic media can be thought of as a "supernormal stimulus," meaning that it is produced to elicit quick and heightened sexual responses. Real-life sexual experiences can seem less stimulating or exciting in comparison, which can lead to less interest in sex with one's partner and actual declines in sexual frequency and satisfaction. Some viewers find it difficult to become sexually aroused without the fast-paced, highly erotic psychological high from pornography. With pornography, the consumer is more in control of the sexual content (e.g., viewing choices, rewinding, or fast-forwarding), whereas with a real partner a healthy sexual encounter involves negotiation and mutuality. Compulsive pornography consumption can lead to unrealistic expectations that put undue **pressure** on one's partner, such as assuming that one's partner will always be ready for sex and in whatever manner one desires.

With all this in mind, it is unsurprising that committed partners/spouses (usually women) of compulsive porn viewers tend to experience

- negative emotional reactions (anger, depression, humiliation);
- a sense of betrayal, feeling like they must compete with the looks and sexual responsiveness of fantasy sex partners, inadequacy and loneliness;
- being objectified (thought of and treated like just an object of pleasure) and coerced to engage sexually in ways they are not necessarily comfortable with;
- frequent suspicion of and lack of trust in their partner/spouse; and
- a lack of general intimacy and sexual fulfillment in the relationship.

Being unhappy in the relationship adds **pressure** to decide what is reasonable to demand from a partner, how long to remain in the relationship, and potentially how to help protect children from a contentious environment. Children notice such contention and sometimes witness a parent viewing pornography or demeaning someone as a sexual object. This can cause great discomfort in the home and concerns about the health and future of the family unit.

How Can Technology/Social Media Compulsions Influence Family Stress?

Who doesn't enjoy a good video game now and then? Or feel a little tingle when someone (especially many someones) transmits an affirming emoji in response to an opinion or picture we post on social media? Who hasn't been a bit annoyed when a seemingly automatic, eager response to a dinging notification completely torpedoes a face-to-face conversation? Experts and parents alike have expressed concern over apparent obsessions with technology. Terms such as "pathological technology use" and "gaming disorder" have arisen to describe compulsive behavior and outcomes related to technology use—particularly related to electronic leisure technology.

As with other compulsions, a **preoccupation** with our screens can reach points at which we feel lost without them and neglect important priorities in our lives. Too much technological leisure can have negative consequences for individuals and families.[16] For example, school-aged and adolescent children with high amounts of video gaming or other screen time (e.g., television, internet/app scrolling) tend to be more psychologically distant during daily routines and family time, engage in more aggressive behavior, have a lower grade point average, get less physical exercise, socially withdraw more from others, and experience less family support. What does "high amount" mean? One large study found that adolescents who had more than 2 hours a day of screen time also had more psychosomatic complaints (physical symptoms—like muscle or stomach aches—that have psychological causes). Whether screen time causes these issues or these issues put children at greater risk for more screen time is somewhat unclear, though children who already had ADHD (which is often associated with screen time) have experienced worsening ADHD symptoms when their increased screen time was tracked over time.

Overall, the idea seems reasonable that a compulsion toward excessive screen time would disrupt important developmental tasks and put children at risk for negative outcomes. But children are not alone in such vulnerability. **Couples** in which a partner seems compelled to spend unrestrained amounts of time with online video games seem to struggle with communicating, intimacy, relational aggression, and isolation from other sources of support.[17] Such compulsions suggest that the pleasure and reward centers of the brain undergo some similar processes as discussed regarding substances—cravings form that are easily triggered and are difficult to ignore.

Some elements of social media also likely play into our susceptibility to developing compulsions, particularly the validating feedback we get from affirming onlookers.[18] (Can I get a thumbs up, anyone?)

Or, perhaps you are tired of social media taking the blame for society's problems. Sure, the problems and causes can be oversimplified. Plenty of people with an active social media presence appear to live healthy lives. Nevertheless, social media can tempt us to think or act in ways that put us at risk for emotional and psychological challenges.[19] For example, people can portray **inauthentic identities** that contribute to unrealistic expectations of reality. We might judge ourselves harshly because we don't measure up to how we perceive others, leading to anxiety and self-doubt. At the same time, skewed presentations of the world can also increase our **paranoia**; fears and dangers can be exaggerated and our natural biases can make popular ideas among our social group seem more believable (see Chapter 2 on cognitive biases). Seeing the impact of virtual mobs ganging up on someone can also increase paranoia. We might also learn to be too concerned about what **other people think about us**. The feedback we get from our online offerings can nudge us toward obsessing over ratios of positive to negative feedback instead of investing in meaningful contributions to our family and beyond. We can feel pressure to present our lives as worthy of all the attention we might seek—a competition with other online profiles that depict interesting daily lives.

We should not be too surprised that young teenagers in particular are less happy the more they engage with social media, even when tracking changes in social media use and their happiness over time.[20] Young adults have also demonstrated this pattern. Parents feel the extra pressure of addressing the negative impacts of technological compulsions, which can be especially challenging when the children are unable or willing to recognize the impacts and need to connect with peers who also rely heavily on technology—*Can I help my child without cutting off social media completely and isolating them?*

Consider also the impact on **family relationships** when more and more members have social media compulsions. How might such relationships be affected when someone is overly obsessed with their virtual relationships, or experience the poorer negative mental health that can result? Think about the arguments and conflicts that might arise when someone who needs personal attention can't compete with the virtual world. Ponder how such preoccupations could detract from attending to the needs of vulnerable family members.

How Do External Contexts Impact Families With Behavior Compulsion Stressors?

As alluded to earlier, in heterosexual relationships, it is more likely that the **man** has the sexual compulsion. Some research suggests that lesbian women are more likely than heterosexual women to have a sexual compulsion but less likely than men as a group. Beliefs and pressures surrounding concepts of masculinity and femininity can contribute to some gender differences in these types of experiences, as might hormonal differences (e.g., testosterone, oxytocin) that can affect sexual arousal, assertiveness, and bonding in relationships.

Gender can also be a factor in how technological leisure impacts children and families.[21] Boys and men in particular are more likely to spend excessive time with video games. Males who struggle with school, employment, or social relationships can feel extra tempted to escape into the gaming world and exacerbate the challenges they are trying to avoid. Teenage girls appear especially vulnerable to the impacts of social media compulsions (see the table in Figure 10.2 regarding hours of daily social media and depression symptoms[22]). With the propensity for females to **ruminate** with one another about their stressors, mixed with an especially strong pressure for adolescent and young adult females to outperform everyone in school and the workplace, social media provides a powerful combination for social contagions of depression, self-harm, eating disorders, and inaccurate self-diagnoses of medical, psychological, and identity conditions (e.g., Tourette's syndrome) to thrive.

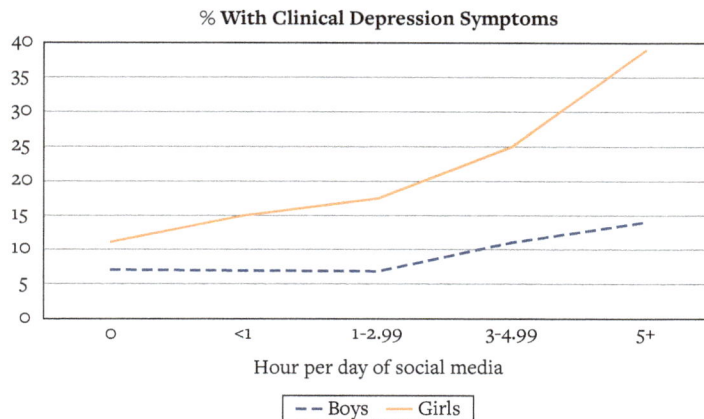

% With Clinical Depression Symptoms

Hour per day of social media

-- Boys   — Girls

FIGURE 10.2 % With Clinical Depression Symptoms

Belief systems related to **religion** and **culture** can also influence how behavioral compulsions are understood and how people cope with them. A conservative religion or religious-inspired culture could contribute to feelings of shame and guilt that for some motivate them to seek change while for others might further damage self-worth and sabotage recovery. How much tolerance a spouse has toward the offending spouse's behavior (especially related to sex) could also be impacted by larger cultural contexts.

What Does All This Mean for You?

Take a few moments to ponder the following:

- How have you been feeling while engaging with this information? Why?
- How much can you personally relate to?
- What other examples have come to mind that illustrate similar or diverse ways that families experience substance problems?
- What hope do families have to cope with substance abuse problems? Can such families ever flourish?

Reminders for Helpers

As a person of influence, you can help guide people through the coping processes and ideally help foster a **flourishing** life. However, take care to avoid letting your personal **interpretations** push you toward assuming too much about somebody else's circumstances, perceptions, and motivations. Always be ready to address issues that might be hard for you to face because of your own history.

Draw upon the elements of the **FIM framework** and other family stress concepts. Remember, **coping** refers to an action or response based on available or new resources and perceptions related to stressors. Families have either successfully **managed** a stressor's pressure through **adjustment coping** or reached crisis in which **adaptive coping** is needed to reestablish some level of **general family functioning**. **Resources** and **perceptions** are key concepts to focus on when confronting family stress. **Review the master table** in Chapter 4 as a guide for exploring the following ideas on how to help families with stressors.

What Are Some Ways to Encourage Effective Family Coping?

Drawing primarily from citations and insights noted in the chapter thus far, we will explore **suggested resources and noteworthy perceptions** that can contribute to successful coping and more optimal family functioning.

How Can You Help Families With Compulsive Substance and Behavioral Stressors?

A key **resource** for helping family members deal with stressors owing to parental, partner, or child substance abuse is **social/emotional support**. People more easily burn out when they are alone. As mentioned, family members can feel embarrassment and shame, which can close them off from social connections. They may need help conquering the stigma associated with substance problems. In some cases, children may need a place to stay or an extra adult figure in their home if parents become partially or fully unavailable because of seeking treatment or supporting a co-parent in treatment. Keep in mind that some families have less access to professional support because of where they live or barriers to travel, how much it costs, and childcare and other responsibilities.

Common ways that **family members think about** family substance problems include depressive cognitions (e.g., *It is getting harder and harder to cope with everything*), responsibility beliefs (e.g., *But it kind of is my fault though ... like I guess I shouldn't get in the way*), and thoughts around trust (e.g., *I cannot help feeling suspicious at times and questioning every move or phone call or message*).[23] Family members may need help in dealing with thoughts of uncertainty about the future and their own capacities, realistic and helpful ways of perceiving responsibility for the stressors, and dealing with the pain of losing trust in a loved one.

A harm-reduction approach to SUD treatment has been growing in popularity, which in short honors the assumed right of people to use substances and to continue to use a substance as long as harm toward others is reduced and eventually eliminated (*harm* meaning financial, physical, emotional damage—but not simply disappointment or anger).[24] Family members could be helped by learning to hold several **paradoxical beliefs** at the same time related to the substance problems:

- It is possible to both demand change in the behavior of the substance-using family member while not demanding complete abstinence from the substance.
- One can still feel overwhelmed while at the same time acknowledging that change is incremental and takes time.
- It is normal to feel anger and frustration toward the substance-using family member while understanding the slow process of change.

Some suggestions for **helping children** while parents go through SUD recovery include the following:[25]

- Explain substance compulsions/addiction and recovery to children in ways they can understand, emphasizing that they are not the cause of parents' behavior.
- Help parents understand that older children may not fully embrace the recovery process right away and to honor their children's choices.
- Encourage adults and youth to join support groups.
- Help normalize (e.g., express that there is nothing to be embarrassed about) the usefulness of therapy for helping the family work through new rules, roles, and boundaries.
- Be aware that some children learned roles to help compensate for a parent with a substance problem, which made the children feel important, so giving up that role may be difficult and cause some resentment.

Other examples of the relevance of substance and behavioral compulsion **perceptions** are sprinkled throughout this chapter. Any come to mind? Family members' perceptions (or beliefs) about the motivations, causes, and the ability of the person with the compulsion affect how family members feel about the person with the problem and how they think the problem should be addressed. As noted, perceptions can be based in part on foundational philosophical and ideological perspectives. Encouraging family members to **become more aware** of their perceptions and to **analyze their usefulness** could help them construct more helpful ways of making sense of their circumstances. *Does my thinking about the stressor this way bring feelings of hope or of discouragement? Does that belief produce more empathy or more resentment? Is that assumption about the motivation of the person with the compulsion based on reality?* It may not always be clear what reactions are best for a given situation, but people should realize the power of their perceptions.

Accurate information about substances, SUD, and various behavioral compulsions can also contribute to helpful perceptions of a family's situation. Minimizing any **stigma** they feel might help them confront and share their feelings and perceptions and seek additional help. Family members often prefer that the compulsion completely stop and are especially supportive of individual counseling for the family member with "the problem." However, they can be leery about participating in family counseling and suspicious of treatments that involve substances (when applicable), such as methadone, that help counter cravings for and the sensations of the original substance, particularly opioids. In short, educating families about important treatment components can help inform their perceptions of their circumstances and help them identify useful coping resources.

A spouse who compulsively views pornography may need help understanding how doing so affects the other spouse, which is partially influenced by each spouse's **perceptions**. The pornography compulsion may have little to do with how one feels about one's spouse or even sexual attraction toward that spouse. It might bring some relief to express and to hear this sentiment. Nevertheless, because such conversations can induce feelings of shame and guilt, which tend to feed a compulsion, the offending spouse may need help finding healthier ways to cope with knowing the pain that is caused by acting on the compulsion.

Parents might need help understanding and educating their children about the risks of excessive **videogame and social media** usage. Parents with greater technological literacy and competence can better monitor their children's technology use and better guide them through making decisions and negotiating limits to screen time/social media. Furthermore, families might benefit by avoiding an all-or-nothing approach to technology—that is, placing no limits and thus putting children at risk for the negative effects of excessive exposure, versus complete restriction that places children at risk for social isolation, especially during adolescence. To the extent that a behavioral compulsion by a child or adult is fed by an excessive need to soothe pain or inadequacy, or as an attempted coping mechanism for other difficult stressors, resources like **social support**, positive **coping skills**, and sources that help build one's **self-worth** continue to be relevant. Professional counseling might also be warranted.

Finally, because **trauma** and **adverse childhood experiences** can be such key factors in fueling compulsions, families might need encouragement to seek professional intervention that targets the trauma specifically. Various therapies are used to help people heal from trauma, and it can take some time and experimentation to find a good therapeutic match for a given individual or family. **Mindfulness**-based principles and exercises (see Chapter 2) are increasingly recommended for trauma survivors and can be conveniently implemented to potentially improve our moods and outlook. For example, Andrea Brandt, a marriage and family therapist, offers the following exercise for adults to help undergo an essential step in healing—processing emotions connected to the trauma (because we may not have been able or allowed to process them when the trauma occurred).[26] You might find these useful for minor intervention approaches that you use in helping someone with a traumatic past, including yourself, if applicable. Starting off with a "smaller" trauma is recommended.

1. **Ground it:** In a peaceful place, focus on the here and now and relax.
2. **Recall it:** Reexperience in your mind an experience that provoked (or should have) an emotional reaction. Be as detailed as possible, and move to the next step once the emotions arise.
3. **Sense it:** While relaxing (deep breaths), notice any physical responses in your body, describe them to yourself.
4. **Name it:** Label each sensation with an emotion (you may need to prepare ahead of time by reviewing the various types of emotions one can experience).
5. **Love it:** Accept everything that you feel—embrace the feelings as part of being human and love yourself for having them.
6. **Feel and experience it:** Sit and let the emotions flow; observe and acknowledge them, welcoming any discomforts they might bring. Follow any urges to cry or emote in other ways.

7. **Receive its message and wisdom:** Look for any insight that the emotions give you about past incidents. Consider journaling your thoughts.
8. **Share it:** Find someone you feel comfortable sharing your experience with. Consider writing a letter to someone who hurt you but not mailing it. The writing or sharing process is key.
9. **Let it go:** Imagine releasing the impact of the trauma. You might consider a variety of physical rituals people have used to do so, like burning a letter or throwing something symbolic into the sea.

One should always be **cautious** about becoming overwhelmed by long-held, pent-up emotions from serious trauma, and be willing to reach out to professionals trained in facilitating such processes. Hence, begin with something more minor if you are doing it on your own or recommending it to someone else. This exercise could feel unpleasant at first but is designed to eventually replace lasting impacts of trauma with more hopeful feelings about the present and future. Overall, it illustrates that trauma can linger and interfere with our emotions and emotional expression, and inhibit our connections with other people, inducing our families.

Do You Want to Learn More?

As usual, we have only touched on a portion of information related to this topic. **What really sparked your interest? What do you wish was covered more thoroughly?** Consider taking some time to further deepen your understanding of addiction, compulsions, and family stressors. The following are a variety of resources that you might find helpful, and some references directly or indirectly referred to in this chapter. Just watch yourself, or you may find you have developed a compulsion for learning (well, that might not be such a bad thing).

Videos

(Use links or do searches with the key words provided)
- Jamie's New Start (3 mins). As found on "Family-Focused Treatment: Healing Parents and Children Together" by Volunteers of America. https://www.voa.org/family-focused-treatment
- Wasted: Exposing the Family Effect of Addiction (15 mins). Sam Fowler, TEDx. https://www.ted.com/talks/sam_fowler_wasted_exposing_the_family_effect_of_addiction
- Lessons From the Child of an Addict (8 mins). Emily Smith, TEDx. https://www.youtube.com/watch?v=TXNrrcmsWYY
- The Ripple Effect of Addiction (9 mins). Brennan Harlow. https://www.youtube.com/watch?v=6AqjvLAGEQQ
- Family Roles and Codependency: Addiction Codependency in Families (7 mins). Family First Intervention. https://family-intervention.com/family-roles/codependency/
- What Is Harm Reduction (4 mins)? As found on "Harm Reduction" by the U.S. Department of Health & Human Services. https://www.hhs.gov/overdose-prevention/harm-reduction

- Using the Family First Act to Help Families With Substance Use Disorders (58 mins). Webinar by the Annie E. Casey Foundation. https://www.aecf.org/blog/using-the-family-first-act-to-help-families-with-substance-use-disorders

Websites

- Drouin, M. (2022, February 2018). 5 ways our constant scrolling is messing with our minds: The constant lens of the internet changes the way we think and act. *Psychology Today*. https://www.psychologytoday.com/us/blog/love-online/202202/5-ways-our-constant-scrolling-is-messing-our-minds
- Gottman, J., & Gottman, J. (n.d.). An open letter on porn. The Gottman Institute. https://www.gottman.com/blog/an-open-letter-on-porn
- National Institute on Drug Abuse (2016, March). Principles of substance abuse prevention for early childhood: A research-based guide. https://www.drugabuse.gov/publications/principles-substance-abuse-prevention-early-childhood/table-contents
- Substance Abuse and Mental Health Services Administration (SAMHSA). (2022, April 6). Harm reduction. https://www.samhsa.gov/find-help/harm-reduction
- Substance Abuse and Mental Health Services Administration (SAMHSA). (2022, May 10). Medication-assisted treatment (MAT). https://www.samhsa.gov/medication-assisted-treatment
- U.S. Department of Health & Human Services. (2021, October 27). What is the U.S. opioid epidemic? https://www.hhs.gov/opioids/about-the-epidemic/index.html

Readings (Articles, Books, Book Chapters)

- Di Sarno, M., De Candia, V., Rancati, F., Madeddu, F., Calati, R., & Di Pierro, R. (2021). Mental and physical health in family members of substance users: A scoping review. *Drug and Alcohol Dependence*, 219(1). https://doi.org/10.1016/j.drugalcdep.2020.108439
- McDonagh, D., Connolly, N., & Devaney, C. (2019). "Bury don't discuss": The help-seeking behaviour of family members affected by substance-use disorders. *Child Care in Practice*, 25(2), 175–188. https://doi.org/10.1080/13575279.2018.1448258
- Nayak, S. M., Huhn, A. S., Bergeria, C. L., Strain, E. C., & Dunn, K. E. (2021). Familial perceptions of appropriate treatment types and goals for a family member who has opioid use disorder. *Drug and Alcohol Dependence*, 221. https://doi.org/10.1016/j.drugalcdep.2021.108649
- Orben, A., Przybylski, A. K., Blakemore, S. J., & Kievit, R. A. (2022). Windows of developmental sensitivity to social media. *Nature Communications*, 13,1649. https://doi.org/10.1038/s41467-022-29296-3
- Orford, J., Cousins, J., Smith, N., & Bowden-Jones, H. (2017). Stress, strain, coping and social support for affected family members attending the National Problem Gambling Clinic, London. *International Gabling Studies*, 17(2), 259–275. https://doi.org/10.1080/14459795.2017.1331251

Notes

1   Baumgartner, J. C., & Radley, D. C. (2021). The drug overdose toll in 2020 and near-term actions for addressing it. Commonwealth Fund. https://doi.org/10.26099/GB4Y-R129

2   National Institute on Drug Abuse. (2021, December 15). Monitoring the future. https://www.drugabuse.gov/drug-topics/trends-statistics/monitoring-future

3   Monitoring The Future. (n.d.). Publications. http://www.monitoringthefuture.org/pubs.html

4   U.S. Department of Health and Human Services (HHS), Office of the Surgeon General. (2016, November). Facing addiction in America: The surgeon general's report on alcohol, drugs, and health. https://addiction.surgeongeneral.gov/sites/default/files/surgeon-generals-report.pdf

5   Di Sarno, M., De Candia, V., Rancati, F., Madeddu, F., Calati, R., & Di Pierro, R. (2021). Mental and physical health in family members of substance users: A scoping review. *Drug and Alcohol Dependence, 219*(1). https://doi.org/10.1016/j.drugalcdep.2020.108439; Godleski, S., & Leonard, K. E. (2019). Substance use and substance problems in families: How families impact and are impacted by substance use. In Fiese, B. H., Celano, M., Deater-Deckard, K., Jouriles, E. N., & Whisman, M. A. (Eds.), *APA handbook of contemporary family psychology: Applications and broad impact of family psychology* (pp. 587–602). American Psychological Association. http://dx.doi.org/10.1037/0000100-036; Horváth, Z., Orford, J., Velleman, R., & Urbán, R. (2020). Measuring coping among family members with substance-misusing relatives: Testing competing factor structures of the coping questionnaire (CQ) in England and Italy. *Substance Use & Misuse, 55*(3), 469–480. https://doi.org/10.1080/10826084.2019.1685547

6   Lewis, V., & Allen-Byrd, L. (2007). Coping strategies for the stages of family recovery. In J. L. Fischer, M. Muslow, & A. W. Korinek (Eds.). *Familial responses to alcohol problems* (pp. 105–124). Routledge.

7   Monitoring the Future. (n.d.). Publications. http://www.monitoringthefuture.org/pubs.html

8   Hill, K. G., Ialongo, N. s., Leve, L., Olds, D. L., & Stotland, N. (20-16). Principles of substance abuse prevention for early childhood: A research-based guide. Nih.gov. https://nida.nih.gov/sites/default/files/early_childhood_prevention_march_2016.pdf

9   Horváth, Z., Orford, J., Velleman, R., & Urbán, R. (2020). Measuring coping among family members with substance-misusing relatives: Testing competing factor structures of the coping questionnaire (CQ) in England and Italy. *Substance Use & Misuse, 55*(3), 469–480. https://doi.org/10.1080/10826084.2019.1685547; Orford, J., Cousins, J., Smith, N., & Bowden-Jones, H. (2017). Stress, strain, coping and social support for affected family members attending the National Problem Gambling Clinic, London. *International Gabling Studies, 17*(2), 259–275. https://doi.org/10.1080/14459795.2017.1331251

10 Monitoring the Future. (n.d.). Publications. http://www.monitoringthefuture.org/pubs.html; National Institute on Drug Abuse. (n.d.). *Sex and gender differences in substance use.* National Institute on Drug Abuse. Retrieved August 16, 2022, from https://nida.nih.gov/publications/research-reports/substance-use-in-women/sex-gender-differences-in-substance-use

11 Monitoring the Future. (n.d.). Publications. http://www.monitoringthefuture.org/pubs.html

12 Cerezo, A., Williams, C., Cummings, M., Ching, D., & Holmes, M. (2020). Minority stress and drinking: Connecting race, gender identity and sexual orientation. *The Counseling Psychologist, 48*(2), 277–303. https://doi.org/10.1177/0011000019887493

13 Monitoring the Future. (n.d.). Publications. http://www.monitoringthefuture.org/pubs.html

14 Orford, J., Cousins, J., Smith, N., & Bowden-Jones, H. (2017). Stress, strain, coping and social support for affected family members attending the National Problem Gambling Clinic, London. *International Gabling Studies, 17*(2), 259–275. https://doi.org/10.1080/14459795.2017.1331251

15 Gottman, J., & Gottman, J. (n.d.). An open letter on porn. The Gottman Institute. https://www.gottman.com/blog/an-open-letter-on-porn; Willoughby, B. J., Leonhardt, N. D., & Augustus, R. A. (2021). Curvilinear associations between pornography use and relationship satisfaction, sexual satisfaction, and relationship stability in the United States. *Computers in Human Behavior, 125*, 10966. https://doi.org/10.1016/j.chb.2021.106966; Willoughby, B. J., Leonhardt, N. D., & Augustus, R. A. (2021). Associations between pornography use and sexual dynamics among heterosexual couples. *The Journal of Sexual Medicine, 18*, 178–192. https://doi.org/10.1016/j.jsxm.2020.10.013

16 Asaduzzaman, K. P., Lee, E., Janssen, I., & Tremblay, M. S. (2022). Associations of passive and active screen time with psychosomatic complaints of adolescents. *American Journal of Preventive Medicine.* https://doi.org/10.1016/j.amepre.2022.01.008; Cherney, K. (2022, March 10). Video games and ADHD: The latest in research. Healthline.com. https://www.healthline.com/health/adhd/video-games-adhd-latest-research; Mak, K., Lai, C., Watanabe, H., Kim, D., Bahar, N., Ramos, M., Young, K. S., Ho, R. C. M., Aum, N., & Cheng, C. (2014). Epidemiology of internet behaviors and addiction among adolescents in six Asian countries. *Cyberpsychology, Behavior and Social Networking, 17*(11), 720. https://doi.org/10.1089/cyber.2014.0139; Park, T. Y., Kim, S., & Lee, J. (2014). Family therapy for an internet-addicted young adult with interpersonal problems. *Journal of Family Therapy, 36*(4), 394–419. https://doi.org/10.1111/1467-6427.12060; Shuai, L., He, S., Zheng, H., Wang, Z., Qiu, M., Xia, W., Cao, X., Lu, L., Zhang, J. (2021). Influences of digital media use on children and adolescents with ADHD during COVID-19 pandemic. *Global Health, 17*(1), 48. https://doi.org/10.1186/s12992-021-00699-z; Zorbaz, S. D., Ulas, O., & Kizildag, S. (2015). Relation between video game addiction and interfamily relationships on primary school students. *Educational Sciences: Theory & Practice, 15*(2), 489–497. https://doi.org/10.12738/estp.2015.2.2090

17 Northrup, J. C., & Shumway, S. (2014). Gamer widow: A phenomenological study of spouses of online video game addicts. *American Journal of Family Therapy, 42*(4), 269–281. https://doi.org/10.1080/01926187.2013.847705

18 Kilburn, E. (2020, September 21). Why are we so addicted to social media? Welldoing.org. https://welldoing.org/article/why-are-we-so-addicted-to-social-media

19 Drouin, M. (2022, February 2018). 5 ways our constant scrolling is messing with our minds: The constant lens of the internet changes the way we think and act. *Psychology Today.* https://www.psychologytoday.com/us/blog/love-online/202202/5-ways-our-constant-scrolling-is-messing-our-minds

20 Orben, A., Przybylski, A. K., Blakemore, S. J., & Kievit, R. A. (2022). Windows of developmental sensitivity to social media. *Nature Communications, 13,*1649. https://doi.org/10.1038/s41467-022-29296-3

21 Cherney, K. (2022, March 10). Video games and ADHD: The latest in research. Healthline.com. https://www.healthline.com/health/adhd/video-games-adhd-latest-research; Schlott, R., (2022, March 12). How TikTok has become a dangerous breeding ground for mental disorders. *New York Post.* https://nypost.com/2022/03/12/tiktok-has-become-a-dangerous-mental-disorder-breeding-ground; Stentiford, L., Koutsouris, G., & Allan, A. (2021). Girls, mental health and academic achievement: A qualitative systematic review. *Educational Review.* http://doi.org/10.1080/00131911.2021.2007052

22 Orben, A., & Przybylski, A.K. (2019). The association between adolescent well-being and digital technology use. *Nat Hum Behav, 3,* 173–182. https://doi.org/10.1038/s41562-018-0506-1

23 Wilson, S. R., Lubman, D. I., Rodda, S., Manning, V., & Yap, M. B. H. (2018). The personal impacts of having a partner with problematic alcohol or other drug use: Descriptions from online counselling sessions. *Addiction Research & Theory, 26*(4), 315–322. https://doi.org/10.1080/16066359.2017.1374375

24 Denning, P., & Little, J. (2017). *Over the influence, second edition: The harm reduction guide to controlling your drug and alcohol use.* The Guildford Press; Substance Abuse and Mental Health Services Administration. (n.d.). Harm reduction. https://www.samhsa.gov/find-help/harm-reduction

25 Lewis, V., & Allen-Byrd, L. (2007). Coping strategies for the stages of family recovery. In J. L. Fischer, M. Muslow, & A. W. Korinek (Eds.). *Familial responses to alcohol problems* (pp. 105–124). Routledge.

26 Brandt, A. (2018, April 2). 9 steps to healing childhood trauma as an adult. *Psychology Today.* https://www.psychologytoday.com/us/blog/mindful-anger/201804/9-steps-healing-childhood-trauma-adult

Image Credits

Fig. 10.1a: Source: Adapted from John E. Schulenberg et al., "Monitoring the Future National Survey Results on Drug Use, 1975-2020: Volume II, College Students and Adults Ages 19-60," p. 79. 2020.

Fig. 10.1b: Source: Adapted from John E. Schulenberg et al., "Monitoring the Future National Survey Results on Drug Use, 1975-2020: Volume II, College Students and Adults Ages 19-60," p. 97. 2020.

Fig. 10.2: Source: Adapted from Amy Orben and Andrew K. Pryzbyski, "The Association Between Adolescent Well-Being and Digital Technology Use," Nature Human Behaviour, vol. 3, 2019.

CHAPTER 11

Fear, Loss, and Family Stress

In Victorian times, the grieving process often included having photos taken of dead loved ones. The photos were displayed in the home, worn inside lockets, and even sent to relatives and friends.[1]

Chapter Preview

- Grief is a normal response to loss, though some people experience complications that prolong intense grief.
- Our views on life and death influence how we make meaning of and adjust to loss.
- Details about the "who," "when," "how," and "why" regarding the death of a loved one impact the nature of family stress and coping.
- Losses of a parent, sibling, spouse, or child can have some similar and some distinct impacts on families.
- Culture, religion, and other contexts help explain risks for certain types of losses (e.g., suicide) and mourning processes.
- School shootings and terrorist attacks exploit fear to maximize stress.
- Post-traumatic stress disorder is a common outcome for people exposed to terrorizing events, even if just through media exposure.
- Military deployment includes several stages that challenge families to adapt to stressful changes.
- Meaning-making is a seemingly integral process toward coping with the loss of a family member and relies on intentional processing of our perceptions.

What Is This Topic About?

How does **fear** influence your thoughts, feelings, and behavior? Psychologists, philosophers, and poets have much to say about fear. Besides fears of public speaking, spiders, and (for some reason) clowns, at the foundation of our fears seems to be distress about ceasing to exist, or essentially

death.[2] Part of our fears and angst about death could be rooted in the fact that we have so little **control** over it. Death of a family member is also a top human fear. Perhaps you know someone who, upon learning that a commuting family member hasn't arrived yet, jumps straight to the conclusion that the loved one was in a car accident, shot in gang crossfire, or suffered from a sudden heart attack. While constantly living with such fears is exhausting and difficult on our bodies, some people's worries are more justified by their stressful surroundings.

Experiencing the death of a loved one has also long been considered one of the most, if not the most, **stressful life events**.[3] Families that are inadequately prepared or able to cope with the loss experience **crisis**. The stressor of losing a family member can also dramatically affect our **identity**—*I am now a widow instead of a spouse. I am no longer a parent. I used to be a sibling.* Losing a family member can require that we rework our **family rules**, **roles**, and **boundaries**—*He was always the calm one to help us feel reassured. Now, who can I confide in?* Sometimes our financial circumstances are threatened by such a loss—*Who will raise me now? Without life insurance, how are we supposed to make ends meet?*

After the death of a loved one, family members go through a **bereavement** period—a time of grief and mourning.[4] **Grief** is an emotional, mental, social, or even physical reaction to a loss such as death. Anger, sadness, despair, anxiety, guilt, and self-isolation are common forms of grief reactions, but experiencing grief is a normal reaction to loss and not considered a disorder like depression.[5] Grief can also be **anticipatory**—we typically begin grieving when we learn of someone's terminal illness; we react to the realization that our anticipated future together will be cut short. **Mourning** commonly refers to an adaptation process after a loss that often includes cultural customs and rituals that guide what are considered to be appropriate types of coping. It typically includes a yearning to be with the person again and perhaps some denial of their permanent absence, a phase of disorganization and sadness and perhaps anger, and a time of reorganization. Why might someone be angry about the death of a loved one?

Certain situations can contribute to a higher risk of coping problems, such as **disenfranchised grief**—a loss that is not socially or culturally validated to the same extent that a grieving person perceives the loss.[6] For example, the loss of a stepparent, an ex-spouse, an abusive partner, and a miscarried fetus might not seem like a big deal to certain friends and coworkers, leading to a lack of empathy and support (or added criticism) that can interfere with mourning and lead to social isolation and loneliness. A lack of information or clarity about a loss can also complicate the mourning process. As you recall from other chapters, **boundary ambiguity** occurs when there is a mismatch between a person's physical and psychological presences. A certain type of loss—known as **ambiguous loss**—leads to boundary ambiguity, such as having a child who has been missing for several years, or an elderly parent with dementia.[7] In such cases, grieving usually begins even though the person is still somewhat present—either psychologically or physically—but the ambiguity makes it difficult if not impossible to fully grieve and mourn.

Some people experience prolonged grieving that interferes with daily living for many months or years. **Complicated grief** (**CG**) is a common term for describing grief that deviates from what is considered culturally normal, usually regarding the length or intensity of the grief and how much it impedes social, occupational, and other types of functioning.[8] When strong feelings that often occur at the beginning of the mourning process—intense yearning, emotional pain, preoccupied thoughts about the person, difficulty accepting the loss and seeing a future without the person—persist for many months or years, they interfere with a person's ability to progress and experience joy in life. One might even feel suicidal.

Apparently, only a small fraction of people (perhaps 10% to 15%) experience CG, but it isn't always clear when someone has it. Experts disagree on its symptoms and cultures differ on what is perceived to be a normal grief response to death.[9] What's more, even resilient people can cope with loss a little differently from one another, and the specific situations surrounding the loss can have a major impact on the pressure we feel—like a sudden loss of one's only child compared to the peaceful loss of a 90-year-old cousin. Determining **whether grief has gone too far** is a major challenge for family members, and this difficulty can contribute to hesitation to seek professional intervention when needed.

Fear and loss apply to numerous topics, but our focus is on issues related to the threat or reality of a family member's death. In this chapter, we explore loss within the general family relationships context and then within the specific applications to school shootings, terrorism, and military deployment.

What Are the Assumptions?

Do you have religious beliefs about an **afterlife**? If so, you have no reason to fear death, right? Perhaps not. Stacks of studies show that being religious can either decrease, increase, or make no difference in our fears of death.[10] How can that be? It seems that specific beliefs about the nature of God (e.g., loving? strict? forgiving? vengeful?), about the qualifications for a pleasant afterlife experience, and whether we think we are meeting such qualifications tends to make a difference in religious' people's feelings about death. Nevertheless, it appears that compared to non-believers, believers are less likely to experience prolonged grief after the death of a loved one and are more likely to see death as being positive. What death—and life—**means** to individuals, families, and cultures can vary substantially and makes up an important part of how we anticipate and respond to it.

Pew Research data indicate that **conservatives** are much more likely than **liberals** to believe in heaven; compared to religious liberals, religious conservatives are more confident in their belief in God, place a greater importance on their religion, and attend religious services more frequently.[11] This pattern suggests that political ideology can intertwine with perspectives on death and on ways of living that could shape or reflect how people make sense of family loss. Whether anything inherent in the political ideologies leads to different perspectives on death seems unclear, but they inform some divergent ideas about how to address specific causes or consequences of family loss. For example, after a school shooting, politicians on the right tend to focus strongly on mental illness and family structure as primary causes for the act, while also seeking to protect the rights of law-abiding citizens to own guns. Politicians on the left focus more on preventing or minimizing damage caused by likely killers through heavier governmental restrictions on access to guns (or certain types of guns), and on avoiding stigmatizing people with mental illness or certain family forms, arguing that most people in such cases are not violent. Think about how such priorities reflect moral foundations of **care**, **liberty**, **fairness**, and **authority** and contribute to diverse perspectives within and across families.

As you **engage with** the rest of the chapter, remember the key elements of family stress theories (e.g., stressors, resources, perceptions, coping, and crisis) and consider the following:

- Why might some families with similar losses become closer while others become strained?
- How do the various pieces of information throughout the chapter fit together to help explain why each family might be affected differently by the death of a loved one?
- How can we prepare for the unexpected death of a loved one without becoming paranoid or overprotective?
- What experiences have you had or observed that help you relate to specific concepts?
- How might the ideological perspectives influence how people (including you) think about potential causes of and solutions to violent/terroristic-type deaths?

Part A. Family Loss Stressors

What Is Stressful About the Death of a Family Member?

Consider that pressures on families can differ based on the circumstances in which a loss occurs. What might make the loss especially stressful? Deaths perceived as more tragic and painful push us to manage our emotional and psychological systems and can tax our abilities to cope with the loss and avoid CG. Physical and relational pressures also accompany family loss. For example, the loss of a loved one can require surviving family members to communicate the loss to friends and family, make funeral and burial arrangements, decide how to divide up or dispose of family heirlooms and address property and space issues (e.g., what to do with a deceased child's bedroom or a deceases spouse's clothing), and perhaps face personal disputes about inheritance issues. Typically, families need to adjust some family routines and patterns—including rules, roles, and boundaries. The tendency to celebrate birthdays, anniversaries, and other family-oriented recurring holidays or events means families have regular and everlasting reminders of their loss, which can interfere with the ability to fully function and fully focus on immediate tasks and responsibilities.

Think about the differences between a 7-year-old whose father was just killed in a random act of violence and a 67-year-old whose father just died in his sleep. How might these two scenarios affect families differently? A key to understanding what is stressful about family loss is accounting for the specific, interconnected details of "**who**," "**when**," "**how**," and "**why**." Such circumstances contribute to the **meanings** we make from and the pressures we experience regarding family loss. For example, consider the following:

- Deaths that happen after a drawn-out illness or major disability create stress well before the actual loss. The energy and other resources invested in years of **care-giving** can diminish the capacity of caregivers to address the additional family loss stressors.

- A sudden, unexpected death means that family members have little opportunity to anticipate and prepare for the loss, and it can shock their psychological system.[12] If the death was violent, it can cause added fear and anxiety for surviving family members who might question their own sense of safety—*Could that happen to me?* Families of homicide victims usually have more distressing grief, which can be compounded by media attention and testimony in court cases that cause family members to relive their trauma.[13]

- Death by **suicide** is usually traumatizing and adds enormously to family stress.[14] Because most suicides are by people who struggle with significant mental illness, family members might already feel embarrassed or stigmatized regarding their struggling family member, and the **stigma** of a suicide is even greater. Families struggle with intense feelings of regret and guilt about their own perceptions of how they possibly contributed to the suicide. Others might subtly (or not-so-subtly) blame the family for the suicide, making it especially difficult for families to openly express their feelings and find support. Some family members feel anger toward the deceased for putting the family through such pain, which can also increase feelings of guilt—*I shouldn't be angry at someone who was in so much pain.* Families can feel a deep sadness that someone they love and cared for felt such hopelessness. The "why" is not always clear, and young family members in particular can struggle to understand the loss.

The following sections are organized around the "who" and "when" (i.e., developmental stages) to address additional specific pressures of family loss, while integrating some content about the "how" and "why" that also play such important roles in how we interpret and cope with family losses. For some national context, the chart in Figure 11.1 illustrates the top five causes of death in the United States in 2019 according to the Centers for Disease Control and Prevention. (In 2020, deaths from COVID-19 became the third leading cause at nearly 350,831 deaths).[15] Notice how death rates vary by marital status—what's going on there?

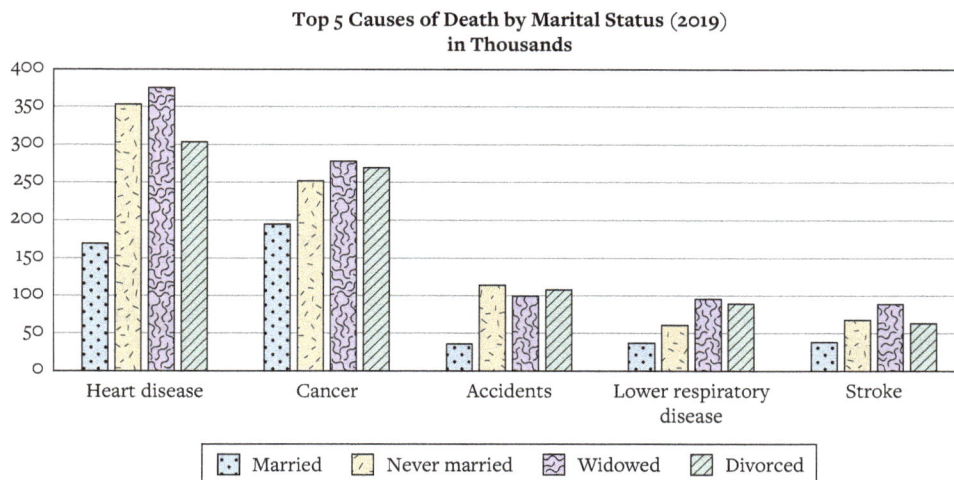

FIGURE 11.1 Top Five Causes of Death by Marital Status (2019)

How Does the Loss of a Parent Influence Family Stress?

While losing a parent under most circumstances is stressful, the loss of an elderly parent is a **normative expectation** and feels less tragic than it otherwise could. Furthermore, consider how the loss might feel when a parent had been painfully disabled for a decade and needed full-time assistance from an adult child. As noted in Chapter 9, such a circumstance is often burdensome, so we might expect the death to provide some sense of relief for the caregiving family members. Yet, primary caregivers could struggle with losing a role that brought them a sense of purpose and satisfaction and with the loss of an intimate connection. Bereaved children might struggle with regret or guilt if the parent-child relationships had lingering problems that seemingly could have been resolved if they had only tried harder before it was too late. The loss of an aging parent sometimes means that adult children become the oldest living generation in the family, pushing them to focus more on their own mortality. This can cause some angst and trigger some changes in how people feel about themselves and use their time, for better or worse.

Conversely, losing a parent as a young child is typically **unexpected** and highly distressing. Children are at heightened risk for CG, sometimes expressed through physical symptoms (e.g., head or stomachaches, difficulty sleeping), for a variety of reasons, including the following:[16]

- **Dependency:** Children rely on others to care for them, and losing a parent usually diminishes the level of care they receive. Having a second parent in mourning over the loss of a spouse or partner can diminish the second parent's availability to the child, and that parent might also be preoccupied with adjusting to changing family roles and other pressures associated with the loss. A child might also avoid sharing their feelings openly to seemingly spare their remaining parent additional stress, which can give the false impression that a child is adjusting well to or is in denial about the loss. Children could also become more independent and take on greater responsibilities around the house and in caring for siblings, elevating risks for parentification.

- **Developmental stage:** Children, especially at a young age, have a lesser ability to understand the causes and consequences of the death. They are potentially prone to drawing inaccurate conclusions about how they might have caused the death, and to overgeneralize their confusion and fear to other aspects of their lives or other people—like fearing that someone else will abandon them. Young children have difficulty fully verbalizing their concerns and might express themselves through what appears to be misbehavior. Children can also regress developmentally—being clingy, throwing tantrums, and bedwetting—which can frustrate and further exhaust parents and other caregivers.

- **Peers:** Older children particularly lean heavily on their peers for support, few of which may be able to understand what it feels like to lose a parent. Thus, teens especially can struggle with isolation and loneliness, especially when others around them are uncomfortable with the topic or how to bring it up. Children's internalizing and externalizing behavior as attempts to cope with the loss can also erode peer support. Isolation and rejection put them at greater risk for using illicit substances.

When a child loses a parent it usually means that someone else in the family is impacted by the same loss but from a different perspective. That parent was potentially someone's spouse, sibling, child, and so forth. Consider how this single loss has both **shared and unshared meanings and impacts** across family members, and how such differences contribute to each person's mourning.

How Does the Loss of a Sibling or Spouse Influence Family Stress?

Though siblings and spouses are different types of family members, both types are typically an **intragenerational** (within generation) **loss**. For adults, siblings and spouses provide more peer-like support than might a parent or child. **Siblings**, however, can have a much longer relationship history than spouses, and usually have shared childhood memories. Such memories can foster closeness but could also include issues of favoritism and rivalry that impact how the loss is experienced. Interviews with adults who had lost a sibling illustrate how individual and family identity can be affected by the loss.[17] For instance, **birth order** can change—losing the identity of being a younger sibling while becoming the oldest sibling could change how the person feels and is viewed by the family. Becoming an only child can function similarly. Some siblings talked about feeling like they had "lost their innocence" (i.e., had to grow up quickly) or that the presence of a hospital or sirens triggered emotional responses and memories. Some also reported that they were able to strengthen other family relationships as they leaned on one another throughout bereavement.

Younger children who lose a sibling could be at risk of **neglect** from grieving parents' preoccupation with intense pain and adjustment.[18] Parents can also stifle (perhaps unknowingly) a child's grief by disallowing open discussion of the loss, sometimes to avoid having to face the subject. Some parents become understandably **overprotective** of their remaining children, possibly impeding a child's progress toward healthy development. Even children who had little if any contact with a deceased sibling can be affected by the loss. For example, interviews with adolescents and adults who had lost an infant sibling suggested that the impact of such a loss can last indefinitely.[19] Some of that impact seemed due to **disenfranchised grief**—people having dismissed their grief because the infant was so young (or was a stillbirth). On the plus side, these surviving siblings had also learned to be more compassionate and empathic people. Interestingly, those who were born after the death of an infant sibling seemed impacted by how the loss affected the family environment in which they were born: those from families that were open about the death were prone to report feeling loved and special while growing up, while those from families with little acknowledgment of the loss were prone to feel either invisible or overprotected.

A **spouse or life partner** tends to be one's primary source of support or a best friend, especially for men, so the loss can feel debilitating. Having combined lives for decades can make the loss feel particularly disorienting as one's relational identity changes and complementary routines and responsibilities are no longer shared the same way, if at all.[20] Some widowed adults struggle with the question of whether to form another couple relationship, perhaps feeling guilty if they do. Other expected reactions, depending on the circumstances, include

- fear about living alone or being a single parent;
- concerns about finances;

- guilt over perceptions of not having done enough to prevent the death, or to have remedied problems in the relationship;
- guilt about feeling relief that extended caregiving has ended; and
- focusing more on one's own eventual death.

How Does the Loss of a Child Influence Family Stress?

Perhaps you have heard it said that "parents aren't supposed to outlive their children." The pain of losing a child seems to be as **emotionally intense** as things can get, even to levels that surprise parents and others.[21] Injuries and suicide are the top causes of childhood death, and the perception that one has failed to **protect** a child from harm—perhaps the most fundamental parenting task—strikes at the heart of grieving parents. Somewhat similar to events explored in prior chapters—namely, having a miscarriage or first learning of a child's serious disability, parents who lose a child have to readjust their visions and dreams of the future. The loss can make life—at least for a while—feel impossible or pointless to manage. Mourning can last for years, and some grief might never leave. However, it is estimated that a minority of cases, perhaps 10% to 25%, will result in long-term emotional instability characteristic of CG. Parents usually reach a point at which they can think back fondly on good memories without being overwhelmed with pain.

I suspect you have noticed that we as humans tend to **idealize** our loved ones who have passed.[22] Think about how that could influence the remaining siblings. Can they live up to the near-mythical accounts of the deceased sibling? Parents might also be tempted to push their dreams for their lost child onto another child, pressuring that sibling to live someone else's life. These kinds of pressures can drive children to feel inadequate and to rebel, creating more issues for the family to tackle. Similarly, parents can harm their couple relationships by placing unrealistic expectations and demands on their partners (e.g., *You manage everything while I mourn*; *you have to take the pain away*), though some couples strengthen their bond as they actively work to support one another through tragedy.

How Do External Contexts Contribute to Experiencing Family Loss?

The "who," "when," "how," and "why" described earlier contain elements of external contexts that impact family mourning and stress. Furthermore, as part of the "who," some research indicates that **gender** is relevant to loss and grief.[23] For example, women tend to struggle more with grief, which could at least be partially explained by the fact that women are more likely to be family caregivers, and greater caregiving distress prior to the death of family members can correspond with longer grief symptoms. Also, females who lose a female sibling tend to have more difficulty than siblings of other gender combinations.

Ethnic and religious cultures can vary dramatically in expectations and rituals surrounding death and bereavement. For example, generally in Islamic cultures, bodies are buried quickly without a viewing, loud crying or wailing is to be avoided, and mourning should usually last for three days during which family and the community bring meals and offer other support to the bereaved.[24] Widows, however, have a mourning period of 4 months and 10 days in which they stay inside their homes as much as possible (at least in part to avoid anyone who could be a potential mate) while also receiving significant support. Being an **immigrant** might hamper one's ability to fully participate in cultural bereavement rituals. For example, Mandaean (Middle Eastern religious sect) refugee families in Australia have been unable to practice cultural burial rites because of certain hospital policies, which added distress to their mourning.[25]

Suicide is a complicated topic but it appears that it can be influenced by **culture**.[26] White men, particularly of middle age and older, make up about 70% of suicide deaths, whereas Black men seem especially unlikely to die by suicide (Black males are more likely to die by homicide than are other groups). Rural areas in the United States tend to have higher suicide rates, and some attribute this to regional values of rugged self-sufficiency (especially for White men), lesser availability of mental health resources, and a higher prevalence of guns (over half of male suicides involve using a firearm). Asian Americans are less likely than other groups to seek help for suicidal thoughts and motives for suicide are especially driven by family-related shame. **Minority stress** is also a predictor of suicide, including gender and sexual minorities especially living in less accepting environments (see Chapter 3).

Improve Your Learning

Without peeking, take a moment to review in your mind (or say out loud) the key concepts from this chapter (this is a proven learning technique). Then review the "Chapter Preview" section at the top and compare. Skim Part A of the chapter with extra attention to the **bolded words**. Skip to the end of the chapter to find more learning resources.

Part B. Terrorizing and Military Deployment Stressors

In this part of the chapter, we apply concepts discussed in Part A to some specific contexts of fear and loss. Here we address losses linked to terrorizing acts and military deployment. School shootings and acts of terrorism create mass fear that impacts societies at large, and military deployment sometimes occurs in response to terrorism, particularly from foreign sources, which adds fear and other pressures for military families.

What Is Stressful About Terrorizing Threats and Acts That Impact Families?

Threats and acts of violence can be traumatizing when they activate our fears of pain and death, putting us on frequent high alert. To **terrorize** someone is to magnify those fears and feelings of distress, often to immobilize us, to scare us away from somewhere, or simply to create psychological harm. Even though the risks of being killed in a mass shooting or terrorist attack are far lower than other causes of death (e.g., car accidents, drowning, choking on food), we seem to think much differently about someone deliberately seeking to cause harm. Why do you think that is? Similarly, the loss of a family member due to a terrorizing act profoundly influences how families experience the loss and related stress.

How Do School Shootings Impact Family Stress?

While mass shootings happen in a variety of contexts, ones that occur in neighborhoods and especially schools are particularly relevant to family stress. In prior chapters we have discussed some of the stressors that occur in violent neighborhoods; losing a family member to homicide or gang crossfire would understandably cause anger and despair while reinforcing fear and hopelessness in a community. Losing a child in a school shooting can lead to similar feelings, especially for the child's family, though school shootings cause major family stress well **beyond the communities** in which they occur.

We all hear about it when someone takes a gun to a school and shoots at others. That it becomes a source of intense public discussion and debate suggests that it is universally perceived as especially disturbing. Why is that? Certainly, the fact that children are involved as victims—and sometimes the shooter—taps into our desires to protect the innocent and vulnerable. Furthermore, parents yield control of their children's welfare to schools, trusting that their children will return home safely (aside from an occasional scraped knee or hurt feelings). Parents need to believe that their children are safe. When children are violently injured or killed in school, parents far and wide can't help but imagine their own children in a similar situation.

Children who directly witness a shooting are at risk for various emotional, psychological, and behavioral challenges; even mere exposure to **media** reports of school shootings, especially after the occurrence of multiple similar incidents, causes anxiety and stress.[27] Thus, besides the pressure to manage one's **fears as a parent**, parents have pressure to help their children—especially younger children—make sense of a complicated situation and feel comfortable about going to school.[28] For parents, trying to determine what and how much information is developmentally appropriate for their children is challenging. Children's nightmares and obsessive thoughts about death or safety place additional pressure on parents. As with any stressor, couples who already have relationship problems are prone to struggle even more in their relationships if they don't cope well under such circumstances.

A survey of educators and parents in Colorado after a school shooting in a nearby district revealed some insightful thoughts and concerns that can result from a school shooting.[29] Pay special attention to how their perceptions feed into their fears.

- "I send my children to school each day expecting that they'll be safe there. ... When a shooting happens, though, I'm reminded that their safety could very well be an illusion."
- "I worry that every day I kiss my kids goodbye, it will be for the last time."
- "My preference would be for her to not go back [to school] this year."
- "I think about the location of her classroom in comparison to the front doors and exits."
- "My 5-year-old has nightmares for a week every time they have a lockdown drill. I hear her screaming 'don't hurt me' in her sleep."
- "There is not one morning that goes by when I drop off my little girl that I don't think about how there could be a shooter. It adds to a family's stress level in a world that is already stressful enough. Not to mention the incredible levels of anxiety it causes in many children."

The interviewed adults also reported hearing students discuss the possibility of switching to homeschooling; one student expressed feeling like he might be seeing a parent for the last time when he says goodbye before school. While these parental and student concerns might seem unrealistic, what matters most is that their **perceptions of danger** are the main sources of worry and stress, and those perceptions are powerful.

How Does Terrorism Impact Family Stress?

Though the term "terrorism" can be used very broadly, what we all probably think of first is a major act of **public violence perpetrated by people with political motives**. Such cases have commonalities with school shootings, particularly regarding the generation and impact of fear throughout a community and beyond. Much of the high-profile terrorism of recent decades in the United States and other Western countries has been associated with perpetrators from the Middle East with proclaimed Islamic roots, such as 9/11, though domestic terrorist acts have also left a legacy of destruction (e.g., the Oklahoma City bombing). Of course, losing a family member to a terrorist act causes families horrific pain.

As with school shootings, terrorist attacks can make us **question our beliefs** about everyday safety and the disposition of people—*Maybe the world is more dangerous than I thought. Those people are filled with hate.* After an attack, people tend to report developing more negative and fearful views about the world, though some feel more hopeful when seeing acts of heroism and communities coming together with acts of mutual support.[30] Parents have their hands full trying to help themselves and their children make sense of the terrorist threats or acts and feel safe enough to have some normalcy in life. Families directly affected by terrorist attacks can also face financial pressures through medical costs and in some cases damages or losses to family businesses.[31]

As described in Chapter 7, **post-traumatic stress disorder** (**PTSD**) generally refers to having persistent, disturbing feelings (e.g., fear, anger, sadness) and thoughts tied to a traumatic event, often accompanied by nightmares or flashbacks and feeling disconnected from others. Reminders of the event can trigger such reactions long after the event occurs. PTSD is a common outcome of terrorism for those who lose a loved one, are involved in but survived the attack, and witness the attack directly or indirectly (through media exposure).[32] In events like 9/11, some families confront PTSD because of their involvement in the aftermath of terrorism. **First responders** (e.g., law enforcement, paramedics, firefighters) are exposed directly to death and destruction and can become traumatized and develop negative coping behaviors, such as substance misuse.[33] Such consequences also create stress and relationship strain for their family members in addition to their concerns about first responders' safety. Some first responder spouses struggle with survivor guilt when thinking about those who lost their partners in a terrorist attack. Overall, the impact terrorist attacks have on families is seemingly multiplied given the constant and global media coverage that they attract. Does that mean such attacks shouldn't be reported?

How Does Military Deployment Impact Family Stress?

Imagine being a young child, living on a military base with a parent, while the other parent is fighting battles in a foreign land. Then you see a news report about American soldiers killed in a bombing attack and contacting the deployed parent is impossible. How would you feel? Imagine being the spouse of the deployed parent—how would you comfort your child? How would you comfort yourself? Having or being a parent or spouse deployed in a warzone or other dangerous military initiatives activates our fears about loss and impacts various family patterns and relationship processes. The loss of a family member in a military operation is tragic like in other circumstances, though military families often find meaning and comfort in their patriotism and the cause for which their loved one paid the ultimate price.

Research suggests that children with a parent in the military have higher rates of internalizing and externalizing symptoms, less secure attachments, and more problems with peers; parents in the military tend to have higher rates of depression, PTSD, divorce, and suicide, particularly related to **deployment** (parent separated from family for a military operation).[34] Parents with such mental health challenges tend to be less sensitive and appropriately responsive to children's needs and to have poorer marital functioning; their children are consequently at greater risk for negative outcomes. While more deployment exposure (higher percentage of their relationship history that spouses are separated due to deployment) isn't always predictive of the caregiving parent's level of depression, PTSD, or alcohol use, it has been more reliably related to poorer **family functioning** in the realms of emotional involvement, family communication, problem-solving, and marital stability.

Deployment does not necessarily mean that a parent is involved in combat. However, even in times of peace, the nature of military deployment creates distinct pressures that can put families at risk for crisis. Furthermore, even when a family member isn't killed, military families experience other types of losses through separation. (Anything come to mind?) Table 11.1 summarizes key points about the **five stages of military deployment**.[35] See if you can come up with specific examples that illustrate the types of pressures family members experience in each stage. Think about which stage might be most stressful, and why.

TABLE 11.1 Five Stages of Military Deployment and Corresponding Pressures

Stages	Tasks	Pressures for Deployed Parent (Soldier)	Pressures for Family at Home
Predeployment	Preparing to leave	Anticipate missing family, worry about family's future welfare, anticipate personal risks of mission	Anticipate missing soldier, worry about soldier's safety, worry about parenting alone
Deployment	Leaving and adjusting to a new location in the field	Feel powerless to help with parenting, adjusting to new routines, facing risks of mission	Disruption of daily routines; adjusting household rules, roles, and boundaries; risks for parentification
Sustainment	Remaining deployed for several months or longer	Missing family, barriers to family communication, unable to help with pressures back home	Missing soldier, barriers to family communication, concerns about continued welfare of soldier

Redeployment	Preparing to return home	Anticipation of reuniting with family, concerns about how changes in the soldier (e.g., PTSD) might affect the family	Anticipation of reuniting with soldier, concerns about how changes in the family might affect the soldier
Post-deployment	Returning and adjusting to being home	Adjusting to a different structure of routines and potential loss of status (e.g., from an officer to just a parent), becoming an active parent and spouse, dealing with possible impact of any PTSD, injury, or other distress (e.g., guilt about killing) on home life	Disruption of daily routines; adjusting household rules, roles, and boundaries (e.g., sharing control over household with soldier, possible parentified child loses status); dealing with soldier's possible PTSD or injury; not able to relate to the deployment experience

Adapted from: Freytes, I. M., LaLaurin, J. H., Zickmund, S. L., Resende, R. D., & Uphold, C. R. (2017). Exploring the post-deployment reintegration experiences of veterans with PTSD and their significant others. *American Journal of Orthopsychiatry, 87*(2), 149–156. http://dx.doi.org/10.1037/ort0000211; Military.com (2022). The emotional cycle of deployment: Military family perspective. https://www.military.com/spouse/military-deployment/emotional-cycle-of-deployment-military-family.html

The deployment cycle might remind you a bit of complex family structural stressors (see Chapter 8) in that structural transitions elevate risks of negative family outcomes. In this case, transitions can be relatively brief and include the same people, but consider how multiple transitions relatively close together create a certain type of pressure. How might parent-child relationships be affected when only one parent is around for several months? Also, think about how the concepts of **boundary ambiguity** and **ambiguous loss** can apply to military families. Finally, ponder how the general lifestyle of military families can contribute to family stress. For example, military families can move frequently, which often interferes with children making friends and having continuity in school.[36]

How Do External Contexts Contribute to Experiencing Terrorizing and Military Stressors?

Gender appears to be linked in certain ways to terrorizing acts.[37] Whether in response to school shootings or general terrorist attacks, girls and women tend to be at higher risk for PTSD. They also tend to report feeling more vulnerable to attacks and having less control over whether they get hurt. Boys appear to struggle more with conduct disorders after acts of terror. Males are also responsible for nearly all school and mass shootings, which often becomes a cause for much debate about cultural meanings of masculinity, the role of violent video games and media, and natural influences on male aggression.

    Immigrants and refugees have reported heightened levels of PTSD and other psychological disturbances following terrorist attacks.[38] Some immigrants have dealt with harassment after incidents such as 9/11 or the Boston Marathon bombing based on their association with Islamic culture, and others experienced triggered memories of similar mass violence in their native countries. Generally speaking, acts of mass violence add pressure on those who feel like outsiders to be on high alert because they fear being blamed or punished for the act just because of who they are. They can also feel extra pressure to represent their heritage or religion as positively as possible to counter the momentum of negative stereotypes.

Some say that the **military** is a unique culture in itself. While family welfare appears to be a high priority, preparedness for military missions will ultimately dominate any other needs. Military families that include officers and are of higher socio-economic status (SES) and education level tend to report less distress.[39] Such families likely have greater resources and more military experience that help counter the challenges of deployment.

What Does All This Mean for You?

Your insights can be valuable to your personal life, your family relationships, and your professional roles. Take a few moments to ponder the following:

- How have you been feeling while engaging with this information? Why?
- How much of this topic can you personally relate to?
- Who do you tend to blame when you hear about a homicide, suicide, or mass violence? Why?
- What opinions do you have about death or terrorizing acts that might differ from other peoples' opinions?
- What other examples have come to mind that illustrate similar or diverse ways that families cope with fear and loss stressors?

Reminders for Helpers

As a person of influence, you can help guide people through the coping processes and ideally help foster a **flourishing** life. However, take care to avoid letting your personal **interpretations** push you toward assuming too much about somebody else's circumstances, perceptions, and motivations. Always be ready to address issues that might be hard for you to face because of your own history.

Draw upon the elements of the **FIM framework** and other family stress concepts. Remember, **coping** refers to an action or response based on available or new resources and perceptions related to stressors. Families have either successfully **managed** a stressor's pressure through **adjustment coping** or reached crisis in which **adaptive coping** is needed to reestablish some level of **general family functioning**. **Resources** and **perceptions** are key concepts to focus on when confronting family stress. **Review the master table** in Chapter 4 as a guide for exploring the ideas below of how to help families with stressors.

What Are Some Ways to Encourage Effective Family Coping?

Drawing primarily from citations and insights noted in the chapter thus far, we will explore **suggested resources and noteworthy perceptions** that can contribute to successful coping and more optimal family functioning.

How Can You Help With Fear and Loss Stressors?

For families who have a terminally ill member, **palliative** or **hospice care** are helpful resources for adjusting to the eventual loss.[40] Palliative care includes a focus on healing an illness, while hospice care addresses situations when the illness won't be cured. Both provide comprehensive care to patients and families, working to create the highest quality end-of-life circumstances. However, families can't always afford such services, and insurance doesn't necessarily cover them. **Support groups** are also helpful in confronting anticipatory and reactive grief by giving families the opportunity to express themselves, hear advice from others who truly relate to their circumstances, and avoid too much isolation. Families might need help learning about the various available services and encouragement to use them.

As with many other stressors, having **social support** helps people find the strength to manage their lives in challenging circumstances and to feel heard and validated. Bereavement experts commonly emphasize the importance of facing and expressing one's grief, though some argue that switching between periods of addressing the feelings and avoiding the feelings helps people learn to both accept the loss and begin a new life without the deceased person.[41] Participating in family, religious, or cultural **rituals** (e.g., funerals, gravesite visits, viewing photographs, and home movies together) are ways for surviving family members to express and process their feelings. Why so much emphasis on feelings?

Feelings reflect our **subjective reality**—our perceptions and interpretations, which we know are vitally important for coping. Certainly, the circumstances surrounding a death contribute to our thoughts and feelings about it. *Was it avoidable? Was it intentional? Who caused it? Was it motivated by hate? Did they die before their time?* Some psychological scholars point out that we naturally need to comprehend how things are connected, usually in ways that seem like a story, to provide order in life.[42] The **meaning-making process** regarding the loss of a loved one involves making sense of the loss, accepting it, finding a positive way to look at it, and realigning one's identity and relationships to the new reality. Such meanings matter for how losses affect us. For example, the meaning parents make out of the loss of a child appears to more strongly predict the level of their grief than the amount of time since the loss (i.e., time to heal) and the nature of the cause of death. Adopting a perspective of seeing life as imperfect yet precious has helped parents benefit from a violent death of a child. Finding meaning in a loss seems to help people avoid CG. Does "accuracy" of meaning really matter here?

In short, family losses seem to push us to construct new ways of thinking about life and our identities and relationships. We seek to make peace with the loss and continue forward with some sense of hope while maintaining just enough of a connection to the deceased that allows us to remember the person without becoming immobilized in other aspects of our lives. This process can take years, especially when identities and routines have become intertwined (e.g., a long marriage), and people might need help with **cognitive and behavioral coping strategies** that contribute to the meaning-making process and regulate powerful emotions. Keep in mind that our constructed stories are also informed by cultural contexts and what is deemed to be normal and appropriate regarding the death of a loved one.

Children also make meaning out of a loss, and we should enable their participation in rituals and allow them to express themselves in ways that might differ from adults. Activities that involve art, drama, music, and writing can be particularly helpful.[43] Though it is important to be open with children, they can become overwhelmed when the circumstances surrounding a death are traumatizing. Some things that parents might need help with in guiding their children through bereavement include the following (and parents may also need help doing some of these things for themselves):[44]

- Understanding the developmental stages of their children and recognizing signs of CG
- Helping children learn to anticipate and prepare for triggers that cause grief to resurface
- Recognizing what they as parents model to their children about grief and mourning, and teaching children helpful coping skills
- Despite their own grief and stress, keeping daily routines as similar and consistent as possible so children maintain some comforting structure
- Becoming more attentive to the possibility of children overhearing details too sensitive for their age, and realizing that children are prone to overhear things more often than adults realize; also keeping in mind that some children become driven to seek out more information about things that they perceive to be forbidden
- Asking children questions to discover any misguided perceptions they might have about the loss, such as being the cause of it or that life is ruined; learning to help their children reframe their perceptions more positively (but not unrealistically)
- Empowering children to let go of things they cannot control and funnel their energies toward things they can control, such as participating in efforts to increase social awareness of certain illnesses or to provide service to others who are similarly in mourning
- Especially in cases of terrorizing events, addressing their own feelings first so they are able to comfort their children without becoming overwhelmed, setting limits on time and certain content regarding media exposure (including social media) to the event, and developing safety plans and assuring children of their safety in school and other public places

An overarching challenge for parents is finding a helpful balance between appreciating the inherent vulnerabilities that children have while also honoring their resiliency and strength. Sometimes parents are **overprotective** or **overreactive** and reinforce a sense of fragility in their children who thus might learn to view their world as more dangerous and hopeless than it really is, and themselves as more powerless than they really are. In interviews a few years after a terrorist attack, parents described the growth they observed in their children since the attack.[45] They mentioned how they saw an increase in their children's appreciation of family relationships (through affection and communication), compassion and empathy, toughness and courage, political engagement, reflectiveness about their personal values (e.g., what really matters in life), and mindfulness of the little things that make life enjoyable. Of course, children need nurture and security to thrive and develop self-confidence for facing tragedy.

Research on military families has generated various suggestions for **coping with deployment**.[46] For example, regular communication between the deployed parents and the nondeployed parent, active problem-solving, and religious participation lessened the likelihood that a stressful deployment would result in PTSD. Furthermore, the effects of PTSD on family relationships can be minimized when families have good communication skills, work to be supportive and bonded to one another, and have parents who form alliances with other parents to create a supportive network. While the military typically offers services for struggling families, some parents—particularly fathers—might need help overcoming **stigma** associated with help-seeking behavior. Other specific suggestions include the following:

- During **predeployment**, families should discuss what separation will be like. They should decide how each member wants to communicate with the deployed parent and how often. Parents should be aware (and not overreact) that children might become distant before deployment to help ease into the separation process. Signing up for a support group can help families coordinate activities with one another and avoid isolation.
- During **deployment/sustainment**, communicate in agreed-upon ways while also adapting to unforeseen circumstances. Make communication a positive and bonding experience, sharing deep feelings and offering assurances for the future.
- When families **reunite**, be prepared for a challenging adjustment period (i.e., plan for it ahead of time). Talk about how to adjust communication. Be sensitive to the mental health needs of family members and pursue help as needed.[47]

Improve Your Learning

Without peeking, take a moment to review in your mind (or say out loud) the key concepts from this chapter (this is a proven learning technique). Then review the "Chapter Preview" section at the top and compare. Skim Part B of the chapter with extra attention to the **bolded words**.

Do You Want to Learn More?

We have only touched on a portion of information related to some elements of this topic. **What really sparked your interest? What do you wish was covered more thoroughly?** Consider taking some time to further deepen your understanding of personal and professional issues related to helping families cope with stressors. The following are a variety of resources that you might find helpful, and some references directly or indirectly referred to in this chapter. Have no fear and deploy your study skills.

Videos

(Use links or do searches with the key words provided)
- When My Parent Passed Away (4 mins). BuzzFeedVideo. https://www.youtube.com/watch?v=elE6iSytJks
- The Moment My Sibling Passed Away (3 mins). BuzzFeedVideo. https://www.youtube.com/watch?v=-PH46MxWQYI
- The Last Mother's Day for Avery Neill (6 mins). *The News & Observer.* (Death of a child and sibling) https://www.youtube.com/watch?v=2rBrOJeePBI
- This Doctor Wants to Humanize Death (22 mins). *The New York Times.* (Losing a child to illness) https://www.youtube.com/watch?v=DHBgTFHjPXI
- We Don't "Move On" From Grief. We Move Forward With It (15 mins). TED, Nora McInerny. (Death of a spouse) https://www.youtube.com/watch?v=khkJkR-ipfw
- Uncoupled—Dealing With The Death of a Spouse (25 mins). Alberta Health Services. https://www.youtube.com/watch?v=_NL9FaBoKYs
- Suicide: What I Wish I Could Tell You Today (5 mins). Participant. https://www.youtube.com/watch?v=PDUsyfJvcj8
- What I Learned From My Husband's Suicide (13 mins). TEDxOgden, Lori Prichard. https://www.youtube.com/watch?v=Jb_1IklnhaU
- I Was Almost a School Shooter (7.5 mins). TEDxBoulder, Aaron Stark. (Includes suicidal ideation) https://www.youtube.com/watch?v=azRl1dI-Cts
- Families of 9/11 Victims Still Angry 20 Years Later (7 mins). ABC News. https://www.youtube.com/watch?v=dnvoN-SSzyQ
- Military Families Struggle to Re-acclimate After Deployment (3 mins). CBS. https://www.youtube.com/watch?v=Vc1oonj3qXI
- How to Successfully Transition From Military to Civilian Life (10 mins). TEDxOakland, Brian O'Connor. (Military culture) https://www.youtube.com/watch?v=61RTfaU6Grs

Websites

- Centers for Disease Control and Prevention. (n.d.). Facts about suicide. https://www.cdc.gov/suicide/facts/index.html
- Cuhna, J. P. (2020, September 30). How does suicide affect loved ones? emedicinehealth. https://www.emedicinehealth.com/how_does_suicide_affect_loved_ones/article_em.htm
- Fagan, C. (2022, May 25). Another school shooting: What parents can do to help kids cope. Psycom. https://www.psycom.net/trauma/school-shooting-survivor-trauma
- Meadows, S. O., Tanielian, T., & Karney, B. (n.d.). How military families respond before, during and after deployment. Rand Corporation. https://www.rand.org/pubs/research_briefs/RB9906.html

- Military.com (2022). The emotional cycle of deployment: Military family perspective. https://www.military.com/spouse/military-deployment/emotional-cycle-of-deployment-military-family.html
- Pew Research Center (n.d.). Political ideology among adults who believe in heaven. https://www.pewresearch.org/religion/religious-landscape-study/political-ideology/among/belief-in-heaven/believe/

Readings (Articles, Books, Book Chapters)

- Cacciatore, J. (2017). *Bearing the unbearable: Love, loss, and the heartbreaking path of grief.* Wisdom Publications.
- Ferow, A. (2019). Childhood grief and loss. *European Journal of Educational Sciences*, 06. https://doi.org/10.19044/ejes.s.v6a1
- Kochen, E. M., Jenken, F., Boelen, P. A., Deben, L. M. A., Fahner, J. C., van den Hoogen, A., Teunissen, S. C. C. M., Geleijns, K., & Kars, M. C. (2020). When a child dies: A systematic review of well-defined parent-focused bereavement interventions and their alignment with grief- and loss theories. *BMC Palliative Care*, *19*(1), 28. https://doi.org/10.1186/s12904-020-0529-z
- Maciejewski, P. K., Maercker, A., Boelen, P. A., & Prigerson, H. G. (2016). "Prolonged grief disorder" and "persistent complex bereavement disorder," but not "complicated grief," are one and the same diagnostic entity: An analysis of data from the Yale Bereavement Study. *World Psychiatry: Official Journal of the World Psychiatric Association* (WPA), *15*(3), 266–275. https://doi.org/10.1002/wps.20348
- Neimeyer, R. A., Klass, D., & Dennis, M. R. (2014). A social constructionist account of grief: Loss and the narration of meaning. *Death Studies*, *38*(6–10), 485–498. https://doi.org/10.1080/07481187.2014.913454

Notes

1   Lovejoy, B. (2017, January 3). "Mirrors with memories": Why did Victorians take pictures of dead people? Mental Floss. https://www.mentalfloss.com/article/90118/mirrors-memories-why-did-victorians-take-pictures-dead-people

2   Albrecht, K. (2012, March 22). The (only) 5 fears we all share. *Psychology Today.* https://www.psychologytoday.com/us/blog/brainsnacks/201203/the-only-5-fears-we-all-share; Chapman University. (n.d.). The division on the study of American fears. https://www.chapman.edu/wilkinson/research-centers/babbie-center/survey-american-fears.aspx

3   Cohen, S., Murphy, M., & Prather, A. A. (2019). Ten surprising facts about stressful life events and disease risk. *Annual Review of Psychology*, *70*, 577–597. https://doi.org/10.1146/annurev-psych-010418-102857; Spurgeon, A., Jackson, C. A., & Beach, J. R. (2001). The life events inventory: Re-scaling based on an occupational sample. *Occupational Medicine*, *51*(4), 287–293. https://doi.org/10.1093/occmed/51.4.287

4   MedicineNet. (2007, September 13). Loss, grief, and bereavement. https://www.medicinenet.com/script/main/art.asp?articlekey=83860

5   Maciejewski, P. K., Maercker, A., Boelen, P. A., & Prigerson, H. G. (2016). "Prolonged grief disorder" and "persistent complex bereavement disorder," but not "complicated grief," are one and the same diagnostic entity: an analysis of data from the Yale Bereavement Study. *World Psychiatry: Official Journal of the World Psychiatric Association* (WPA), *15*(3), 266–275. https://doi.org/10.1002/wps.20348

6   Psych Central (n.d). All about disenfranchised grief. https://psychcentral.com/health/disenfranchised-grief?c=1585339728199#causes

7   Boss, P. (2002). *Family stress management: A contextual approach* (2nd ed.). SAGE Publications.

8   Nakajima S. (2018). Complicated grief: Recent developments in diagnostic criteria and treatment. *Philosophical transactions of the Royal Society of London. Series B, Biological sciences, 373*(1754), 20170273. https://doi.org/10.1098/rstb.2017.0273

9   Maciejewski, P. K., Maercker, A., Boelen, P. A., & Prigerson, H. G. (2016). "Prolonged grief disorder" and "persistent complex bereavement disorder," but not "complicated grief," are one and the same diagnostic entity: an analysis of data from the Yale Bereavement Study. *World Psychiatry: Official Journal of the World Psychiatric Association* (WPA), *15*(3), 266–275. https://doi.org/10.1002/wps.20348

10   Bassett, J. F., & Bussard, M. L. (2021). Examining the complex relation among religion, morality, and death anxiety: Religion can be a source of comfort and concern regarding fears of death. *Omega: Journal of Death and Dying, 82*(3), 467–487. https://doi.org/10.1177/0030222818819343; Ellis, L., & Wahab, E. A. (2013). Religiosity and fear of death: A theory oriented review of the empirical literature. *Review of Religious Research, 55*, 149–189. https://doi.org/10.1007/s13644-012-0064-3; Feldman, D. B., Fischer, I. C., & Gressis, R. A. (2016). Does religious belief matter for grief and death anxiety? Experimental philosophy meets psychology of religion. *Journal for the Scientific Study of Religion, 55*(3), 531–539. https://doi.org/10.1111/jssr.12288

11   Pew Research Center. (n.d.). Political ideology among adults who believe in heaven. https://www.pewresearch.org/religion/religious-landscape-study/political-ideology/among/belief-in-heaven/believe/

12   Ferow, A. (2019). Childhood grief and loss. *European Journal of Educational Sciences, 06*. https://doi.org/10.19044/ejes.s.v6a1

13   Rynearson, E. K. (2012). The narrative dynamics of grief after homicide. *OMEGA—Journal of Death and Dying, 65*(3), 239–249. https://doi.org/10.2190/OM.65.3.f

14   Cuhna, J. P. (2020, September 30). How does suicide affect loved ones? Emedicinehealth. https://www.emedicinehealth.com/how_does_suicide_affect_loved_ones/article_em.htm; Goldstein, T. R., Birmaher, B., Axelson, D., Goldstein, B. I., Gill, M. K., Esposito-Smythers, C., Ryan, N. D., Strober, M. A., Hunt, J., & Keller, M. (2009). Family environment and suicidal ideation among bipolar youth. *Archives of Suicide Research, 13*(4), 378–388. https://doi.org/10.1080/13811110903266699; Yoder, K. A., & Hoyt, D. R. (2005). Family economic pressure and adolescent suicidal ideation: Application of the family stress model. *Suicide and Life-Threatening Behavior, 35*(3), 251–264. https://doi.org/10.1521/suli.2005.35.3.251

15   Centers for Disease Control and Prevention. (n.d.). Leading causes of death. https://www.cdc.gov/nchs/fastats/leading-causes-of-death.htm

16   Bergman, A.-S., Axberg, U., & Hanson, E. (2017). When a parent dies—a systematic review of the effects of support programs for parentally bereaved children and their caregivers. *BMC Palliative Care, 16*(1). https://doi.org/10.1186/s12904-017-0223-y; Ferow, A. (2019). Childhood grief and loss. *European Journal of Educational Sciences, 06*. https://doi.org/10.19044/ejes.s.v6a1

17   Funk, A. M., Jenkins, S., Astroth, K. S., Braswell, G., & Kerber, C. (2018). A narrative analysis of sibling grief. *Journal of Loss and Trauma, 23*(1), 1–14. https://doi.org/10.1080/15325024.2017.1396281

18   Ferow, A. (2019). Childhood grief and loss. *European Journal of Educational Sciences, 06*. https://doi.org/10.19044/ejes.s.v6a1

19   Jonas-Simpson, C., Steele, R., Granek, L., Davies, B., & O'Leary, J. (2015). Always with me: Understanding experiences of bereaved children whose baby sibling died. *Death Studies, 39*(4), 242–251. https://doi.org/10.1080/07481187.2014.991954

20   Healgrief.org. (n.d.). Grieving the death of a spouse. https://healgrief.org/grieving-the-death-of-a-spouse/; Neptune Society (n.d.). Coping with the loss of a spouse or partner. https://www.neptunesociety.com/resources/coping-with-the-loss-of-a-spouse-or-partner

21   Kochen, E. M., Jenken, F., Boelen, P. A., Deben, L. M. A., Fahner, J. C., van den Hoogen, A., Teunissen, S. C. C. M., Geleijns, K., & Kars, M. C. (2020). When a child dies: A systematic review of well-defined parent-focused bereavement interventions and their alignment with grief and loss theories. *BMC Palliative Care, 19*(1), 28. https://doi.

org/10.1186/s12904-020-0529-z; Wender, E., & Committee on Psychosocial Aspects of Child and Family Health. (2012). Supporting the family after the death of a child. *Pediatrics, 130*(6), 1164–1169. https://doi.org/10.1542/peds.2012-2772

22 Wender, E., & Committee on Psychosocial Aspects of Child and Family Health. (2012). Supporting the family after the death of a child. *Pediatrics, 130*(6), 1164–1169. https://doi.org/10.1542/peds.2012-2772

23 Fletcher, J., Mailick, M., Song, J., & Wolfe, B. (2013). A sibling death in the family: Common and consequential. *Demography, 50*(3), 803–826. https://doi.org/10.1007/s13524-012-0162-4; Kim, Y., Carver, C. S., Spiegel, D., Mitchell, H., & Cannady, R. S. (2017). Role of family caregivers' self-perceived preparedness for the death of the cancer patient in long-term adjustment to bereavement. *Psycho-Oncology, 26*(4), 484–492. https://doi.org/10.1002/pon.4042

24 eCondolence. (n.d.). Islam: Periods of mourning. https://www.econdolence.com/learning-center/religion-and-culture/islam/islam-periods-of-mourning/

25 Nickerson, A., Bryant, R. A., Brooks, R., Steel, Z., Silove, D., & Chen, J. (2011). The familial influence of loss and trauma on refugee mental health: A multilevel path analysis. *Journal of Traumatic Stress, 24*(1), 25–33. https://doi.org/10.1002/jts.20608

26 Chu, J., Hoeflein, B. T. R., Goldblum, P., Bongar, B., Heyne, G. M., Gadinsky, N., & Skinta, M. D. (2017). Innovations in the practice of culturally competent suicide risk management. *Practice Innovations, 2*(2), 66–79. https://doi.org/10.1037/pri0000044; Chu, J., Maruyama, B., Batchelder, H., Goldblum, P., Bongar, B., & Wickham, R. E. (2020). Cultural pathways for suicidal ideation and behaviors. *Cultural Diversity and Ethnic Minority Psychology, 26*(3), 367–377. https://doi.org/10.1037/cdp0000307.supp; El Ibrahimi, S., Xiao, Y., Bergeron, C. D., Beckford, N. Y., Virgen, E. M., & Smith, M. L. (2021). Suicide distribution and trends among male older adults in the U.S., 1999–2018. *American Journal of Preventive Medicine, 60*(6), 802–811. https://doi.org/10.1016/j.amepre.2020.12.021

27 Fagan, C. (2022, May 25). Another school shooting: What parents can do to help kids cope. Psycom. https://www.psycom.net/trauma/school-shooting-survivor-trauma; Garfin, D. R., Holman, E. A., & Silver, R. C. (2015). Cumulative exposure to prior collective trauma and acute stress responses to the Boston marathon bombings. *Psychological Science, 26*(6), 675–683. https://doi.org/10.1177/0956797614561043; Santilli, A., O'Connor Duffany, K., Carroll-Scott, A., Thomas, J., Greene, A., Arora, A., Agnoli, A., Gan, G., & Ickovics, J. (2017). Bridging the response to mass shootings and urban violence: Exposure to violence in New Haven, Connecticut. *American Journal of Public Health, 107*(3), 374–379. https://doi.org/10.2105/AJPH.2016.303613

28 Aubrey, A. (2022, May 26). What to say to kids about school shootings to ease their stress. National Public Radio. https://www.npr.org/sections/health-shots/2022/05/26/1101306073/what-to-say-to-kids-about-school-shootings-to-ease-their-stress

29 Meltzer, E., Gorski, E., & Cramer, P. (2019, May 9). *"Nothing makes me feel safe." How Colorado educators and parents are processing yet another school shooting.* Chalkbeat Colorado. https://co.chalkbeat.org/2019/5/8/21108129/nothing-makes-me-feel-safe-how-colorado-educators-and-parents-are-processing-yet-another-school-shoo

30 Nordanger, D. Ø., Hysing, M., Posserud, M., Lundervold, A. J., Jakobsen, R., Olff, M., & Stormark, K. M. (2013). Posttraumatic responses to the July 22, 2011, Olso Terror among Norwegian high school students. *Journal of Traumatic Stress, 26*(6), 679–685. https://doi.org/10.1002/jts.21856

31 Prieto-Rodriguez, J., Rodriguez, G. J, Salas, R., & Suarez-Pancliello, J. (2009). Quantifying fear: The social impact of terrorism. *Journal of Policy Modeling, 31*(5), 803–817. https://doi.org/10.1016/j.jpolmod.2008.07.004

32 Comer, J. S., Furr, J. M., & Gurwitch, R. H. (2019). Terrorism exposure and the family: Where we are, and where we go next. In B. H. Fiese, M. Celano, K. Deater-Deckard, E. N. Jouriles, & M. A. Whisman (Eds.), *APA handbook of contemporary family psychology: Applications and broad impact of family psychology* (p. 571–585). American Psychological Association. https://doi.org/10.1037/0000100-035

33 Menendez, A. M., Molloy, J., & Magaldi, M. C. (2006). Health responses of New York City firefighter spouses and their families post-September 11, 2001 terrorist attacks. *Issues in Mental Health Nursing, 27*(8), 905–917. https://doi.org/10.1080/01612840600842642

34 Baptist, J., Barros, P., Cafferky, B., & Johannes, E. (2015). Resilience building among adolescents from National Guard families: Applying a developmental contextual model. *Journal of Adolescent Research, 30*(3), 306–334. https://doi.org/10.1177/0743558414558592; Lester, P., Aralis, H., Sinclair, M., Kiff, C., Lee, K., Mustillo, S., & MacDermid

Wadsworth, S. (2016). The impact of deployment on parental, family and child adjustment in military families. *Child Psychiatry and Human Development, 47*, 938–949. https://doi.org/10.1007/s10578-016-0624-9; Meadows, S. O., Tanielian, T., & Karney, B. (n.d.). How military families respond before, during and after deployment. Rand Corporation. https://www.rand.org/pubs/research_briefs/RB9906.html

35 Freytes, I. M., LaLaurin, J. H., Zickmund, S. L., Resende, R. D., & Uphold, C. R. (2017). Exploring the post-deployment reintegration experiences of veterans with PTSD and their significant others. *American Journal of Orthopsychiatry, 87*(2), 149–156. http://dx.doi.org/10.1037/ort0000211; Military.com (2022). The emotional cycle of deployment: Military family perspective. https://www.military.com/spouse/military-deployment/emotional-cycle-of-deployment-military-family.html

36 Lincoln, A. J., & Sweeten, K. (2011). Considerations for the effects of military deployment on children and families. *Social Work in Health Care, 50*(1), 73–85. https://doi.org/10.1080/00981389.2010.513921

37 Cohen, L. K., & Levy, I. (2020). Risk perception of a chronic threat of terrorism: Differences based on coping types, gender and exposure. *International Journal of Psychology, 55*(1), 115–122. https://doi.org/10.1002/ijop.12552; Lowe, S. R., & Galea, S. (2017). The mental health consequences of mass shootings. *Trauma, Violence, & Abuse, 18*(1), 62–82. https://doi.org/10.1177/1524838015591572; Nordanger, D. Ø., Hysing, M., Posserud, M., Lundervold, A. J., Jakobsen, R., Olff, M., & Stormark, K. M. (2013). Posttraumatic responses to the July 22, 2011 Olso Terror among Norwegian high school students. *Journal of Traumatic Stress, 26*(6), 679–685. https://doi.org/10.1002/jts.21856; Pfefferbaum, B. J., DeVoe, E. R., Stuber, J., Schiff, M., Klein, T. P., & Fairbrother, G. (2005). Psychological impact of terrorism on children and families in the United States. *Journal of Aggression, Maltreatment & Trauma, 9*(3–4), 305–317. https://doi.org/10.1300/J146v09n03_01

38 Kinzie, J. D. (2005). Some of the effects of terrorism on refugees. *Journal of Aggression, Maltreatment & Trauma, 9*(3–4), 411–420. https://doi.org/10.1300/J146v09n03_12; Nordanger, D. Ø., Hysing, M., Posserud, M., Lundervold, A. J., Jakobsen, R., Olff, M., & Stormark, K. M. (2013). Posttraumatic responses to the July 22, 2011 Olso Terror among Norwegian high school students. *Journal of Traumatic Stress, 26*(6), 679–685. https://doi.org/10.1002/jts.21856

39 Hollingsworth, W.-G. L., Dolbin-MacNab, M. L., & Marek, L. I. (2016). Boundary ambiguity and ambivalence in military family reintegration: Boundary ambiguity and ambivalence. *Family Relations, 65*(4), 603–615. https://doi.org/10.1111/fare.12207

40 Kim, Y., Carver, C. S., Spiegel, D., Mitchell, H., & Cannady, R. S. (2017). Role of family caregivers' self-perceived preparedness for the death of the cancer patient in long-term adjustment to bereavement. *Psycho-Oncology, 26*(4), 484–492. https://doi.org/10.1002/pon.4042; National Institute on Aging. (2021, May 14). What are palliative care and hospice care? https://www.nia.nih.gov/health/what-are-palliative-care-and-hospice-care

41 Nakajima S. (2018). Complicated grief: Recent developments in diagnostic criteria and treatment. *Philosophical transactions of the Royal Society of London. Series B, Biological Sciences, 373*(1754), 20170273. https://doi.org/10.1098/rstb.2017.0273

42 Neimeyer, R. A., Klass, D., & Dennis, M. R. (2014). A social constructionist account of grief: Loss and the narration of meaning. *Death Studies, 38*(6–10), 485–498. https://doi.org/10.1080/07481187.2014.913454

43 Ferow, A. (2019). Childhood grief and loss. *European Journal of Educational Sciences, 06*. https://doi.org/10.19044/ejes.s.v6a1

44 Callanan, M. A. (2014). Diversity in children's understanding of death: COMMENTARY. *Monographs of the Society for Research in Child Development, 79*(1), 142–150. https://doi.org/10.1111/mono.12087; DeVoe, E. R., Klein, T. P., Bannon, W., & Miranda-Julian, C. (2010). Young children in the aftermath of the World Trade Center attacks. *Psychological Trauma: Theory, Research, Practice, and Policy, 3*(1), 1–7. https://doi.org/10.1037/a0020567; Fagan, C. (2022, May 25). Another school shooting: What parents can do to help kids cope. Psycom. https://www.psycom.net/trauma/school-shooting-survivor-trauma; Ferow, A. (2019). Childhood grief and loss. *European Journal of Educational Sciences, 06*. https://doi.org/10.19044/ejes.s.v6a1

45 Glad, K. A., Kilmer, R. P., Dyb, G., & Hafstad, G. S. (2019). Caregiver-reported positive changes in young survivors of a terrorist attack. *Journal of Child and Family Studies, 28*, 704–719. https://doi.org/10.1007/s10826-018-1298-7

46 Olson, J. R., Welsh, J. A., Perkins, D. F., & Ormsby, L. (2018). Individual, family, and community predictors of PTSD symptoms following military deployment: Predictors of PTSD symptoms. *Family Relations, 67*(5), 615–629. https://doi.org/10.1111/fare.12343; Rossetto, K. R. (2015). Developing conceptual definitions and theoretical

models of coping in military families during deployment. *Journal of Family Communication, 15*, 249–268. https://doi.org/10.1080/15267431.2015.1043737

47 Knobloch, L. K., Basinger, E. D., Wehrman, E. C., Ebata, A. T., & McGlaughlin, P. C. (2016). Communication of military couples during deployment and reunion: Changes, challenges, opportunities, and advice. *Journal of Family Communication, 16*, 160–179. https://doi.org/10.1080/15267431.2016.1146723; Sahlstein, E., Maguire, K. C., & Timmerman, L. (2009). Contradictions and praxis contextualized by wartime deployment: Wives' perspectives revealed through relational dialectics. *Communication Monographs, 76*, 421–442. https://doi.org/10.1080/03637750903300239

Image Credits

Fig. 11.1: Source: Adapted from https://www.cdc.gov/nchs/data/hestat/mortality/mortality_marital_status_10_17.htm.

CHAPTER 12

Large-Scale Disasters and Family Stress

The Central China flood of 1931, caused by heavy rains (over 24 inches in one month) combined with snow melt, inundated nearly 70,000 square miles of land and killed an estimated 2 to 3.7 million people.[1]

Chapter Preview

- As with terrorizing violence, large-scale disasters create fear and loss that increase family stress.
- The extent to which a hazardous event with natural origins becomes a "disaster" depends in part on human preparedness and response capacities.
- Disaster survivors and first responders are at heightened risk for post-traumatic stress disorder and other psychological challenges.
- The severity of a natural disaster is one of several key characteristics that determine how potentially stressful it will be.
- Pre-disaster circumstances, level of a disaster's disruption, and post-disaster circumstances combine to impact families in various ways.
- Belonging to an integrated, trustworthy community can significantly boost resiliency to a natural disaster's impact.
- The COVID-19 pandemic produced stressors related to every chapter of the textbook, providing us with an opportunity to review concepts and topics.
- Families felt pressures regarding their health and safety because of the virus; they also felt pressures regarding social isolation, relationship outcomes, and everyday living patterns because of restrictive quarantines.
- Large-scale disasters often disrupt social support and challenge families to make meaning from their experiences that keep them optimistic and hopeful.

What Is This Topic About?

Perhaps you are still reflecting on the pains of family loss and anxiety associated with mass shootings and terrorist attacks. But wait, there's more! (Don't get ahead of yourself though, it's not all bad.) This chapter extends themes of **fear** and **loss** to other large-scale stressors—namely, **natural disasters** and widespread disease, such as a **pandemic**. These events typically create major **disruptive damage** to human property or health. While some environmental disasters indirectly impact human health and mortality by contributing to the overall state of regional or global conditions (e.g., climate, wildlife), our emphasis will be on the relatively direct and easily identifiable consequences disasters have for families. Large-scale disasters tend to occur from major storms (e.g., hurricanes, tornados, rain), extreme temperatures (e.g., heat waves, freezing conditions), drought, earthquakes/tsunamis, wildfires, mudslides/avalanches, volcanic eruptions, or pandemics.

Large-scale disasters can greatly impact the everyday lives of families, communities, and those who assist with the aftermath (e.g., first responders and their families). They also influence the broader **society** by triggering potential help-oriented responses (e.g., donations), causing worry about future disasters harming our own loved ones, and pushing us to question our philosophies about life, death, humanity, and divinity. As you well know by now, the way we perceive and make sense of stressor events is an important part of how we cope with the pressures they create.

What Are the Assumptions?

What is the difference between an earthquake that destroys several buildings and a terrorist's bomb that does the same? In the last chapter, we noted that the intentionality to do harm impacts us differently than a fluke accident. Similarly, what we tend to label as "natural" or "an act of God" seems to have different meanings from what has traditionally been called "man-made" (or human-caused) disasters. However, the label "natural disaster" is somewhat controversial.[2]

Some argue that a "disaster" is an interaction of a **hazardous event**—including an act of nature—with human contexts of vulnerability and capacity, potentially creating major **disruption**. Hence, a natural hazard is only disastrous when it majorly interferes with functional living. For example, an earthquake is less likely to be a disaster when structures are built to withstand earthquakes and when people effectively practice personal safety procedures—like avoiding windows and protecting their heads. Of course, some events can overwhelm our best preparation. Others argue that the label "natural disaster" simply emphasizes that at least a major component of the event has nonhuman origins (though not necessarily from beings of another planet, I assume).

Views on the causes of "natural" events could be somewhat connected to **political ideology**. Some religious-based conservatism, especially in more traditional and less industrialized cultures, seems to lean toward seeing a divine hand in the causes of natural disasters—perhaps to send a sign or to punish disobedience. Modern environmentalism tends to align more with liberal politics, though ideological differences might be magnified by political polarization (see Chapter 6).[3] Liberals appear quicker than conservatives to highlight human-caused elements of a natural disaster, which might reflect the general tendency to value the **care** foundation (avoiding harm to animals and nature) and a specific application of the **sanctity** foundation—a lean toward more highly valuing what is "natural" (e.g., food production, ingredients in cleaners). Conservatives are generally less trusting of large-scale government interventions, including some environmental policies and federal approaches to intervening after a disaster, for the sake of **liberty** and to protect the **stability** of economic institutions from overregulation. In practice, large-scale disasters often unify humanity, and the political ideologies of most families probably have little effect on supporting sufferers.

The COVID-19 pandemic appears to have tapped into political polarization that perhaps further blurs lines between ideology and political party. Politicians and citizens alike engaged in abundant, passionate debate about causes of and solutions to the pandemic.[4] The nationwide quarantine and some state-specific restrictions in parts of 2020 and 2021 were especially contentious, with Republicans seeming to push for less restriction on personal and business decisions and Democrats seeming to push for more. Some ideological disagreements were likely functions of differing views on the power of government and how the perceived risks associated with slowing the economy and closing schools compared to the perceived risks of not doing so. However, polarizing perceptions of the dangers of the virus and of vaccinations could arguably be more about faithfully aligning with one's political party (and associated media) than about genuine differences in underlying moral foundations. Disagreements over pandemic-related issues could have played out in families across the country (and the world).

As you **engage with** the rest of the chapter, remember the key elements of family stress theories (e.g., stressors, resources, perceptions, coping, and crisis) and consider the following:

- How can families effectively prepare for minimizing the impact of large-scale disasters?
- How possible is it for families to actually flourish in the face of large-scale disasters?
- How do the various pieces of information throughout the chapter fit together to help explain why each family might be affected differently by large-scale disasters?
- What experiences have you had or observed that help you relate to specific concepts?
- How might the ideological perspectives influence how people (including you) think about potential causes of and solutions to large-scale disaster stressors for families?

Part A. Natural Disaster Stressors

What Is Stressful About Natural Disasters?

What type of natural disaster worries you the most? Severe storms and floods are the most common natural disasters in the United States, but some regions of the country are especially prone to earthquakes, forest fires, extreme temperatures, or drought.[5] Hurricanes are usually the most deadly and expensive natural disasters—the 1900 hurricane in Galveston, Texas, took the lives of up to an estimated 12,000 people.[6] Hurricane Katrina, which hit the New Orleans area in 2005, was the most expensive natural disaster with an estimated cost of $180 billion in recovery efforts. Other top 10 deadliest nonhurricane natural disasters in the United States include the following:

- **The heatwave of 1936 across most of the country:** It destroyed crops and took years for soil to recover; up to 5,000 people died.
- **The San Francisco earthquake in 1906:** It destroyed about 80% of the city, causing around 3,000 deaths.
- **The Johnstown flood of 1889 in Pennsylvania:** A dam burst after heavy rains; up to 60-foot-high swells of water washed through homes and other buildings at up to 45 mph, killing over 2,000 people.
- **The Peshtigo forest fire in Wisconsin and Michigan in 1871:** It killed around 2,000 people and burned over 1 million acres of forest. A mass grave was created for about 350 bodies because nobody survived who could identify them.

Post-traumatic stress disorder (PTSD) is perhaps the most commonly investigated psychological outcome of natural disasters, with depression, anxiety, anger, and psychological distress also high on the list.[7] Losing a loved one or highly valued objects or ambitions (e.g., a dream home, family heirlooms and pictures, living in a certain area forever) tend to promote **grief**, can lead to **social isolation**, and increase the risks of **substance problems**. Individual psychological challenges and draining physical demands can contribute to weakened or strained social and family relationships.

While overall it appears that trauma from a natural disaster is usually less serious than trauma from interpersonal violence or abuse, natural disasters can still have devastating effects for families that last for months or even years.[8] In certain circumstances, such as losing a family member to a flood or fire, the experience would be as painful and stressful as anything (see Chapter 11). Various other characteristics of a natural disaster contribute to the attributes and levels of family stress, as is explored in the next section.

What Contributes to the Stress of a Natural Disaster?

Considering the specific **characteristics** of a disaster helps us anticipate or understand the pressures and challenges associated with experiencing it. Table 12.1 (next page) is similar to the one appearing in Chapter 1 but adapted to highlight the specific characteristics of a hurricane. Think about how the details of a hurricane could have different impacts on family stress. You could do the same for an earthquake, a forest fire, and so forth.

TABLE 12.1 Characteristics of Stressor: A Hurricane

Characteristic	Focus of Characteristic	Example Application
Severity	How intense or major is the stressor?	Depends on the size and strength of storm, high potential for great intensity.
Location of Source	Did the stressor occur within the family or outside the family?	Outside the family (unless magic is real).
Pace of Onset	How gradually or suddenly did the stressor occur?	Hurricane warnings can come several days in advance, but the severity is often speculative.
Duration	How long did the stressor last?	Hurricanes often last 12 to 24 hours, but the anticipation and aftermath can last much longer.
Predictability	How easy is it to anticipate the stressor?	Easier in areas where hurricanes are common, but severity is often speculative.
Amount of Choice	How much choice did someone have about this stressor occurring?	Level of choice depends largely on how much choice someone has in living where they do.
Cumulation	Is this a single stressor or a pileup of multiple stressors?	Hurricanes can damage property and injure and kill people; a series of storms can occur.
Issues of Quantity	Is the stressor related to having too little or too much of something?	Too much wind and water.
Clarity	Are the facts surrounding the stressor clear or confusing/ambiguous?	Severity is often speculative, and sometimes predictions are wrong.
Potential Trigger	Is the stressor itself the real cause of stress or does it trigger memories or feelings of the real source of stress?	The storm can be the key stressor but could also trigger memories of trauma from past disasters.

As noted in the table, the **severity** of a hurricane is not always predictable. Why would that matter? In the Galveston, Texas, hurricane of 1900, residents had apparently grown complacent about storm warnings because they had already been through several storms that caused little damage. You might have heard of other cases in which people were warned to leave a pre-disaster area but decided not to. The uncertainty surrounding many natural disasters tends to make them particularly stressful[9]—*What exactly are we preparing for?* Our **perceptions** of risk can play a large role in how well we prepare for a natural disaster, and, of course, some people may struggle to prepare because of poverty and the lack of resources.

Large-scale disasters are prone to create **long-term**, **comprehensive pressures** that pile up and potentially overwhelm families. For example, families might experience power outages, home damage, physical injury, transportation limitations, food shortages, exposure to toxins, community chaos (e.g., theft, violence), employment and educational disruption, and health-care limitations.

The need to comfort fearful children and elderly parents adds other pressures to the pile. Besides the characteristics of the natural disaster itself, risks for negative individual and family outcomes are also often related to the following:[10]

- **Pre-disaster circumstances:** People, especially children, with a history of other trauma experiences (e.g., family violence, war, natural disasters) tend to be at greater risk for PTSD when hit with a natural disaster. Adolescents with a history of more delinquent behavior tend to struggle with internalizing and externalizing behavior after a disaster, and people who already struggle with anxiety tend to be more traumatized afterward. Parents whose profession is threatened by the disaster (e.g., farmers during a drought or flooding) are likely to be especially distressed. Having strained financial resources also increases vulnerability given the additional economic challenges that come along with a natural disaster. Strained family relationships can lead to even more relationship problems during and after a disaster.
- **Damages and disruption:** Overall, families most strongly affected by a natural disaster experience longer term trauma symptoms. Greater losses, property damages, and disruption to daily routines—including schooling, sleep quality, and social interaction—add to the enduring effects of the disaster. Of note, adolescents who had their homes damaged or destroyed by a wildfire were also prone to demonstrate more pro-social behavior afterward, suggesting that stress creates opportunities for people to step up and demonstrate helpful behavior.
- **Post-disaster circumstances:** Children being separated from their parents during and after a disaster is highly distressing, and children who experience more stressors and less social support are more likely to be traumatized by the disaster. Families that struggle with emotional cohesion and overall functioning are more vulnerable to poorer coping and negative outcomes. Children tend to mirror their parents' level of distress, and parental overprotectiveness or inadequate parental support tends to put children at higher risk for trauma symptoms. Living in a temporary shelter throws off daily routines, contributes to a lack of privacy, and can expose children to conflicts that come from overcrowding. Perceiving a weak sense of community in one's environment has also corresponded to greater distress.

Of course, some human-caused disasters have similar qualities to and consequences of natural disasters. For example, building fires, chemical spills, and airplane crashes in populated areas can cause stressful evacuations and other disruptions to daily life and threaten injury and family losses. How might such disasters differ from natural disasters in how people make meaning of their damages and losses?

Who Else Is Impacted by Natural Disasters?

Similar to terrorist attacks such as 9/11 (see Chapter 11), natural disasters are also stressful for **first responders** and their families.[11] Some firefighters in Australia continued to have disruptive flashbacks for over 2 years after major brushfires had occurred. Women who participated in rescue efforts after an earthquake in Turkey were more likely than other women to report deterioration in family relationships afterward, perhaps because of **secondary trauma** (see Chapter 2) or family members feeling neglected. First responders in general who have more direct exposure to devastating injury and losses tend to struggle more with trauma symptoms; they are also more likely to use substances to cope with anxiety and insomnia and to seek out psychological counseling. Psychological distress increases when there are fears of having been exposed to dangerous chemicals during rescue efforts.

Where do families go when their town is destroyed? With Hurricane Katrina, the population of the New Orleans area dropped by about 300,000 people, most of whom relocated to the Baton Rouge area.[12] The impact on **receiving towns** can tax the infrastructure, including dramatic increases in traffic and commute times, calls to emergency services, occupation of hospital beds, overcrowding in restaurants and stores, wait time for services (e.g., doctor/dental, cell phone, insurance), costs of living, shortages in goods, and fears of increasing criminal activity. Reports of both hostile and welcoming attitudes existed toward the survivors. Consider how families from a receiving town and families who relocated there might experience the same pressures differently. What might make it more likely for a town in such circumstances to unite and willingly adapt to the influx of disaster victims?

How Do External Contexts Impact Families Experiencing Natural Disasters?

Studies regularly show that **girls** and **women** have higher rates of PTSD and similar symptoms after experiencing a natural disaster compared to males.[13] Women generally take on a heavy load of caring for others who are impacted by a disaster, which can contribute to secondary trauma or compassion fatigue. Women also tend to deal with stress by connecting with other people, and natural disasters often create barriers to social support—people living close by are also preoccupied with managing the same disaster. Debates will continue about whether gender differences in mental health outcomes are caused primarily by information processing and emotional regulation differences related to physiology (e.g., chromosomes, hormones), by coping tendencies related to one's relative physical size and strength (e.g., men physically confronting or outrunning dangers, women leaning on groups for self-defense), or by cultural socialization based on ideology or arbitrary traditions.[14] The precise combination of such factors is difficult to determine.

A person's **age** is also relevant to the impact of natural disasters.[15] Children are more like to have trauma (or worse trauma) symptoms compared to adults, and younger children struggle more than older children. Lesser emotional maturity and life experience and greater dependence on reliable and available caregivers likely contribute to younger children's vulnerability to negative outcomes. Cognitive and emotional processing capacities also influence children's coping. Very young children use imagination to make sense of their experiences, including attributing human characteristics to disasters—*The cloud angry!* Pre-schoolers struggle to perceive things from perspectives other than their own; they are at risk of seeing themselves as causing disasters in some way. Older children can use their emerging abstract thinking to have deeper reflection and more empathy for others and to use helpful cognitive coping strategies (see Chapter 2). Older adolescents rely heavily on peers for social support, which could be an asset when parents are preoccupied with other concerns.

Ethnic heritage is inconsistently related to the risk of trauma symptoms.[16] Research tends to either find very similar outcomes for various ethnic groups or that ethnic minority families struggle somewhat more with the impacts of natural disasters. **Minority stressors** (see Chapter 3) arguably contribute to higher baseline levels of stress and fewer resources, making some individuals and families more vulnerable to experiencing **crisis** because of a disaster. After Hurricane Floyd (in 1999, affecting much of the eastern coast of the United States), Black fourth-graders were more likely than their White peers to cognitively cope with stress by blaming others for the disaster. Such a strategy could be based on a history of victimization by the racial majority, perhaps as a mechanism for finding meaning that motivates certain responses. Interestingly, a study of Black youth who survived a forest fire showed that the youth who were more highly acculturated—as measured by strongly identifying with their own ethnicity *and* with others around them—were less likely to have traumatic symptoms than their less acculturated peers.

Natural disasters tend to affect large geographical areas, so the qualities of **communities** can influence the impacts of such disasters on families.[17] Feeling a sense of **belonging**, **mutual commitment**, and **mutual trust** within one's community has led to greater life satisfaction after a major natural disaster, as has satisfaction with the government's response to address deteriorated living conditions. Consider how it might feel if people around you or the government seemed not to care about your welfare after a disaster. Fear and mistrust can lead to excessive community conflict after a disaster. Conversely, the Vietnamese community in New Orleans—originally formed by religious refugees (Catholic)—has a long history of communal **resilience**, including with Hurricane Katrina. Though this group tended to already have more mental health risks than the general population of the area (attributed largely to minority stressors), they appeared to recover from the hurricane better than other communities. Its success seems to be rooted in a strong ethnic identity, strong community networking, having leadership roles in the Catholic Church and other organizations, values of self-sufficiency and communal support, and a legacy of having overcome other challenges. How well would your local community work together to recover from a natural disaster?

Improve Your Learning

Without peeking, take a moment to review in your mind (or say out loud) the key concepts from this chapter (this is a proven learning technique). Then review the "Chapter Preview" section at the top and compare. Skim Part A of the chapter with extra attention to the **bolded words**. Skip to the end of the chapter to find more learning resources.

Part B. COVID-19 (or Pandemic) Stressors

On December 12, 2019, several people in Wuhan, China, showed symptoms of what would come to be known as the respiratory disease COVID-19 (caused by the new SARS-CoV-2 virus).[18] On March 11, 2020, the World Health Organization declared COVID-19 a worldwide **pandemic**—a large-scale disease outbreak. A few days later, schools, restaurants, and other public places begin to shut down across the country, and universities typically sent students home to continue their education online. These events marked the beginning of what many simply refer to as **the quarantine** or **lockdown**. Anxiety and depression levels increased to unusually high levels for families, especially during quarantine, along with higher rates of childhood behavioral problems and poorer overall mental and physical health for adults and children.[19] By the end of May 2020, over 100,000 deaths in the United States had been attributed to COVID. Many more would come.

What Is Stressful About the Pandemic?

The global COVID-19 pandemic placed numerous and often intense kinds of pressures on families, many of which have been addressed in this book. More **vulnerable** families, like those with less cohesion, more overall stress, and a history of mental health challenges, were more prone to struggle with pandemic stressors, making the **coping** process and potential for **flourishing** more difficult.[20] The stress of the pandemic was intensified by the major level of uncertainty (or **ambiguity**) associated with it—*What is COVID? How dangerous is it? How does it spread? How long will this last? When will businesses reopen? How safe and effective is the vaccine? What new variants might arise?* Planning for the future seemed impossible at times. Though not the only pandemic to have ever occurred, it will serve as our case study for investigating this type of **family stressor** within the **FSS integrated model (FIM) of family stress and crisis framework** (Chapter 1) and other related content.

Consider how personal concerns about anyone in the family catching COVID provoked anxiety that could intensify family conflict or disconnection. Furthermore, how self- or government-imposed social restrictions intended to contain the spread of disease confined families to their homes in ways that induced new interaction patterns. Not everyone embraced such a quarantine, and many felt trapped and socially isolated, especially when schools and workplaces closed. Negativity in the home (e.g., arguing, feeling annoyed or driven crazy) corresponded with depressive and anxious symptoms that seemed to only get worse over time.[21] Spouses, parents, and children who received less affection than desired experienced more loneliness and depression.[22]

Having more people constantly **sharing space** often made caregiving more complicated.[23] Increases in both **negative** and **positive** interaction throughout the first year of the pandemic or beyond were common.[24] Some families were more able or willing to enjoy more time together—to seemingly make up for lost time in their otherwise busy lives. Some parents came to understand their children better and discovered that teenagers can actually be pleasant to have around. Numerous parents across the world reported feeling more confident in their parenting abilities. Overall, healthy family engagement appeared to lessen the negative consequences of pandemic stress, as did additional sleep and exercise, particularly for older children—though extra screen time for children tended to have the opposite effect.

The remainder of the chapter is organized around the other chapters of this book while, as usual, highlighting elements of personal/professional application (Chapter 2) and diverse external contexts (Chapter 3).

How Is the Pandemic Related to Economic Stress (Chapter 4)?

By late April 2020, the U.S. **unemployment** rate peaked at 14.8%, the highest since the great depression in the 1930s. Nearly 50 million people lost their jobs because their employers were unable to maintain business.[25] Government funding helped counter some of the losses, but as you would expect, many families experienced significant pressure from job insecurity and financial uncertainty. Many family-run businesses were vulnerable to closing (and did), causing certain distress over losing a legacy of hard work and investment.

The intersection of **work and family** was a prominent pressure during quarantine. As seen in the table in Figure 12.1, Pew Research data from 2020 illustrates some of the challenges faced by employed parents.[26] Working from home seemed to be a mixed blessing—it provided some additional flexibility and opportunity for family time, but the work and family realms might more easily interfere with one another. Some mothers who had quit their jobs to focus on their children voiced frustration with the inability to take children to the library, on playdates, and to other stimulating public places despite putting work on hold.[27]

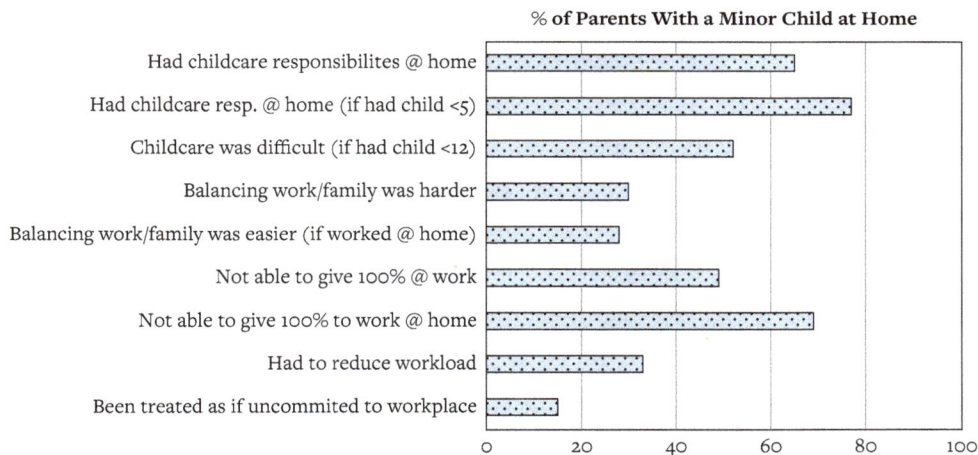

FIGURE 12.1 % of Parents With a Minor Child at Home

Dealing with **schools** was another pandemic by-product that influenced work-family pressures.[28] School closings caused many parents to work more of their hours from home to monitor their children. With online schooling, parents faced countless frustrations with technology, child motivation, and children missing face-to-face social interaction with their peers—including extra-curricular activities. Some children struggled with online learning and fell behind, and behavioral problems seemed to increase as children had to readjust to schools opening back up, giving parents even more to worry about.

How Is the Pandemic Related to Family Fertility Stressors (Chapter 5)?

The pandemic typically interfered with **infertility** treatment and **adoption** services.[29] Slowing down of nonessential medical procedures might have resulted in more resources for patients with COVID, but it was disheartening for prospective parents to put their dreams on hold. Similarly, the pandemic slowed adoption processes in part because of procedural challenges (e.g., understaffed agencies and courtrooms, halting international adoptions, prioritizing other legal services) and in part because of an apparent lessening supply of adoptable babies. Some adoption lawyers have speculated that the quarantine and college campus closings contributed to fewer young women having unintended pregnancies.

Those who overcame or lacked fertility barriers were also affected by the pandemic in various ways.[30] For example, consider the following:

- Little information was available about the impact of COVID on **pregnancy**, and conflicting advice only added to stressful uncertainty.
- Some research suggests that **babies born** during the heart of the pandemic tended to have poorer verbal, motor, and cognitive skills (including lower IQs) compared to those born between 2011 and 2019, on average. Differences are suspected to be due to stress during pregnancy and childrearing, and lack of child stimulation during quarantine.
- Preschoolers also demonstrated various **developmental delays** coming off of quarantine. Some had been unable to continue early intervention services and fell further behind, while others who might qualify for the services went undiagnosed.
- On the flip side, reports from around the world, including the United States, indicate an upswing in the number of girls experiencing **early puberty** (e.g., 5-year-olds developing breasts and 7-year-olds menstruating). Experts speculate that lockdowns contributed to more obesity, a sedentary lifestyle, greater stress, and more exposure to chemicals that disrupt the hormonal system (e.g., from food, water, personal care items, and electronic devices). Early puberty is generally a risk factor for depression, eating disorders, antisocial behavior, and substance use problems for girls, adding yet more pressure on busy families.

How Is the Pandemic Related to Intergenerational Challenges and Polarization (Chapter 6)?

How eager were you to experience life away from the nest and explore what college life had to offer? Imagine after just a few months of school, having found a social niche and established some daily habits, that you must leave campus within a few days and continue your courses online. What would that transition be like? If you lived with your parents, would they treat you like a teenager again? Would the posters in your bedroom make you feel like you took a step backward? Would you long for more privacy? Would you miss campus life and all the resources—including academic and mental health supports—it had to offer? On top of that, you are heavily restricted from going out in public. Is that a pretty picture?

Research on **college students** who returned to live with parents during early campus closures suggests that negative family relationship factors—conflicted interaction, feeling less welcome, and having less autonomy from parents—were key factors in perceived declines in students' mental health.[31] Students who struggled to feel more like an adult, based on their parents' treatment and their own sense of identity, especially reported negative family issues during quarantine. As noted in Part A, political ideology fueled much debate about the danger of the virus, the effectiveness of mask wearing, and the necessity to restrict businesses (or the length of time for doing so); adult children and their parents who disagreed on such issues might find it especially difficult to share extended close proximity without engaging in polarizing exchanges. However, some students reportedly enjoyed their family time and togetherness, and appreciated the opportunity to improve family relationships.

How Is the Pandemic Related to Intimate Partner Abuse and Child Maltreatment (Chapter 7)?

You might wonder if the stresses of being cooped up day after day with the same people, combined with worries about a potentially fatal disease, finances, and mental health, would lead to more violence; the data is complicated.[32] While some sources show significant decreases in reports of child abuse and couple violence, other sources suggest that actual incidents increased during the pandemic, especially during quarantine. For example, a review of nine pediatric trauma centers indicated about a 300% increase in the number of child abuse victims over the age of 4. Abuse numbers are difficult to obtain and rely heavily on effective reporting mechanisms. Because schoolteachers are a major source of child abuse reports, school closings could have contributed to some declines in reporting. Domestic violence overall appeared to have increased by about 8% across the United States during quarantine. One thing to keep in mind is that parents and partners with a history of abusive behavior were much more likely than others to have been abusive during quarantine; how common it was for family members to first become abusive *because* of the quarantine is difficult to know, but it could have been relatively rare.

How Is the Pandemic Related to Family Structural Complexity (Chapter 8)?

Would you expect the pandemic to increase or decrease the **divorce** rate? You might be right. In some ways, pandemic stressors could make marriages more fragile; in some ways marriages could benefit from more time together and couples uniting against COVID (and maybe against their children). Early evidence suggests that both were occurring.[33] Both marriage and divorce rates seem to have dropped in 2020 and to have recovered or perhaps increased since. Time may tell what the overall net impact of the pandemic was on marriage, but for those couples who were already headed toward divorce, the quarantine might have been like pouring gasoline on a fire. Imagine two people who struggle with getting along having little chance to have a break from one another and limited access to others for encouragement and support. Add all the other pressures mentioned that come with a pandemic and **tensions** likely intensify. Quarantined children might have witnessed more parental conflict and talk of divorce than they otherwise would have. As with adoption, the legal system tended to slow down and prolong divorce procedures, which could contribute to a temporary lowering of the divorce rate.

The pandemic added to **co-parenting** challenges for separated and divorced parents, including the following issues:

- Communicating and agreeing about strategies to minimize the risk of getting COVID and whether to eventually have children immunized
- Arguing about doing one's fair share of helping with remote schooling
- Renegotiating and managing schedules that are no longer dictated by school hours but also affected by changes to employment patterns
- Having barriers to travel to exchange children, especially for those who rely on public transportation

Such challenges were not necessarily unique to complex family structures, but living apart, possibly having other adults with influential opinions contributing to disagreement (e.g., step-parent figures), and lingering bitterness between former spouses could threaten much-needed cooperation during such uncertain times.

How Is the Pandemic Related to Disability Stress (Chapter 9)?

Families with disabled children or adults experienced extra pressure because of the lessening of services provided to assist with their circumstances.[34] Some families **perceived** that providers were using COVID as an excuse to make cutbacks. School closings also meant that many children involved with special education lost access to various therapies, and some parents worried that their disabled children might be given less priority than typically abled children if they were to need medical attention. Caregivers of frail, elderly adults were extra burdened by fears of loved ones catching COVID, hearing it was most fatal for older and health-compromised individuals; caregivers of high-risk categories also had to worry about getting sick and being unable to provide essential care. Many caregivers felt guilt and worry as they left the side of a needy family member and returned to work once restrictions lessoned, also wondering if they would bring the virus home with them and endanger their household. For families with a disabled member living in a care facility, restrictions that minimized or eliminated visits also caused some distress, anxiety, and loneliness among family members.

How Is the Pandemic Related to Addiction and Compulsion (Chapter 10)?

Changes in substance use problems appeared to coincide with the pandemic.[35] National Center for Health Statistics revealed a 25% increase in alcohol-related deaths among individuals 16 years or older in 2020 compared to 2019. Rates for people ages 25 to 44 were close to 40%. Compared to May 2019, the number of **overdose** deaths in May 2020 was 58% higher, and the year ended with over 20,000 more overdose deaths than the prior year (which had been a record high). It would seem that substances became an increasingly common coping mechanism for pandemic stress. As with other types of services already mentioned, the limiting of addiction services and treatments during quarantine, along with less access to social support, likely intensified the substance-related compulsions and their consequences.

Some evidence suggests that **adolescent alcohol use** declined in 2020 but the use of nicotine products and misuse of prescription drugs appeared to increase. Adolescents who experienced more distress and family problems (e.g., financial stress, parental substance use) during the pandemic especially were likely to turn to substance use. How do you think being home together as families influenced these trends?

How Is the Pandemic Related to Fear and Loss (Chapter 11)?
"Fear" and "loss" are fitting descriptors of a pandemic. Well over 300,000 deaths in the United States by the end of 2020 have been directly attributed to COVID; as of July 2022, that number had reached about 1.02 million (and 6.34 million worldwide). Additional deaths also occurred—many from heart disease, Alzheimer's, and diabetes—that have been attributed to limited health-care access, lower prioritization to non-COVID-related health care, and problematic behavioral coping that contributed to weight gain and poor nutritional intake.[36] Suicide rates were expected to increase because of pandemic stress, but preliminary evidence suggests a slight decline, though hospitalizations due to suspected suicide attempts by 12- to 25-year-olds seemed to have increased into 2021, especially for females.[37] While some continue to debate whether we generally overreacted or underreacted to COVID threats and risks associated with the vaccines, countless families felt the pressures of concern for the health of their loved ones, and millions lost a family member who might otherwise have lived longer.

The pandemic also altered how many families were affected by fear and loss.[38] For example, consider the following:

- Children were likely exposed to much more media and family member communication related to death. This could result in more fear and anxiety but also be an opportunity for families to discuss the topic.
- Having a family member placed in the intensive care unit was frequently linked to families experiencing PTSD symptoms several months later. Being restricted from visiting a dying loved one was especially distressing.
- Relying on virtual funeral services potentially altered the grieving process of family members in unknown ways. Families with technology barriers might have missed out completely on customary grieving rituals that help them process the loss.

How Do External Contexts Impact Families During a Pandemic?

Examples of external contexts are scattered throughout Part B. To elaborate further on **gender**, research frequently shows that women were at greater risk for the negative impacts of pandemic stress.[39] As we discovered with other fear and loss stressors, including natural disasters, girls and women tended to experience more depression and anxiety during the pandemic; eating disorders also increased. Employed mothers especially had their typical routines disrupted. Industries that largely employ women were generally more adversely affected by the pandemic, resulting in greater job losses for women (at least initially) and greater reduction of work hours. While stressed about the economic circumstances, mothers were also disproportionally affected by work and family challenges (including with children's schooling). On the other hand, it appears that more men died from COVID than did women, and at least some of the gap was related to social and occupational influences.[40]

As you would expect, families of lower socioeconomic status tended to struggle more during the pandemic.[41] They were more likely to experience job loss or cutbacks in hours, struggle with childcare arrangements, have limited access to reliable internet and related devices, and experience depression and anxiety. Children from more impoverished areas experienced greater learning loss in the 2020–2021 school year, regardless of how school instruction was delivered.

Black and Hispanic families also tended to disproportionately struggle with the pandemic given their higher rates of poverty and minority stressors, including being more likely to get, be hospitalized from, and die from COVID. Many such families had members with less flexible jobs that may have increased their risk of exposure to the virus. Asian American families were sometimes targets of discriminatory behaviors because of the virus originating in China.[42] Conversely, some families with minority identities—including sexual and gender minorities—felt that their resilience through other challenges helped them handle isolation and marginalization throughout the pandemic, despite experiencing greater rates of mental health problems (especially lesbian, gay, bisexual, and transgender youth).[43] Some religious minority groups in the United States, particularly of Hindu and Muslim faiths, were distressed when swift cremation or burial of deceased family members—in accordance with their religious traditions—was impeded because of understaffing and contact restrictions of mortuary services.[44]

What Does All This Mean for You?

Your insights can be valuable to your personal life, your family relationships, and your professional roles. Take a few moments to ponder the following:

- How have you been feeling while engaging with this information? Why?
- Has your family experienced any natural disasters or unique elements of the pandemic? What was it like?
- What opinions do you have about the pandemic and lockdowns that might differ from other peoples' opinions, including from family members?
- What other examples have come to mind that illustrate similar or diverse ways that families cope with large-scale stressors?

Reminders for Helpers

As a person of influence, you can help guide people through the coping processes and ideally help foster a **flourishing** life. However, take care to avoid letting your personal **interpretations** push you toward assuming too much about somebody else's circumstances, perceptions, and motivations. Always be ready to address issues that might be hard for you to face because of your own history.

Draw upon the elements of the **FIM framework** and other family stress concepts. Remember, **coping** refers to an action or response based on available or new resources and perceptions related to stressors. Families have either successfully **managed** a stressor's pressure through **adjustment coping** or reached crisis in which **adaptive coping** is needed to reestablish some level of **general family functioning**. **Resources** and **perceptions** are key concepts to focus on when confronting family stress. **Review the master table** in Chapter 4 as a guide for exploring the ideas below of how to help families with stressors.

What Are Some Ways to Encourage Effective Family Coping?

Drawing primarily from citations and insights noted in the chapter thus far, we will explore **suggested resources and noteworthy perceptions** that can contribute to successful coping and more optimal family functioning.

How Can You Help With Large-Scale Disaster Stress?

A large-scale disaster typically implies that families cannot just rely on themselves but also on community and government efforts to rebuild or fortify infrastructures and services. But that can take some time, and being able to draw on family strengths can increase resilience, particularly when families are isolated or otherwise restricted from outside contact. Hopefully, you have noticed that **social support** and **coping strategies** are repeatedly mentioned **resources** for addressing family stressors. Natural disasters and especially pandemics can create barriers to the social supports and services families are used to. Families might need help finding other ways to express their concerns and receive encouragement, perhaps through support groups and virtual forms of communication. Ideally, families can generate support within the home and unite against devastating setbacks or paralyzing fears.

Helping people analyze the effectiveness of their coping strategies can lead to better outcomes. Examples of coping strategies reported during large-scale disasters include the following:[45]

- Children often cope with disasters by numbing their emotions, ruminating about their concerns, or withdrawing from others—all of which tend to increase anxiety in the long run.
- Adolescents have resisted family efforts to reach out to community agencies for help because it confirms their vulnerability, causes traumatic memories to resurface, and is socially humiliating.
- Wives who blamed marital conflicts on the stress of the pandemic were better able to minimize the deterioration of the relationship.
- Older adults were able to soothe themselves after a major hurricane by comparing themselves with others with worse losses, expressing gratitude and optimism, and focusing on their psychological strengths.
- Being able to reduce one's fear of COVID appeared to improve people's mental health but also seemed to make them less cautious about preventing infection. Finding a way to emphasize the control one has to minimize the risks of dangers while not disregarding their seriousness seems to be a more fruitful combination.

Along with their essential role in cognitive coping strategies, **perceptions** also contribute to coping as part of the overall **meaning** people make from their experiences with large-scale disasters.[46] Attributing the causes of disasters in some way to one's self—something children especially might do—contributed to greater distress. People who believe in a just world—that people tend to get what they deserve and are treated fairly—are generally more optimistic, hopeful, and trusting and experience fewer negative mental health outcomes in the face of large-scale disasters. Do you see any downsides to this worldview?

Improve Your Learning

Without peeking, take a moment to review in your mind (or say out loud) the key concepts from this chapter (this is a proven learning technique). Then review the "Chapter Preview" section at the top and compare. Skim Part B of the chapter with extra attention to the **bolded words**.

Do You Want to Learn More?

We have only touched on a portion of information related to some elements of this topic. **What really sparked your interest? What do you wish was covered more thoroughly?** Consider taking some time to further deepen your understanding of personal and professional issues related to helping families cope with stressors. The following are a variety of resources that you might find helpful and some references directly or indirectly referred to in this chapter. Flood your mind and let your excitement quake as you become infected with the joy of continuous learning.

Videos

(Use links or do searches with the key words provided)
- Research Finds Natural Disasters Lead to PTSD in Kids (1.5 mins). Global News. https://www.youtube.com/watch?v=8FubKEPgxjM
- 20 Times Mother Nature Got Angry on Camera (33 mins). Amerikano. https://www.youtube.com/watch?v=bFjAU5snYYQ
- The Impact of Natural Disaster-Related ACES on Children's Mental Health (3.5 mins). KidsXpress. https://www.youtube.com/watch?v=-13ovDDq8jw
- How Natural Disasters Can Impact Your Mental Health (5 mins). CBS News. https://www.youtube.com/watch?v=_xJnG5pPjsA
- Finding a New Normal: Life After a Natural Disaster (3 mins). CDC. https://www.youtube.com/watch?v=rgDiRHy-1lo
- Families, Caregivers Traumatized by COVID-19 Visiting Restrictions at Care Homes (9 mins). CBC News: The National. https://www.youtube.com/watch?v=iu3vhcwsgvc

- My Entire Family Survived COVID-19. Here's What I Wish I Knew Earlier (3.5 mins). *Good Morning America*. https://www.youtube.com/watch?v=Xyf1ruAeF6c
- Quarantine Stereotypes (9 mins). Dude Perfect. https://www.youtube.com/watch?v=eZUKSxE2UZg

Websites

- CDC. (2022, May 12). Basics of COVID-19. Centers for Disease Control and Prevention. https://www.cdc.gov/coronavirus/2019-ncov/your-health/about-covid-19/basics-covid-19.html
- CDC. (n.d.). COVID-19. https://www.cdc.gov/coronavirus/2019-nCoV/index.html
- Helliwell, J. F., Layard, R., Sachs, J. D., De Neve, J.-E., Aknin, L. B., & Wang, S. (Eds.). (2022). *World happiness report 2022*. Sustainable Development Solutions Network. https://worldhappiness.report/ed/2022/
- Mikles, N. (2021, May 4). Indians forced to change death rituals as COVID-19 rages. HowStuffWorks. https://people.howstuffworks.com/culture-traditions/funerals/india-change-death-rituals-news.htm
- WebMD. (n.d.). Why men and women handle stress differently. https://www.webmd.com/women/features/stress-women-men-cope

Readings (Articles, Books, Book Chapters)

- Chmutina, K., & von Meding, J. (2019). A dilemma of language: "Natural disasters" in academic literature. *International Journal of Disaster Risk Science*, 10(3), 283–292. https://doi.org/10.1007/s13753-019-00232-2
- Crandall, A., Daines, C., Hanson, C. L., & Barnes, M. D. (2022). The effects of COVID-19 stressors and family life on anxiety and depression one-year into the COVID-19 pandemic. *Family Process*. https://doi.org/10.1111/famp.12771
- Hall, S. S., & Zygmunt, E. (2021). "I hate it here": Mental health changes of college students living with parents during the COVID-19 quarantine. *Emerging Adulthood*, 9(5), 449–461. https://doi.org/10.1177/21676968211000494
- Laugharne, J., van der Watt, G., & Janca, A. (2011). After the fire: The mental health consequences of fire disasters. *Current Opinion in Psychiatry*, 24(1), 72–77. https://doi.org/10.1097/YCO.0b013e32833f5e4e
- Lawson, M., Piel, M. H., & Simon, M. (2020). Child maltreatment during the COVID-19 pandemic: Consequences of parental job loss on psychological and physical abuse towards children. *Child Abuse & Neglect, 110*. https://doi.org/10.1016/j.chiabu.2020.104709
- Scaramella, L. V., Sohr-Preston, S. L., Callahan, K. L., & Mirabile, S. P. (2008). A test of the family stress model on toddler-aged children's adjustment among Hurricane Katrina impacted and nonimpacted low-income families. *Journal of Clinical Child & Adolescent Psychology*, 37(3), 530–541. https://doi.org/10.1080/15374410802148202

Notes

1 Pappas, S., & Means, T. (2022, March 3). 10 of the deadliest natural disasters in history. Livescience.Com; Live Science. https://www.livescience.com/33316-top-10-deadliest-natural-disasters.html

2 Chmutina, K., & von Meding, J. (2019). A dilemma of language: "Natural disasters" in academic literature. *International Journal of Disaster Risk Science*, 10(3), 283–292. https://doi.org/10.1007/s13753-019-00232-2

3 Gromet, D. M., Kunreuther, H., & Larrick, R. P. (2013). Political ideology affects energy-efficiency attitudes and choices. *Proceedings of the National Academy of Sciences of the United States of America*, 110(23), 9314–9319. https://doi.org/10.1073/pnas.1218453110

4 Atske, S. (2020, April 16). 2. COVID-19 and the country's trajectory. Pew Research Center—U.S. Politics & Policy. https://www.pewresearch.org/politics/2020/04/16/covid-19-and-the-countrys-trajectory; Cakanlar, A., Trudel, R., & White, K. (2022). Political ideology and the perceived impact of coronavirus prevention behaviors for the self and others. *Journal of the Association for Consumer Research*, 7(1), 36–44. https://doi.org/10.1086/711834

5 Substance Abuse and Mental Health Services Administration (SAMHSA), (2022, April 14). Types of disasters. https://www.samhsa.gov/find-help/disaster-distress-helpline/disaster-types

6 Kassraie, A., & Kassraie, A. (2022). 10 worst natural disasters to strike the U.S. AARP. https://www.aarp.org/politics-society/history/info-2021/costliest-natural-disasters.html; Roller, S. (n.d.). *The 10 worst natural disasters in US history*. History Hit. Retrieved June 23, 2022, from https://www.historyhit.com/the-deadliest-natural-disasters-in-us-history

7 Hirth, J. M., Leyser-Whalen, O., & Berenson, A. B. (2013). Effects of a major U.S. hurricane on mental health disorder symptoms among adolescent and young adult females. *Journal of Adolescent Health*, 52, 765–772. http://dx.doi.org/10.1016/j.jadohealth.2012.12.013; Laugharne, J., van der Watt, G., & Janca, A. (2011). After the fire: The mental health consequences of fire disasters. *Current Opinion in Psychiatry*, 24(1), 72–77. https://doi.org/10.1097/YCO.0b013e32833f5e4e; Rowe, C. L., La Greca, A. M., & Alexandersson, A. (2010). Family and individual factors associated with substance involvement and PTS symptoms among adolescents in greater New Orleans after Hurricane Katrina. *Journal of Counseling and Clinical Psychology*, 78(6), 806–817. https://doi.org/10.1037/a0020808; Sezgin, A. U., & Punamäki, R. (2016). Perceived changes in social relations after earthquake trauma among Eastern Anatolian women: Associated factors and mental health consequences. *Stress and Health*, 32, 355–366. https://doi.org/10.1002/smi.2629; Sprague, C. M., Kia-Keating, M., Felix, E., Afifi, T., Reyes, G., & Afifi, W. (2015). Youth psychosocial adjustment following wildfire: The role of family resilience, emotional support, and concrete support. *Child & Youth Care Forum*, 44, 433–450. https://doi.org/10.1007/s10566-014-9285-7

8 Laugharne, J., van der Watt, G., & Janca, A. (2011). After the fire: The mental health consequences of fire disasters. *Current Opinion in Psychiatry*, 24(1), 72–77. https://doi.org/10.1097/YCO.0b013e32833f5e4e

9 Xie, X., Liu, H., & Gan, Y. (2011). Belief in a just world when encountering the 5/12 Wenchuan earthquake. *Environment and Behavior*, 43(4), 566–586. https://doi.org/10.1177/0013916510363535

10 Langley, A. K., & Jones, R. T. (2005). Coping efforts and efficacy, acculturation, and post-traumatic symptomatology in adolescents following wildfire. *Fire Technology*, 41(2), 125–143. https://doi.org/10.1007/s10694-005-6387-7; Laugharne, J., van der Watt, G., & Janca, A. (2011). After the fire: The mental health consequences of fire disasters. *Current Opinion in Psychiatry*, 24(1), 72–77. https://doi.org/10.1097/YCO.0b013e32833f5e4e; Osofsky, H. J., Osofsky, J. D., Kronenberg, M., Brennan, A., & Hansel, T. C. (2009). Posttraumatic stress symptoms in children after Hurricane Katrina: Predicting the need for mental health services. *The American Journal of Orthopsychiatry*, 79(2), 212–220. https://doi.org/10.1037/a0016179; Rowe, C. L., La Greca, A. M., & Alexandersson, A. (2010). Family and individual factors associated with substance involvement and PTS symptoms among adolescents in greater New Orleans after Hurricane Katrina. *Journal of Counseling and Clinical Psychology*, 78(6), 806–817. https://doi.org/10.1037/a0020808; Scaramella, L. V., Sohr-Preston, S. L., Callahan, K. L., & Mirabile, S. P. (2008). A test of the family stress model on toddler-aged children's adjustment among Hurricane Katrina impacted and nonimpacted low-income families. *Journal of Clinical Child & Adolescent Psychology*, 37(3), 530–541. https://doi.org/10.1080/15374410802148202; Sprague, C. M., Kia-Keating, M., Felix, E., Afifi, T., Reyes, G., & Afifi, W. (2015). Youth psychosocial adjustment following wildfire: The role of family resilience, emotional support, and concrete support. *Child & Youth Care Forum*, 44, 433–450. https://doi.org/10.1007/s10566-014-9285-7

11 Laugharne, J., van der Watt, G., & Janca, A. (2011). After the fire: The mental health consequences of fire disasters. *Current Opinion in Psychiatry*, 24(1), 72–77. https://doi.org/10.1097/YCO.0b013e32833f5e4e; Sezgin, A. U.,

& Punamäki, R. (2016). Perceived changes in social relations after earthquake trauma among Eastern Anatolian women: Associated factors and mental health consequences. *Stress and Health*, *32*, 355–366. https://doi.org/10.1002/smi.2629; Witteveen, A. B., Bramsen, I., Twisk, J. W. R., Huizink, A. C., Slottje, P., Smid, T., & Van Der Ploeg, H. M. (2007). Psychological distress of rescue workers eight and one-half years after professional involvement in the Amsterdam air disaster. *The Journal of Nervous and Mental Disease*, *195*(1), 31–40. https://doi.org/10.1097/01.nmd.0000252010.19753.19

12 Kamo, Y., Henderson, T. L., Roberto, K. A., Peabody, K. L., & White, J. K. (2015). Perceptions of older adults in a community accepting displaced survivors of Hurricane Katrina. *Current Psychology*, *34*(3), 551–563. https://doi.org/10.1007/s12144-015-9356-4

13 Hirth, J. M., Leyser-Whalen, O., & Berenson, A. B. (2013). Effects of a major U.S. hurricane on mental health disorder symptoms among adolescent and young adult females. *Journal of Adolescent Health*, *52*, 765–772. http://dx.doi.org/10.1016/j.jadohealth.2012.12.013; Osofsky, H. J., Osofsky, J. D., Kronenberg, M., Brennan, A., & Hansel, T. C. (2009). Posttraumatic stress symptoms in children after Hurricane Katrina: Predicting the need for mental health services. *The American Journal of Orthopsychiatry*, *79*(2), 212–220. https://doi.org/10.1037/a0016179; Pfefferbaum, B., Noffsinger, M. A., Wind, L. H., & Allen, J. R. (2014). Children's coping in the context of disasters and terrorism. *Journal of Loss and Trauma*, *19*(1), 78–97. https://doi.org/10.1080/15325024.2013.791797

14 Albert, P. R. (2015). Why is depression more prevalent in women? *Journal of Psychiatry & Neuroscience: JPN*, *40*(4), 219–221. https://doi.org/10.1503/jpn.150205; WebMD. (n.d.). Why men and women handle stress differently. https://www.webmd.com/women/features/stress-women-men-cope

15 Osofsky, H. J., Osofsky, J. D., Kronenberg, M., Brennan, A., & Hansel, T. C. (2009). Posttraumatic stress symptoms in children after Hurricane Katrina: Predicting the need for mental health services. *The American Journal of Orthopsychiatry*, *79*(2), 212–220. https://doi.org/10.1037/a0016179; Pfefferbaum, B., Noffsinger, M. A., Wind, L. H., & Allen, J. R. (2014). Children's coping in the context of disasters and terrorism. *Journal of Loss and Trauma*, *19*(1), 78–97. https://doi.org/10.1080/15325024.2013.791797

16 Pfefferbaum, B., Noffsinger, M. A., Wind, L. H., & Allen, J. R. (2014). Children's coping in the context of disasters and terrorism. *Journal of Loss and Trauma*, *19*(1), 78–97. https://doi.org/10.1080/15325024.2013.791797; Russoniello, C. V., Skalko, T. K., O'Brien, K., McGhee, S. A., Bingham-Alexander, D., & Beatley, J. (2002). Childhood posttraumatic stress disorder and efforts to cope after Hurricane Floyd. *Behavioral Medicine*, *28*(2), 61–71. https://doi.org/10.1080/08964280209596399

17 Helliwell, J. F., Layard, R., Sachs, J. D., De Neve, J.-E., Aknin, L. B., & Wang, S. (Eds.). (2022). *World happiness report 2022*. Sustainable Development Solutions Network. https://worldhappiness.report/ed/2022/; Huang, Y., & Wong, H. (2014). Impacts of sense of community and satisfaction with governmental recovery on psychological status of the Wenchuan earthquake survivors. *Social Indicators Research*, *117*(2), 421–436. https://doi.org/10.1007/s11205-013-0354-3; Laugharne, J., van der Watt, G., & Janca, A. (2011). After the fire: The mental health consequences of fire disasters. *Current Opinion in Psychiatry*, *24*(1), 72–77. https://doi.org/10.1097/YCO.0b013e32833f5e4e; Stain, H. J., Kelly, B., Carr, V. J., Lewin, T. J., Fitzgerald, M., & Fagar, L. (2011). The psychological impact of chronic environmental adversity: Responding to prolonged drought. *Social Science & Medicine*, *73*(11), 1593–1599. https://doi.org/10.1016/j.socscimed.2011.09.016 ; Xu, Q. (2017). How resilient a refugee community could be: The Vietnamese of New Orleans. *Traumatology*, *23*(1), 56–67. https://doi.org/10.1037/trm0000091

18 CDC. (2022a, January 5). CDC museum COVID-19 timeline. Centers for Disease Control and Prevention. https://www.cdc.gov/museum/timeline/covid19.html; CDC. (2022b, May 12). *Basics of COVID-19*. Centers for Disease Control and Prevention. https://www.cdc.gov/coronavirus/2019-ncov/your-health/about-covid-19/basics-covid-19.html

19 Czeisler, M. É., Lane, R. I., Petrosky, E., Wiley, J. F., Christensen, A., Njai, R., Weaver, M. D., Robbins, R., Facer-Childs, E. R., Barger, L. K., Czeisler, C. A., Howard, M. E., & Rajaratnam, S. M. W. (2020). Mental health, substance use, and suicidal ideation during the COVID-19 pandemic – United States, June 24–30, 2020. *MMWR. Morbidity and Mortality Weekly Report*, *69*(32), 1049–1057. https://doi.org/10.15585/mmwr.mm6932a1; Feinberg, M. E., A Mogle, J., Lee, J.-K., Tornello, S. L., Hostetler, M. L., Cifelli, J. A., Bai, S., & Hotez, E. (2022). Impact of the COVID-19 pandemic on parent, child, and family functioning. *Family Process*, *61*(1), 361–374. https://doi.org/10.1111/famp.12649; Press Trust of India. (2022, April 13). Lockdowns doubled risk of mental health symptoms, finds study. NEWS9LIVE. https://www.news9live.com/health/covid-19/lockdowns-doubled-risk-of-mental-health-symptoms-finds-study-164473

20 Dunleavy, B. P. (2022, January 24). Study: Family ties, sleep, activity aided youth mental health during pandemic. UPI. https://www.upi.com/Health_News/2022/01/24/teens-supportive-relationships-pandemic-study/5431643036762;

Fosco, G. M., LoBraico, E. J., Sloan, C. J., Fang, S., & Feinberg, M. E. (2022). Family vulnerability, disruption, and chaos predict parent and child COVID-19 health-protective behavior adherence. *Families, Systems & Health: The Journal of Collaborative Family Healthcare*, 40(1), 10–20. https://doi.org/10.1037/fsh0000649; Hartshorne, J. K., Huang, Y. T., Lucio Paredes, P. M., Oppenheimer, K., Robbins, P. T., & Velasco, M. D. (2021). Screen time as an index of family distress. *Current Research in Behavioral Sciences*, 2(100023), 100023. https://doi.org/10.1016/j.crbeha.2021.100023; Köhler-Dauner, F., Clemens, V., Lange, S., Ziegenhain, U., & Fegert, J. M. (2021). Mothers' daily perceived stress influences their children's mental health during SARS-CoV-2-pandemic-an online survey. *Child and Adolescent Psychiatry and Mental Health*, 15(1), 31. https://doi.org/10.1186/s13034-021-00385-3

21 Crandall, A., Daines, C., Hanson, C. L., & Barnes, M. D. (2022). The effects of COVID-19 stressors and family life on anxiety and depression one-year into the COVID-19 pandemic. *Family Process*. https://doi.org/10.1111/famp.12771

22 Hesse, C., Mikkelson, A., & Tian, X. (2021). Affection deprivation during the COVID-19 pandemic: A panel study. *Journal of Social and Personal Relationships*, 38(10), 2965–2984. https://doi.org/10.1177/02654075211046587

23 Haskett, M. E., Hall, J. K., Finster, H. P., Owens, C., & Buccelli, A. R. (2022). "It brought my family more together": Mixed-methods study of low-income U.S. mothers during the pandemic. *Family Relations*. https://doi.org/10.1111/fare.12684

24 Black, S. (2022, January 4). 'I understand my kid more': How the pandemic changed parenting. *The Guardian*. https://amp.theguardian.com/lifeandstyle/2022/jan/05/i-understand-my-kid-more-how-the-pandemic-changed-parenting; Blackwell, C. K., Mansolf, M., Sherlock, P., Ganiban, J., Hofheimer, J. A., Barone, C. J., Bekelman, T. A., Blair, C., Cella, D., Collazo, S., Croen, L. A., Deoni, S., Elliott, A. J., Ferrara, A., Fry, R. C., Gershon, R., Herbstman, J. B., Karagas, M. R., LeWinn, K. Z., … Wright, R. J. (2022). Youth well-being during the COVID-19 pandemic. *Pediatrics*, 149(4). https://doi.org/10.1542/peds.2021-054754; Kantar.com. (n.d.). Finding the positives of parenting during the pandemic. https://www.kantar.com/inspiration/research-services/finding-the-positives-of-parenting-during-the-pandemic-pf; Kerr, M. L., Rasmussen, H. F., Fanning, K. A., & Braaten, S. M. (2021). Parenting during COVID-19: A study of parents' experiences across gender and income levels. *Family Relations*, 70(5), 1327–1342. https://doi.org/10.1111/fare.12571

25 Bls.gov. (2021, July 8). 6.2 million unable to work because employer closed or lost business due to the pandemic, June 2021: The Economics Daily. U.S. Bureau of Labor Statistics. https://www.bls.gov/opub/ted/2021/6-2-million-unable-to-work-because-employer-closed-or-lost-business-due-to-the-pandemic-june-2021.htm

26 Igielnik, R. (2021, January 26). A rising share of working parents in the U.S. say it's been difficult to handle child care during the pandemic. Pew Research Center. https://www.pewresearch.org/fact-tank/2021/01/26/a-rising-share-of-working-parents-in-the-u-s-say-its-been-difficult-to-handle-child-care-during-the-pandemic

27 Pearson, C. (2021, January 22). Millennial moms have been driven to their breaking point. HuffPost. https://www.huffpost.com/entry/millennial-moms-pandemic-stress_l_600ae2b2c5b6a46978d09117

28 Leonhardt, D. (2022, January 4). No way to grow up. *The New York Times*. https://www.nytimes.com/2022/01/04/briefing/american-children-crisis-pandemic.html; Schreiber, M. (2022, February 25). Eating disorders among teen girls doubled during pandemic, CDC study shows. *The Guardian*. https://amp.theguardian.com/world/2022/feb/24/eating-disorders-teen-girls-doubled-pandemic-cdc

29 Kaur, H., Pranesh, G. T., & Rao, K. A. (2020). Emotional impact of delay in fertility treatment due to COVID-19 pandemic. *Journal of Human Reproductive Sciences*, 13(4), 317–322. https://doi.org/10.4103/jhrs.JHRS_144_20; Yazbek, H. (2021, June 3). Prospective parents looking to adopt have faced pandemic delays. Columbia News Service; Columbia Journalism School. https://columbianewsservice.com/2021/06/03/prospective-parents-looking-to-adopt-have-faced-pandemic-delays/

30 Changoiwala, P. (2022, March 28). Early puberty cases have surged during COVID, doctors say. The Fuller Project. https://fullerproject.org/story/pandemic-girls-early-puberty/; Lewis, H. (2020, March 19). The coronavirus is a disaster for feminism. *Atlantic Monthly*. https://www.theatlantic.com/international/archive/2020/03/feminism-womens-rights-coronavirus-covid19/608302/; Wenner Moyer, M. (2022). The COVID generation: How is the pandemic affecting kids' brains? *Nature*, 601(7892), 180–183. https://doi.org/10.1038/d41586-022-00027-4; Wong, A. (2022, June 15). Pandemic babies are behind after years of stress, isolation affected brain development. *USA Today*. https://www.usatoday.com/in-depth/news/education/2022/06/09/pandemic-babies-now-toddlers-delayed-development-heres-why/9660318002/

31 Hall, S. S., & Zygmunt, E. (2021). Dislocated college students and the pandemic: Back home under extraordinary circumstances. *Family Relations*, 70(3), 689–704. https://doi.org/10.1111/fare.12544; Hall, S. S., & Zygmunt, E. (2021).

"I hate it here": Mental health changes of college students living with parents during the COVID-19 quarantine. *Emerging Adulthood, 9*(5), 449–461. https://doi.org/10.1177/21676968211000494

32 Citroner, G. (2021, October 8). Children at home were more likely to face domestic violence during the pandemic. Healthline Media. https://www.healthline.com/health-news/children-at-home-were-more-likely-to-face-domestic-violence-during-the-pandemic; Lawson, M., Piel, M. H., & Simon, M. (2020). Child maltreatment during the COVID-19 pandemic: Consequences of parental job loss on psychological and physical abuse towards children. *Child Abuse & Neglect, 110.* https://doi.org/10.1016/j.chiabu.2020.104709; Lee, S. J., Ward, K. P., Lee, J. Y., & Rodriguez, C. M. (2021). Parental social isolation and child maltreatment risk during the COVID-19 pandemic. *Journal of Family Violence.* https://doi.org/10.1007/s10896-020-00244-3; Piquero, A. R., Wesley, G. J., Jemison, E., Kaukinen, C., & Knaul, F., M. (2021). Domestic violence during COVID-19: Evidence from a systematic review and meta-analysis. Council on Criminal Justice. https://counciloncj.org/impact-report-covid-19-and-domestic-violence-trends/

33 Goldberg, A. E., Allen, K. R., & Smith, J. Z. (2021). Divorced and separated parents during the COVID-19 pandemic. *Family Process, 60*(3), 866–887. https://doi.org/10.1111/famp.12693; Lebow, J. L. (2020). The challenges of COVID-19 for divorcing and post-divorce families. *Family Process.* https://doi.org/10.1111/famp.12574; Wilson, J. (2021, August 30). Divorce surge driven by COVID-19 pandemic still on the rise in 2021. FormsPal. https://formspal.com/knowledge-base/divorce-during-covid/

34 Beach, S. R., Schulz, R., Donovan, H., & Rosland, A.-M. (2021). Family caregiving during the COVID-19 pandemic. *The Gerontologist, 61*(5), 650–660. https://doi.org/10.1093/geront/gnab049; Horovitz, B., & Horovitz, B. (2021, August 4). Caregivers stressed about returning to work after COVID. AARP. https://www.aarp.org/caregiving/life-balance/info-2021/returning-to-work-stress.html; Meredith, R. (2021, July 24). Covid-19: Children with special educational needs "forgotten" during pandemic. BBC. https://www.bbc.com/news/uk-northern-ireland-57948640; Mitchell, L. L., Albers, E. A., Birkeland, R. W., Peterson, C. M., Stabler, H., Horn, B., Cha, J., Drake, A., & Gaugler, J. E. (2022). Caring for a relative with dementia in long-term care during COVID-19. *Journal of the American Medical Directors Association, 23*(3), 428–433.e1. https://doi.org/10.1016/j.jamda.2021.11.026

35 Baumgartner, J. C., & Radley, D. C. (2021). The drug overdose toll in 2020 and near-term actions for addressing it. Commonwealth Fund. https://doi.org/10.26099/GB4Y-R129; National Institute on Drug Abuse. (2021, December 15). Percentage of adolescents reporting drug use decreased significantly in 2021 as the COVID-19 pandemic endured. National Institute on Drug Abuse. https://nida.nih.gov/news-events/news-releases/2021/12/percentage-of-adolescents-reporting-drug-use-decreased-significantly-in-2021-as-the-covid-19-pandemic-endured; White, A. M., Castle, I.-J. P., Powell, P. A., Hingson, R. W., & Koob, G. F. (2022). Alcohol-related deaths during the COVID-19 pandemic. *JAMA: The Journal of the American Medical Association, 327*(17), 1704–1706. https://doi.org/10.1001/jama.2022.4308; Unprecedented increase in overdose deaths during the COVID-19 pandemic—with substantial regional variation. (2021, June 28). Recovery Research Institute. https://www.recoveryanswers.org/research-post/unprecedented-increase-overdose-deaths-covid-19-substantial-regional-variation/

36 Albert-Deitch, C. (2022, May 11). Doctors say these pandemic side effects are serious problems—and unlikely "to go away anytime soon." CNBC. https://www.cnbc.com/2022/05/11/doctors-say-pandemic-side-effects-are-becoming-serious-health-problems.html; Woolf, S. H., Chapman, D. A., Sabo, R. T., & Zimmerman, E. B. (2021). Excess deaths from COVID-19 and other causes in the US, March 1, 2020, to January 2, 2021. *JAMA: The Journal of the American Medical Association, 325*(17), 1786. https://doi.org/10.1001/jama.2021.5199

37 Yard, E., Radhakrishnan, L., Ballesteros, M. F., Sheppard, M., Gates, A., Stein, Z., Hartnett, K., Kite-Powell, A., Rodgers, L., Adjemian, J., Ehlman, D. C., Holland, K., Idaikkadar, N., Ivey-Stephenson, A., Martinez, P., Law, R., & Stone, D. M. (2021). Emergency department visits for suspected suicide attempts among persons aged 12–25 years before and during the COVID-19 pandemic—United States, January 2019–May 2021. *MMWR. Morbidity and Mortality Weekly Report, 70*(24), 888–894. https://doi.org/10.15585/mmwr.mm7024e1

38 Amass, T., Van Scoy, L. J., Hua, M., Ambler, M., Armstrong, P., Baldwin, M. R., Bernacki, R., Burhani, M. D., Chiurco, J., Cooper, Z., Cruse, H., Csikesz, N., Engelberg, R. A., Fonseca, L. D., Halvorson, K., Hammer, R., Heywood, J., Duda, S. H., Huang, J., … Curtis, J. R. (2022). Stress-related disorders of family members of patients admitted to the intensive care unit with COVID-19. *JAMA Internal Medicine, 182*(6), 624–633. https://doi.org/10.1001/jamainternmed.2022.1118; Anderer, J. (2021, October 4). Virtual funerals become new norm as families adapt during COVID. Studyfinds.org. https://www.studyfinds.org/virtual-funerals-covid; Pelaez, M., & Novak, G. (2020). Returning to school: Separation problems and anxiety in the age of pandemics. *Behavior Analysis in Practice, 13*, 521–526. https://doi.org/10.1007/s40617-020-00467-2

39 Blackwell, C. K., Mansolf, M., Sherlock, P., Ganiban, J., Hofheimer, J. A., Barone, C. J., Bekelman, T. A., Blair, C., Cella, D., Collazo, S., Croen, L. A., Deoni, S., Elliott, A. J., Ferrara, A., Fry, R. C., Gershon, R., Herbstman, J. B., Karagas, M. R., LeWinn, K. Z., ... Wright, R. J. (2022). Youth well-being during the COVID-19 pandemic. *Pediatrics*, 149(4). https://doi.org/10.1542/peds.2021-054754; Hamel, L., & Salganicoff, A. (2020, April 6). Is there a widening gender gap in coronavirus stress? KFF. https://www.kff.org/policy-watch/is-there-widening-gender-gap-in-coronavirus-stress/; Pettigrew, R. N. (2021). An untenable workload: COVID- 19 and the disproportionate impact on women's work-family demands. *Journal of Family and Consumer Sciences*, 113(4), 8–15. https://doi.org/10.14307/jfcs113.4.8

40 Danielsen, A. C., Lee, K. M., Boulicault, M., Rushovich, T., Gompers, A., Tarrant, A., Reiches, M., Shattuck-Heidorn, H., Miratrix, L. W., & Richardson, S. S. (2022). Sex disparities in COVID-19 outcomes in the United States: Quantifying and contextualizing variation. *Social Science & Medicine (1982)*, 294(114716), 114716. https://doi.org/10.1016/j.socscimed.2022.114716.

41 Brown, S. M., Doom, J. R., Lechuga-Peña, S., Watamura, S. E., & Koppels, T. (2020). Stress and parenting during the global COVID-19 pandemic. *Child Abuse & Neglect*, 110(2). https://doi.org/10.1016/j.chiabu.2020.104699; Hicks, D. M., & Faulk, D. (2022, January 20). Study: Instructional mode played no significant role in COVID-19-related learning loss in Indiana public schools in 2020–21. ESchool News. https://www.eschoolnews.com/2022/01/20/study-instructional-mode-played-no-significant-role-in-covid-19-related-learning-loss-in-indiana-public-schools-in-2020-21; Kerr, M. L., Rasmussen, H. F., Fanning, K. A., & Braaten, S. M. (2021). Parenting during COVID-19: A study of parents' experiences across gender and income levels. *Family Relations*, 70(5), 1327–1342. https://doi.org/10.1111/fare.12571; Shevlin, M., McBride, O., Murphy, J., Miller, J. G., Hartman, T. K., Levita, L., Mason, L., Martinez, A. P., McKay, R., Stocks, T. V. A., Bennett, K. M., Hyland, P., Karatzias, T., & Bentall, R. P. (2020). Anxiety, depression, traumatic stress and COVID-19-related anxiety in the UK general population during the COVID-19 pandemic. *BJPsych Open*, 6(6), e125. https://doi.org/10.1192/bjo.2020.109

42 Cheah, C. S. L., Wang, C., Ren, H., Zong, X., Cho, H. S., & Xue, X. (2020). COVID-19 racism and mental health in Chinese American Families. *Pediatrics*, 146(5). https://doi.org/10.1542/peds.2020-021816

43 Gonzalez, K. A., Abreu, R. L., Arora, S., Lockett, G. M., & Sostre, J. (2021). "Previous resilience has taught me that I can survive anything": LGBTQ resilience during the COVID-19 pandemic. *Psychology of Sexual Orientation and Gender Diversity*, 8(2), 133–144. https://doi.org/10.1037/sgd0000501; Hawke, L. D., Hayes, E., Darnay, K., & Henderson, J. (2021). Mental health among transgender and gender diverse youth: An exploration of effects during the COVID-19 pandemic. *Psychology of Sexual Orientation and Gender Diversity*, 8(2), 180–187. https://doi.org/10.1037/sgd0000467

44 Mikles, N. (2021, May 4). Indians forced to change death rituals as COVID-19 rages. HowStuffWorks. https://people.howstuffworks.com/culture-traditions/funerals/india-change-death-rituals-news.htm

45 Langley, A. K., & Jones, R. T. (2005). Coping efforts and efficacy, acculturation, and post-traumatic symptomatology in adolescents following wildfire. *Fire Technology*, 41(2), 125–143. https://doi.org/10.1007/s10694-005-6387-7; Neff, L. A., Gleason, M. E. J., Crockett, E. E., & Ciftci, O. (2022). Blame the pandemic: Buffering the association between stress and relationship quality during the COVID-19 pandemic. *Social Psychological and Personality Science*, 13(2), 522–532. https://doi.org/10.1177/19485506211022813; Smith, A. M., Willroth, E. C., Gatchpazian, A., Shallcross, A. J., Feinberg, M., & Ford, B. Q. (2021). Coping with health threats: The costs and benefits of managing emotions. *Psychological Science*, 32(7), 1011–1023. https://doi.org/10.1177/09567976211024260

46 Lack, C. W., & Sullivan, M. A. (2008). Attributions, coping, and exposure as predictors of long-term posttraumatic distress in tornado-exposed children. *Journal of Loss & Trauma*, 13, 72–84. https://doi.org/10.1080/15325020701741906; Sezgin, A. U., & Punamäki, R. (2016). Perceived changes in social relations after earthquake trauma among Eastern Anatolian women: Associated factors and mental health consequences. *Stress and Health*, 32, 355–366. https://doi.org/10.1002/smi.2629; Xie, X., Liu, H., & Gan, Y. (2011). Belief in a just world when encountering the 5/12 Wenchuan earthquake. *Environment and Behavior*, 43(4), 566–586. https://doi.org/10.1177/0013916510363535

Image Credits

Fig. 12.1: Source: Adapted from https://www.pewresearch.org/fact-tank/2021/01/26/a-rising-share-of-working-parents-in-the-u-s-say-its-been-difficult-to-handle-child-care-during-the-pandemic.

Index

www.ingramcontent.com/pod-product-compliance
Lightning Source LLC
Chambersburg PA
CBHW061343210326
41598CB00035B/5868